Orthopedic Research and Therapy

# Musculoskeletal Pain (Common Clinical Presentations)

# ORTHOPEDIC RESEARCH AND THERAPY

Additional books and e-books in this series can be found
on Nova's website under the Series tab.

ORTHOPEDIC RESEARCH AND THERAPY

# MUSCULOSKELETAL PAIN (COMMON CLINICAL PRESENTATIONS)


MEHMET CENK TURGUT

AND

SERDAR TOY

EDITORS



nova
Medicine & Health
New York

DOI: https://doi.org/10.52305/AHSG3156



**Library of Congress Cataloging-in-Publication Data**

ISBN: 978-1-68507-410-4

*Published by Nova Science Publishers, Inc. † New York*

# Contents

# PREFACE

With the increasing interest in sports and the prolongation of life expectancy, the frequency of musculoskeletal pain is increasing day by day. Musculoskeletal pain, which is included in the differential diagnosis of every physician regardless of branch, can cause serious problems in people's daily lives. People's unresolved pain disrupts their social lives and brings along various psychological problems. When this becomes a vicious cycle, it creates pain that cannot be solved. In this book, the possibilities of recognizing and understanding pain and taking an active role in the treatment process are presented. This book, which offers a deep examination of the physiology and genetics of pain, provides an approach to the causes and treatments of musculoskeletal pain that physicians frequently encounter in their daily clinics. The authors hope that this book, which they have prepared with the contributions of all relevant specialists, will be a book that our physicians will frequently benefit from.

Chapter 1 - Pain is defined as "a localized or generalized unpleasant bodily sensation or complex of sensations that causes mild to severe physical discomfort and emotional distress and typically results from a bodily disorder (such as injury or disease)" in the dictionary (Pain|Definition of Pain by Merriam-Webster, n.d.). Pain is a prevalent reason for outpatient attendance. People who suffer from pain have to struggle with many consequences caused by pain, according to studies. While pain shows its effects in all areas of our lives, it becomes more critical to understand the mechanisms that create pain, and to learn how to manage it. In particular, musculoskeletal pain is one of the most common ailments in society. Musculoskeletal pain generally originates from muscles, bones, tendons, ligaments, and joints. The transmission of the painful stimulus with or without tissue damage from the tissue to the brain is complex. It varies according to the type of pain. G-protein-dependent secondary messengers are activated by inflammatory mediators. In voltage-gated ion channels, action potentials and neurotransmitter release occur. The painful stimulus carried by the ascending pathways is evaluated and answered in different brain parts according to its type and characteristics. Family physicians are the closest health service providers to the community. Therefore, patients prefer to first consult their family doctor about a health problem. Family medicine is one of the disciplines most frequently encountered with pain complaints. Musculoskeletal pain, the most common pain in the community, constitutes many outpatient clinic applications. Because of these reasons, it becomes more important for family physicians to accurately assess pain in primary care. The patient should be managed appropriately by assessing the pain correctly. A multidisciplinary approach should be interiorized when evaluating the patient because the pain has biological, psychological, and social aspects. As a result of a patient evaluation, treatment should be administered if needed, so a positive contribution to the patient's life quality should be provided. If required, the patient should be referred to the relevant specialist.

Chapter 2 - Low back pain is an important reason for hospital admissions. Low back pain affects the families and environment of patients by causing economic losses, decreases in work performance, need for medical care and psychological stress. The authors classify low back pain according to the duration of symptoms as acute, subacute and chronic. The diagnosis and treatment process is shaped according to this classification. The authors can collect the etiology of low back pain under three main headings. These are mechanical low back pain, non-mechanical low back pain and referred pain. Age, weight, occupational, sociocultural and psychosocial factors are important risk factors for low back pain. In the approach to the patient with low back pain, detailed anamnesis, detailed physical examination and imaging methods are used. Although the treatment varies according to the etiology, rest, medical treatments, exercise, physical therapy programs and surgical treatments are the primary approaches.

Chapter 3 - Cervical pain is one of the most common musculoskeletal pain syndromes. Its prevalence is similar to low back pain and it may lead to disability. Intervertebral discs, zygapophyseal joints, cervical nerve roots and referred pain are causes of cervical pain. Neck pain is acute, subacute or chronic; nociceptive or neuropathic. Red flags are important and need to be investigated. Rheumatological diseases such as spondyloarthropathies and rheumatoid arthritis are important besides cervical sprains, strains and myofascial pain. Spondylosis gains importance with aging. Disc hernias should be kept in mind for radicular pain and myelopathy. Taking history and physical examination are two cornerstones for reaching a diagnosis. Radiological imaging and laboratory tests are used when needed. Nonsteroidal anti-inflammatory drugs, rest or exercises, physical therapy modalities or cervical collars are first treatment options. For resistant cases therapeutic injections or cervical spine interventions are considered.

Chapter 4 - Chest pain is the second most common cause of emergency admissions. Patients can describe discomfort in the chest as related to the heart, lungs, great vessels, esophagus, stomach and mediastinum, and abdominal organs. For emergency doctors, the patient examination is crucial in terms of clinical and vital findings, and defining and eliminating life-critical etiologies. Musculoskeletal chest pain (MSCP) forms 25% of admitting emergencies with a chest pain complaint. Though MSCP was observed in approximately 30-45% of patients who performed a percutaneous coronary intervention without any pathology, it should be known that the MSCP finding is not a reason to eliminate coronary disease. Diagnosing, differential diagnosis and treatment of isolated musculoskeletal chest pain (MSCP) will be discussed in this section of the book.

Chapter 5 - Fibromyalgia syndrome is the third most frequent painful musculoskeletal condition after lumbar pain and osteoarthritis, in terms of prevalence. It is a complicated disease that causes severe impairment in quality of life and function, as well as significant financial costs. Although its diagnosis has improved with the development of more precise diagnostic criteria, there may be missed diagnoses of fibromyalgia. Once a diagnosis has been determined, clinicians should enhance patient function and reduce the severity of pain by nonpharmacological and pharmacological treatments. A multi-modal therapy strategy is required due to the various components of the etiology and maintenance of the disease. The rate of disability is shown to be considerably decreased with effective treatment.

Chapter 6 - Osteoarthritis of the hip is a common degenerative arthritis and a common reason for disability. Common etiological factors are femoroacetabular impingement, dysplastic hip, trauma and osteonecrosis. The diagnosis is clinical and radiological. The most common symptoms are decreased range of motion and pain around the hip. Narrowing of joint spaces and osteophytes are the common radiological findings. The first line of treatment is conservative. Lifestyle modifications, weight loss, and physiotherapy are the choices. If these measures fail, then surgical treatment must be done.

Chapter 7 - Femoroacetabular impingement (FAI) is a hip pathology that has been known to orthopedic surgeons for nearly 90 years, but for which gold standards have not yet been established in terms of its mechanism, clinical symptoms, diagnosis, and treatment. Diagnosis is attempted with different examination methods and radiological parameters, and in clinical practice, it is mostly seen in the athlete patient group. Conservative and surgical methods are used in its treatment. There is not yet a consensus on the optimal surgical procedure.

Chapter 8 - Although there is no consensus on the diagnosis of piriformis syndrome, it can generally be defined as sciatic nerve compression by the piriformis muscle. Even though there is no specific maneuver for the diagnosis of piriformis syndrome, physical examination might be helpful in diagnostics. Apart from that, electrodiagnostic tests and alternative radiological imaging techniques can be utilized to diagnose piriformis syndrome. In terms of treatment, while conservative approaches are primary choices, alternative surgical methods can be utilized for patients who are unresponsive to conservative treatment and patients with persistent complaints.

Chapter 9 - Coccydynia is seen in all age groups and both sexes, it is more common in the 40s and five times more common in women than men. Coccydynia describes pain in the coccyx or tailbone. The coccyx is a bone formed by the fusion of 3-5 vertebrae in the distal segment of the vertebral column. The coccyx bone, forming the terminal segment of the vertebral column, has great functional importance as it is the attachment site of many muscles, tendons, and ligaments. Besides, the coccyx bone also serves as positional support to the anus. A direct fall on the coccyx and repetitive microtraumas are the most common causes of coccydynia, but the etiology could not be determined in 30% of coccydynia patients. The Postacchini-Massobrio classification based on sacrococcygeal angulation is the most commonly used classification system in the coccyx fracture classification. Coccydynia patients have pain in the lumbar region and around the coccyx. The pain becomes evident after sitting for a long time or during getting up from sitting. Besides, pain may also increase during defecation or sexual intercourse.

Conservative treatment is primarily applied, and 90% of the patients respond well to conservative treatment. Surgical treatment can be applied in resistant coccydynia patients who are unresponsive to conservative treatment. Coccygectomy is applied as surgical treatment.

Chapter 10 - Restless legs syndrome (RLS) is a neurological disease that negatively affects daily activities and especially causes sleeping problems with a wide variety of symptoms such as pain, numbness, and tingling, a desire to move, and abnormal sensations, especially at night in the distal of both feet. Although there are certain symptoms of the disease, nonspecific symptoms often delay consulting the right outpatient clinic and diagnosis, therefore most of the patients reach the appropriate treatment later. Especially in some age groups, there are major difficulties in both diagnosis and treatment. Although iron deficiency is known to have a major role in pathophysiology, many genetic and environmental factors also have an effect. Even though dopamine agonists are still the first choice in treatment, it is clear that there will be new developments in both diagnosis and treatment in the upcoming period.

Chapter 11 - One of the most common joint diseases in the world is osteoarthritis (OA). Knee osteoarthritis is a common chronic joint disease, which causes limitation of movement and pain. Regional cartilage damage, such as fibrillation and thinning, is observed in OA. All joint tissues such as the synovium, subchondral bone, and joint ligaments but especially cartilage tissue are affected. OA can be classified as primary and secondary. Trauma, infection and biochemical and inflammatory processes are the main causes of secondary OA. The exact cause of primary osteoarthritis is unknown. Age, ethnicity, physical characteristics and genetics are thought to play a role in the development of primary osteoarthritis. All three compartments of the knee can be affected by arthrosis to varying degrees. OA can affect only one compartment, or it can affect three parts of the joint with varying severity. The medial compartment is predominantly affected in about half of the patients.

Chapter 12 - Meniscopathy is a broad concept that encompasses all pathologies of the meniscus. Meniscopathy can be treated with conservative or arthroscopic surgery. It has been determined that the meniscus prevents the formation of arthrosis and has a role in normal knee function. For this reason, in the current treatments of all diseases of the meniscus, there is an attempt to protect the meniscus.

Chapter 13 - Rotator cuff tears are a broad-spectrum disease group that can cause disability with different clinical manifestations, ranging from clinically silent lesions that occur with age against a traumatic or degenerative background to massive retracted tears. The ultimate goal is to prevent disability. At this point, patient- and lesion-specific treatments are needed. Age, tear type, smoking, and the presence of retraction and fatty degeneration affect the treatment results. The aim of this chapter is to evaluate the clinic and treatment of rotator cuff tears in the light of current information.

Chapter 14 - Impingement syndrome is mechanical compression of the rotator cuff tendons under the antero-inferior part of the acromion and in the flexion and internal rotation position of the shoulder. Two mechanical theories have been proposed as to the cause of the space narrowing in SIS. These can be defined as "intrinsic degeneration" and "extrinsic compression." SIS is diagnosed with anamnesis, physical examination and complementary imaging methods. There are 2 options in the treatment of SIS: conservative and surgical. A personal treatment plan is edited for each patient according to pain, functional status and accompanying pathologies.

Chapter 15 - Biceps tendinopathy is a relatively common ailment that typically presents as pain, tenderness, and weakness in the tendon of the long head of the biceps brachii. Pathologies occurring in the insertio part of the muscle shouldn't be hope for. A thorough patient history, physical examination and radiographic evaluation are necessary for diagnosis. Nonsurgical management including rest, nonsteroidal anti-inflamatuvar drugs, physical therapy and injection is approached first in patients with mild disease. Surgical management is indicated for refractory pain or severe disease.

Chapter 16 - Cubital tunnel syndrome is the most common compression neuropathy in the upper extremity after carpal tunnel syndrome. The most common site of compression of the ulnar nerve is the elbow, and this is known as cubital tunnel syndrome. Entrapment of the ulnar nerve in the cubital tunnel can occur in the acute or chronic process. Risk factors include female gender, advanced age, systemic neuropathy (such as diabetes), occupations requiring repetitive or challenging elbow flexion, and sleeping with elbow flexion. Conservative treatment that is applied for 2-4 months can be started in many patients with mild cubital tunnel syndrome. At least 3 months of conservative treatment can be preferred in patients with a motor conduction velocity of more than 40 m/sec along the elbow with electrodiagnostic tests. In patients with chronic symptoms and muscle atrophy, surgical treatment is often required in patients with failed conservative treatment. Surgical options include in situ decompression, subcutaneous transposition, intramuscular transposition, submuscular transposition, and medial epicondyectomy.

Chapter 17 - Carpal tunnel syndrome (CTS) represents the most frequently observed entrapment neuropathy of the upper limb. It is considered to be associated with increased intracarpal pressure and decreased circulation of the median nerve. The CTS pathophysiology generally originates from combined compression and traction mechanisms. The diagnosis of carpal tunnel syndrome is based on electromyography and nerve conduction studies. The treatment of CTS depends on the patient's severity. Conservative treatments are given in mild cases of CTS. It is necessary to perform surgical treatment in advanced cases in which conservative treatment is not beneficial and for which conservative treatment is not first considered. Surgical treatment aims to cut the transverse carpal ligament and relieve the carpal tunnel.

Chapter 18 - Painful stenosing tenosynovitis of the first extensor compartment of the wrist, involving the abductor pollicis longus and extensor pollicis brevis tendons, is called de Quervain's disease. The patient complains of pain and tenderness, usually localized at the radial styloid and aggravated by thumb motion. With a splint or casts that keep the wrist slightly extended with thumb abduction, symptoms may regress, but symptoms tend to recur when the triggering activities are resumed after the cast is removed. Corticosteroid injections together with lidocaine may benefit 50-80% of patients. First extensor compartment release is required if the complaints do not regress with conservative treatment.

Chapter 19 - Epicondylitis of the elbow is a widely encountered pathology seen both laterally and medially. Lateral epicondylitis, often referred to as "tennis elbow," is a very common problem of the extensor origin at the lateral epicondyle resulting from repetitive work- and/or athletic-related microtrauma. Typical symptoms include lateral elbow pain especially during extension of the wrist and decreased grip strength. Medial epicondylitis, also known as "golfer's elbow," is another common pathology, although less frequent when compared to lateral epicondylitis, which occurs due to repetitive valgus stress and common flexor tendon microtrauma. A typical patient complaint is pain on the medial aspect of the elbow, which is aggravated by daily activities and especially wrist flexion. A thorough history and a meticulous physical examination are essential for the epicondylitis diagnosis which is primarily clinical. Initially, imaging modalities are not indicated; however, recalcitrant cases, possible nerve entrapment syndromes, and inflammatory conditions may require imaging. Treatment methods include discontinuation of the exacerbating occupational and athletic activities, physical therapy modalities, exercises and injections. Patients who do not respond to conservative treatment modalities may be eligible for surgical interventions.

Chapter 20 - Achilles tendinopathy is one of the most common overuse pathologies of the foot and ankle, usually presenting with pain and edema around the tendon. Although the etiology is not fully deciphered, it is reported to be multifactorial. Achilles tendinopathy has been shown to be more common in athletes and overweight individuals. Increased involvement in sportive activities worldwide has also led to an increase in the frequency of Achilles tendinopathy. Anatomical classification is used to define two groups: insertional and non-insertional tendinopathy. Histopathological studies of Achilles tendinopathy reported that degenerative signs were encountered as opposed to inflammatory ones. The Achilles tendinopathy diagnosis can be readily made with a detailed anamnesis, a thorough physical examination and imaging aids. Pain is the prominent symptom. Several special tests can also be used during the physical examination. An initial evaluation is usually carried out with plain radiography. However, MRI is the most sensitive modality, and it is thus considered to be the gold standard in imaging. Conservative treatment modalities are considered to be the first-line treatment methods in Achilles tendinopathy. Conservative methods include cryotherapy, NSAID use, activity modification and physical therapy. Cases that do not benefit from conservative methods can be treated surgically. Although surgical results are generally satisfactory, complications such as surgical site infections may be encountered.

Chapter 21 - Plantar heel pain which sometimes seriously disrupts the activities of daily living is one of the main reasons for admission to orthopedic outpatient clinics. Although pain may originate due to rheumatological, inflammatory, neurological, or oncological reasons, the most common cause is plantar fasciitis. History and physical examination are the mainstays of the diagnosis, and imaging tools or electromyography can be used to exclude several reasons for plantar heel pain. The localization or distribution of the pain, the age of the patient, unilateral or bilateral involvement, accompanying symptoms like burning or paresthesia, and some physical examination tests are generally enough to make a prompt diagnosis. Conservative treatment options like oral nonsteroidal anti-inflammatory drugs, shoe modifications, and physical therapy modalities are generally satisfactory to relieve symptoms, and surgery is rarely needed in recalcitrant cases.

Chapter 22 - Sinus tarsi syndrome is a clinical disease characterized by chronic anterolateral ankle soreness, that occurs following severe ankle injuries. As a result of traumatic injuries, the ligaments in the sinus tarsi cavity are damaged. The sinus tarsi cavity is filled with fibrotic tissue remnants and synovitis following ligament injuries. Synovitis and fibrotic tissue deposits accumulate in this space and stimulate the chronic inflammatory process. Patients with sinus tarsi syndrome have ankle sprain caused by the supination/inversion mechanism. Acute ankle sprain typically presents with pain associated with anterolateral ankle swelling, ecchymosis, and tenderness. Conservative treatment is the first treatment method to be applied in sinus tarsi syndrome. If conservative treatments fail, surgical treatment becomes necessary. The aim is to excise the sinus tarsi contents and to clean the fibrotic tissues and synovial hypertrophy.

Chapter 23 - Tarsal tunnel syndrome represents an entrapment neuropathy, which is rare, insufficiently diagnosed and often confused with other clinical conditions. There are contradictions in diagnosing and treating the most frequently observed entrapment neuropathy of the foot. Treatment includes conservative methods such as analgesics and physical therapy and rehabilitation or surgical procedures. In this chapter, the etiology, pathophysiology, diagnostic methods, and treatments of tarsal tunnel syndrome are reviewed by employing a systematic approach.

Chapter 24 - Hallux valgus is a combination of deformities involving complex abnormalities of the first metatarsophalangeal joint. Hallux valgus is defined as an increase in the outward axis of the big toe relative to the axis of the first metatarsal. The main complaint of patients is the formation of a painful lump in the medial of the first metatarsophalangeal joint. Sometimes a lump without pain causes cosmetic complains. Though the deformity generally occurs because of idiopathic reasons, choice of narrow-toed, high-heeled shoes is also among the etiological reasons that contribute to the emergence of the clinic. It has treatment methods from shoe modification to surgical treatment. Hallux rigidus is degenerative arthritis of the first metatarsophalangeal joint. It occurs idiopathically as well as secondary to some ligament tissue diseases. The main complaint of patients is pain. Conservative and surgical treatment methods are available in its treatment.

Chapter 25 - Morton's neuroma is a degenerative neuropathy featuring fibrosis of the common interdigital nerve. Patients typically present with symptoms of forefoot pain that can be associated with burning, tingling or numbness between the toes. Morton's neuroma is primarily a clinical diagnosis; however, radiological assessment is frequently requested to aid or confirm the diagnosis. Surgery is considered if symptoms persist after 3 months of non-operative treatment.

Chapter 26 - Musculoskeletal pain is frequently encountered in the community. In the treatment of musculoskeletal pain, the treatment scheme should be determined after the etiology of the pain has been carefully determined. Age, gender, comorbid diseases, medications used, and onset of pain should be considered in the selection of treatment. Pain management should be individualized on a patient basis. In this section, information about the non-steroidal anti-inflammatory drugs, opioids and adjuvant drugs which are frequently used in the treatment of musculoskeletal pain will be given.

Chapter 27 - Sports injuries can be seen in millions of athletes every year, and therefore the pain caused by these injuries is treated. In these injuries, accurate and effective pain treatment is as important as correct diagnosis. As the athlete's return to sports can be shortened, activity losses due to pain are also prevented. There are many methods for pain management in sports injuries, from rest, medication and medical treatment to surgical interventions. Today, sports-related pain can be successfully treated with appropriate treatment methods.

Chapter 28 - Postoperative analgesia is an important part of the healing process. Adequate analgesia allows early mobilization, reducing complications such as thromboembolism and allowing patients to start their daily lives. Many pharmacological and non-pharmacological (peripheral nerve blocks and neuraxial blocks) methods are used to provide postoperative analgesia. In this chapter, the authors aim to discuss the postoperative analgesia methods in general terms.

Chapter 29 - Musculoskeletal system pain frequency increases with the aging population. Taking a detailed history and physical examination are the most important things for a correct diagnosis. Imaging should be considered as a tool to confirm the diagnosis. A number of imaging modalities are used to evaluate musculoskeletal system diseases. Despite the emergence of new imaging techniques for the assessment of musculoskeletal system pain, conventional radiology remains the cornerstone of diagnostic imaging. Radiography is the most advantageous and cheapest method in evaluating bone abnormalities such as fractures, dislocations, and osteoarthritis. Computed tomography can provide high-resolution, two- and three-dimensional images. Nuclear medicine applications are used in investigating stress fractures, occult fractures, bone tumors, or infections. Magnetic resonance imaging is used to evaluate soft tissue disorders, including ligaments, tendons, cartilage tissue, and masses. Ultrasonography is effective in evaluating effusions, cysts, ligaments, muscles, and tendons. Vascularization can also be identified with the use of Doppler. There is also the possibility to perform aspirations and injections under ultrasonography guidance. It is important to choose the most appropriate imaging method to accelerate the diagnosis and treatment. The imaging method to be preferred also changes depending on the structure of each joint and region investigated and the characteristics of the diseases considered in the differential diagnosis.

Chapter 30 - Polyneuropathies, especially diabetic polyneuropathy, are the most common peripheral nervous system disease that affects adults. Polyneuropathies can be classified in many ways, and axonal damage is a common result of this disease. In many neuropathies, the sensory fibers are primarily affected, and if the damage continues, motor weakness develops. Some neuropathies cause severe pain and are due to damage of the small fibers. The most common cause of this type of pain is distal symmetrical polyneuropathy due to diabetes. Anamnesis and examination findings should be noted in a patient with suspected polyneuropathy. Laboratory findings, electrodiagnostic tests and, if necessary, lumbar puncture or genetic tests are helpful in identifying diagnostic and etiological factors.

Chapter 31 - In muscle diseases, muscle weakness, thinning and sometimes pain or cramps are seen due to the disease of the muscle fibers. Hereditary muscle diseases can be classified into seven categories. Disease forms consist of "Duchenne and Becker; myotonic dystrophy; facioscapulohumeral; Emery-Dreifuss; oculopharyngeal; distal; and limb-girdle." They occur due to mutations in various genes. Although the disorder that causes hereditary muscle diseases is present from birth, the age at which it manifests itself is variable. Some appear from birth, while others begin at a later age. Congenital deficiency of proteins necessary for the proper functioning of the muscles leads to disorders and diseases in the muscles. Muscle diseases that show familial characteristics and cause progressive weakness are called "dystrophy." In some of these, the disease is passed from mother to son (X-linked), and in others, from mother or father to children (autosomal dominant). In others, both the mother and father must be carriers. In this type, the disease occurs in children who inherit the disease gene from both parents, while the parents don't show the disease characteristics (autosomal recessive). In this chapter, hereditary muscle diseases were classified and their phenotypic findings and gene mutations were defined. The genotype-phenotype relationship was revealed and the criteria that could guide the diagnosis were expressed.

Chapter 32 - Pain is the most common complaint in musculoskeletal tumors. It should be addressed appropriately to increase the health quality of life of these patients. There are operative and medical treatment options. The treatment should be individualized according to the patient's general status, stage of the disease, and estimated life expectancy. This chapter will give an overview of the management of pain in musculoskeletal tumors.

Chapter 33 - Neuropathic pain is defined as burning, stinging, pricking, tingling, squeezing, and chills. Metabolic, infectious, autoimmune, inflammatory and trauma-related diseases of the peripheral and central nervous system may cause neuropathic pain. Neuropathic pain occurs in 7 - 10% of the population. The quality of life of neuropathic pain patients was found to be low due to the ineffectiveness of neuropathic pain treatments and misdiagnosis. In neurology practice, the authors see patients with neuropathic pain very often. The patients with neuropathic pain have chronic diseases and multidrug usage. However, the treatment of neuropathic pain is limited to pharmacological treatments in a daily routine. Alternative non-pharmacological therapies are increasingly being offered to patients in recent years.

Chapter 34 - Meralgia paresthetica (MP) is an entrapment neuropathy caused by damage to the lateral femoral cutaneous nerve (LFCN). Typical clinical manifestations of MP are numbness, tingling, pain, and dysesthesia in the anterolateral thigh area. The disease course can be spontaneous or iatrogenic. Reduction of paresthesia after local anesthetic agent injection and nerve conduction tests are the most commonly used diagnostic methods. Conservative methods should be tried first in treatment, and surgery should be chosen for resistant cases.

In: Musculoskeletal Pain (Common Clinical Presentations) ISBN: 978-1-68507-410-4
Editors: Mehmet Cenk Turgut and Serdar Toy 

*Chapter 1*

# THE PHYSIOLOGY OF PAIN AND THE APPROACH TO MUSCULOSKELETAL PAIN IN PRIMARY CARE

***Duygu Ustunol**, MD***
Department of Family Medicine, Sulakyurt State Hospital,
Kırıkkale, Turkey

## ABSTRACT

Pain is defined as "a localized or generalized unpleasant bodily sensation or complex of sensations that causes mild to severe physical discomfort and emotional distress and typically results from a bodily disorder (such as injury or disease)" in the dictionary (Pain|Definition of Pain by Merriam-Webster, n.d.).

Pain is a prevalent reason for outpatient attendance. People who suffer from pain have to struggle with many consequences caused by pain, according to studies. While pain shows its effects in all areas of our lives, it becomes more critical to understand the mechanisms that create pain, and to learn how to manage it. In particular, musculoskeletal pain is one of the most common ailments in society. Musculoskeletal pain generally originates from muscles, bones, tendons, ligaments, and joints.

The transmission of the painful stimulus with or without tissue damage from the tissue to the brain is complex. It varies according to the type of pain. G-protein-dependent secondary messengers are activated by inflammatory mediators. In voltage-gated ion channels, action potentials and neurotransmitter release occur. The painful stimulus carried by the ascending pathways is evaluated and answered in different brain parts according to its type and characteristics.

Family physicians are the closest health service providers to the community. Therefore, patients prefer to first consult their family doctor about a health problem.

* Corresponding Aurthor's E-mail: duyguustunol@gmail.com.

Family medicine is one of the disciplines most frequently encountered with pain complaints. Musculoskeletal pain, the most common pain in the community, constitutes many outpatient clinic applications. Because of these reasons, it becomes more important for family physicians to accurately assess pain in primary care. The patient should be managed appropriately by assessing the pain correctly. A multidisciplinary approach should be interiorized when evaluating the patient because the pain has biological, psychological, and social aspects. As a result of a patient evaluation, treatment should be administered if needed, so a positive contribution to the patient's life quality should be provided. If required, the patient should be referred to the relevant specialist.

## INTRODUCTION

Pain is defined as "An unpleasant sensory and emotional experience associated with, or resembling that associated with, actual or potential tissue damage" by the International Association for the Study of Pain (IASP). In addition, pain is always a personal experience and can be learned from life. Also, IASP states that a sense of pain will be affected by biological, psychological, and social factors (IASP Terminology – IASP, n.d.).

One of the most common reasons for consulting a doctor worldwide is pain. According to studies conducted in the USA, it has been determined that more than 116 million people complain of chronic pain and the number of people with chronic pain is more than the sum of those with heart failure, diabetes, and cancer (Tsang et al., 2008). In a similar study conducted in Europe, it was determined that 19% of adult Europeans have chronic pain complaints, and this situation seriously affects their life quality (Breivik et al., 2006).

It has been stated that the physical and emotional functions of a person are adversely affected because of chronic pain in the study conducted by Turk et al., Also, pain affects different areas of a person's life due to economic problems, including expenditures for pain treatment and the performance loss in business life (Turk et al., 2011).

The effect of pain on life quality has been shown in people who have pain and compared healthy people in a study conducted by McCarberg et al., (2008). In this study, pain sufferers have decreased self-care, less enjoyment of the activities they participate in, decreased sleep quality, problems in interpersonal relationships, an adversely affected sexual life, withdrawal from social relations, poor performance in business life, and emotional problems such as stress, anxiety and anger control disorder (McCarberg et al., 2008).

Pain is a personal experience, and the events that a person has experienced before affect how the pain feels. Understanding the physiological mechanisms that cause pain will contribute to the pain approach and enable more effective pain management. The patient should be evaluated from a biopsychosocial perspective in pain management, and a multidisciplinary approach should be applied. Basic pain physiology and the approach to musculoskeletal pain in primary care are explained in this chapter.

## PHYSIOLOGY OF PAIN

Pain is expressed as an unpleasant and undesirable condition by patients. Pain is part of a complex system that alerts us when there is a problem in our body, whether there is any damage or not, and ensures our survival. The nervous system continuously monitors the presence of tissue damage or conditions that may develop tissue damage. If a stimulus that can cause pain is detected, a neural process occurs, called nociception, that is transmitted to the brain through the activation of neural pathways and pain pathways including transduction and transmission. This process begins with receptors, called nociceptors, which are particularly sensitive to painful stimuli, being stimulated.

Nociceptors are the free endings of nerve fibers. There are two main types of nociceptors: Aδ fibers and C fibers. Aδ fibers are myelinated, 2-5 μm in diameter, with a sharp, rapid, response to primary pain, and have a transmission speed of 5-15 m/s. C fibers are unmyelinated, ‹2 μm in diameter, with a slow, blunt, response to secondary pain and have a transmission speed of 0.5-2 m/s. Three types of nociceptors have been identified according to the way they are activated. These are thermal, mechanical, and polymodal nociceptors. Thermal nociceptors consist of Aδ fibers which are activated at very low or very high temperatures. Mechanical nociceptors consist of Aδ fibers which are activated by high pressure. Polymodal nociceptors consist of C fibers which are activated by mechanical, chemical, and thermal stimuli. Usually, these three receptors work together.

After tissue damage for various reasons, hydrogen ions, 5-hydroxytryptamine (5-HT), cytokines, bradykinin, histamine, prostaglandin, and leukotrienes are released from the damaged tissue as inflammatory mediators. Nociceptors are activated by these inflammatory mediators. Prostaglandins and bradykinin ensure the activation of nociceptors by low-intensity stimuli. Histamine and 5-HT cause the feeling of pain in the nerve endings. While hydrogen ions and 5-HT enter the cell directly through ion channels, other mediators bind to membrane receptors and activate G-protein-dependent secondary messenger systems.

Voltage-gated sodium and potassium channels effect an action potential by transmitting the painful stimulus to the synapse in the dorsal horn. Voltage-gated calcium channels have an essential role in the release of pain-inducing neurotransmitters in synapses. Some of the analgesic drugs work by targeting sodium and calcium channels. It is shown that increased potassium channel activity has a therapeutic benefit in treating persistent pain (Brown & Passmore, 2009).

Nociceptors use glutamate as the primary neurotransmitter. Other neurotransmitters may accompany glutamate. They are classified as peptidergic nociceptors and nonpeptidergic nociceptors according to the neurotransmitters they use. Peptidergic nociceptors use CGRP (calcitonin gene-related peptide) and substance P. Nonpeptidergic nociceptors use IB4 (its binding of a unique lectin), and most synthesize P2X3 purigenic receptors in response to ATP.

The nociceptive primary afferent fiber cell bodies are in the dorsal root ganglion. The fibers enter here and proceed through the dorsal horn of the spinal cord to reach lamina 1 and lamina 2 in the spinal gray matter, where they will synapse. Spinal cord neurons in lamina 1 are usually sensitive to painful stimuli transmitted by the Aδ and C fibers. Lamina 2 is mainly comprised of excitatory and inhibitory interneurons, which respond to nociceptive stimulations. Lamina 5 contains neurons that send a stimulus to the thalamus and brain stem. Also, these neurons receive painful and non-painful stimuli through the Aδ fibers directly and the C fibers indirectly. These neurons in lamina 5 are called wide dynamic range (WDR) neurons. WDR neurons have a role in the referred pain phenomenon, as somatic and visceral neurons aggregate and interact while transmitting a visceral stimulus (Basbaum et al., 2009).

The nociceptive stimulus is transported to the cerebral cortex by the spinothalamic, spinoreticular, spinomesencephalic, cervicothalamic, and spinohypothalamic tracts. These pathways are second-order neurons in pain transmission. Conduction by these pathways causes a feeling of pain. As a result of the spinothalamic tract's injury, the pain sensation in the other half of the body is significantly reduced. The spinothalamic tract originates from laminae 1, 5, 6, and 7 in the dorsal horn and terminates in the thalamus. This tract is the most commonly used route. Third-order neurons are located in the thalamus. Dysfunction of the thalamic tracts may result in pain. For example, central pain is felt in the paralyzed area (thalamic pain) in patients who have had a stroke (Kopf & Patel, 2010).

The thalamus processes information while transmitting it. Nociceptive information is combined and integrated by the thalamus. So, it has an essential role in pain modulation. The trigeminal nucleus and the part of the thalamus that receives pain information receive normal stimuli such as touch and pressure. From here, nerve fibers are sent to the superficial area of the brain that processes sensory information. In areas where nociceptive and normal somatic sensations are clustered and interacting, pain intensity information can be processed as localized pain sensation and a source of pain. For example, after limb amputations, cortical interaction may change and lead to sensations of pain (phantom pain) and non-painful telescopic phenomena (Kopf & Patel, 2010). The posterior nuclei, ventrobasal nuclei, and medial intralaminar nuclei of the thalamus are thought to participate in nociception. It was shown that ventral posterior lateral (VPL) and medial nuclei (VPM), and intralaminar nuclei play a role in the transmission of pain information (Min, 2010).

There is no specific brain region that receives pain information. Pain information is transmitted to different brain regions according to the type of painful stimulus. According to neuroimaging studies, a network that receives information from many pain pathways between somatosensory, limbic, and associative areas has been defined in the brain (Apkarian et al., 2005). A brain activity involving the entire cortex is required to perceived pain consciously.

As part of the limbic system, the cingulate gyrus in the cerebral cortex mainly controls the emotional response to pain. The insular cortex, another part of the limbic system, integrates sensory, emotional, and cognitive components in the pain response. Primary (S1) and secondary (S2) somatosensory areas in the cerebral cortex are specialized for pain's sensory and discriminative components (Apkarian et al., 2005).

If the primary somatosensory (S1) area is damaged, characteristics such as the localization and severity of the painful stimulus cannot be accurately evaluated. The secondary somatosensory area (S2) evaluates the localization and intensity of the painful stimulus less than S1. Somatosensory area injuries may cause hyperalgesia in the contralateral body in some cases. The insular cortex is connected with the primary somatosensory, secondary somatosensory, and cingulate gyrus, which are other areas of pain. The insular cortex is also associated with the amygdala and perirhinal cortex, which belong to the limbic system. This situation plays a role in explaining the emotional response to pain (Bushnell et al., 2013). The pain experience is thus individualized and perceived according to the personality. In addition, responses from the hypothalamus and hippocampus occur.

When the spinothalamic tract transmits the painful stimulus, there is an increase in norepinephrine levels released from neurons in the locus coeruleus. Alpha 2-adrenergic receptors are activated by norepinephrine. So, the sympathetic nervous system is activated to defend against pain. During pain modulation, periaqueductal gray matter (PAG) in the descending system connects with the medullary reticular formation (rostral ventromedial medulla = RVM) and ensures serotonin and norepinephrine release. Serotonin is synthesized in the nucleus raphe magnus and plays an essential role in the antinociceptive system. In response to norepinephrine release, endogenous opioids such as endorphins, enkephalin, and dynorphin are released, and opioid receptors densely located in the dorsal horn lamina 1 and 2 periaqueductal gray matter are inhibited for analgesia (Garland & Ph, 2013).

Changes in brain activities during the assessment of pain intensity were observed to increase in direct proportion to the intensity of the pain. Changes in the same direction were detected in the cerebellum, putamen, thalamus, insular cortex, anterior cingulate cortex, and secondary somatosensory area. In addition, negative changes were detected in the primary somatosensory area, supplementary motor area, and ipsilateral ventral premotor area when pain intensity increased (Coghill et al., 1999).

The pain response changing both the central and peripheral nervous systems is called neural plasticity. In experimental studies, an increase in the excitation time of dorsal horn neurons was observed due to repetitive activation of C fiber nociceptors at a frequency of 0.5-1 Hz. This situation is named the "wind up phenomenon." This phenomenon is also known as short-term reverse synaptic plasticity.

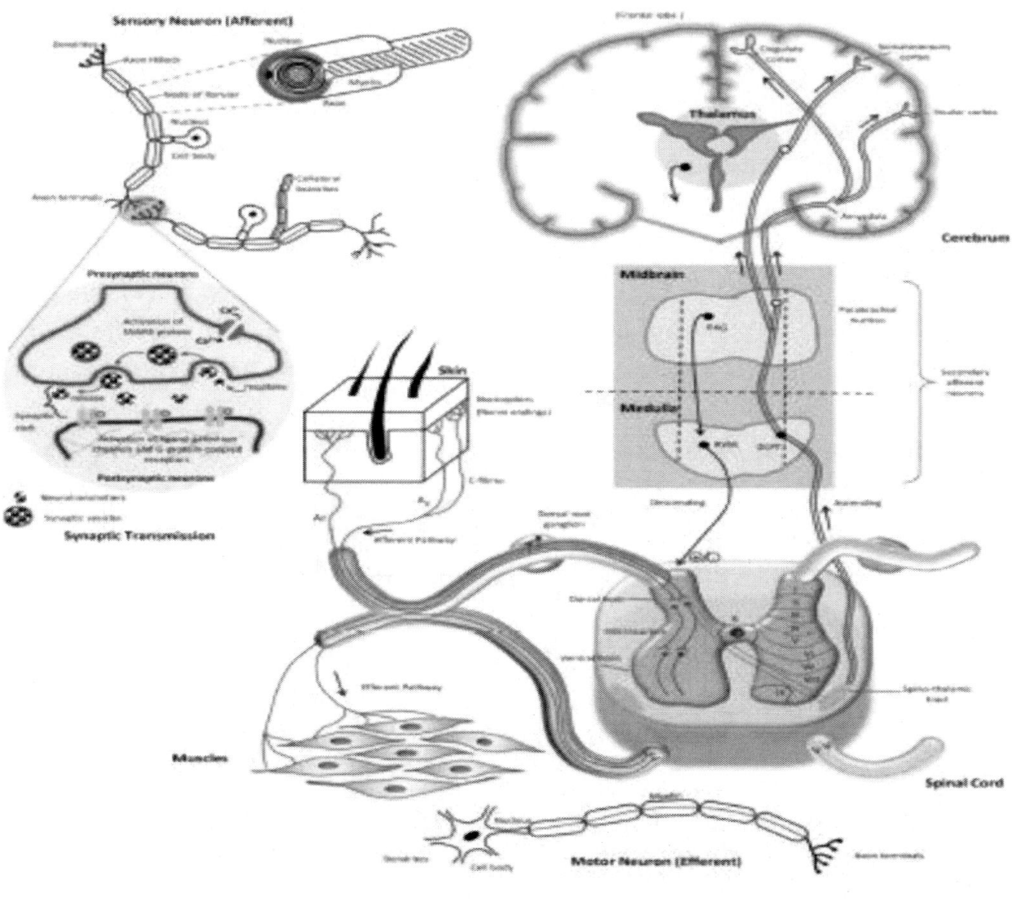


Figure 1. Pain neurotransmitters and pain transmission pathways in the synaptic cleft (Yam et al., 2018).

## APPROACH TO MUSCULOSKELETAL PAIN IN PRIMARY CARE

The pain complaint is a condition that the patient should evaluate by the biopsychosocial approach. The pain experience is multidimensional and affected by the patient's personality, mood, past experiences, and social relationships. The same pain is interpreted differently by different people. However, the same pain may be interpreted differently by the same person at different times (Deniz et al., 2013).

Family physicians are the group of doctors who are the health system's closest point and can be reached easily. So, patients prefer to apply to their family physicians when they feel the slightest pain in their bodies. Evaluation of pain is essential for family physicians who see diseases according to their prevalence in the community. In this section, the approach to musculoskeletal pain in primary care will be explained.

## Pain Assessment

Pain assessment has an essential role in pain management. When a patient presents with a pain complaint, the first issues that should be evaluated after the vital signs are as follows:

1. Pain history
2. Whether the pain is chronic
3. Pain experience.

The onset and timing of the pain, pain location, distribution of pain, pain intensity, pain characteristics, how much the daily activities are affected by pain, the conditions that pain increases or decreases, and whether the patient has a concomitant acute or chronic disease should be asked in the assessment of pain history. The patient should be asked how long the pain has been going on; pains shorter than 6 months should be considered as acute pain and those over 6 months should be considered as chronic pain. The patient should be asked whether there is a change in mood and a willingness to start acting due to pain in evaluating pain experience. However, the person's tolerance to pain and ability to cope with pain, and the presence of pain-related anxiety may affect the person's view of pain. So, patients may state that they are experiencing less pain than they are (Haefeli & Elfering, 2006).

The age and gender of the patient cause differences in the perception and experience of pain. In addition, situations such as exercise capacity, psychological state, social support, family relations, genetic characteristics, and previous diseases or surgeries may cause differences in the interpretation of pain.

Many scales are used in pain assessment, both unidimensional and multidimensional. While unidimensional scales only evaluate pain intensity, multidimensional scales also peruse pain quality. One-dimensional scales are frequently preferred because they are a valid method with ease of use and high patient compliance. Commonly used one-dimensional scales are the visual analytics scale (VAS), numeric rating scale (NRS), verbal rating scale (VRS), and face pain scale. NRS is more sensitive, VRS is less sensitive, but VRS is the easiest to use. VAS provides less information about pain than the other scales (Agaezi Onwuasoanya, 2016).

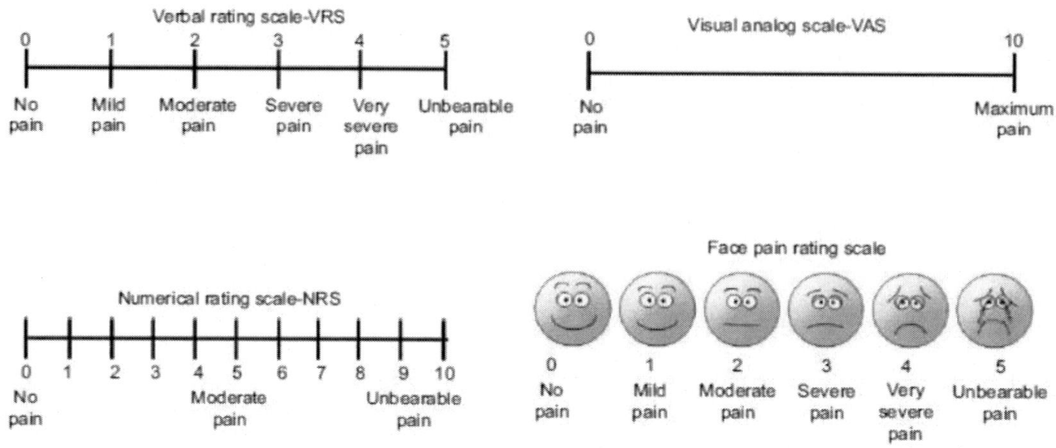


Figure 2. Pain Assessment Scales: numerical rating scale (NRS), verbal rating scale (VRS), visual analog scale (VAS), and face scale (Zubrzycki et al., 2018).

The three most common causes of musculoskeletal pain are daily activities, trauma, and systemic diseases. Patients with pain complaints may show behavioral changes for self-protection, such as continuous rest and avoiding acting due to anxiety and fear. Most musculoskeletal pain occurs due to trauma or daily activities. An underlying severe illness or psychological problem should be considered in the presence of some alarming signs, except traumatic situations. Therefore, an accurate pain assessment has a significant role. For example, patients should be examined further for severe underlying diseases in conditions such as severe fatigue, severe pain at rest, fever, unexplained weight loss, accompanying neurological disorder, a newly developed limitation of joint movements, previous cancer history, and bladder or bowel dysfunction. A traumatized patient should be evaluated with imaging methods. The patient should be supported psychologically and additively to pain treatment if conditions such as self-harm, depression, social isolation, increased anxiety and fear, and social or financial problems are accompanied by pain (MacKichan et al., 2008).

Pain can cause sleep disorders, and also sleep disorders can cause pain to feel differently than it is. Therefore, the patient's sleep pattern and sleep quality should be questioned. The patient should be informed about sleep hygiene.

Patients should have a comprehensive physical examination, and their psychological state should be evaluated. Patients with musculoskeletal pain should especially undergo an extensive neurological and musculoskeletal examination. Movements or positions in which pain increases or decreases should be questioned. Muscle tone, muscle strength, and deep tendon reflexes should be checked. It should be checked whether the movable joints have a normal range of motion.

## Pain Management in Primary Care

A patient-centered approach should be interiorized when pain management is planned. Stepwise treatment should be applied considering the World Health Organization (WHO) recommendations when analgesic treatment is arranged. These recommendations are essential in terms of preventing the abuse of opioid analgesics having a highly addictive potential. Antidepressant treatment can be added to the analgesic treatment by evaluating the patient's psychological state. It has been shown that serotonin and noradrenaline reuptake inhibitors (SNRIs) positively affect treatment, especially in chronic pain of the musculoskeletal system. In addition, tricyclic antidepressants are beneficial in the treatment of chronic musculoskeletal diseases and neuropathic pain (Bergman, 2007).

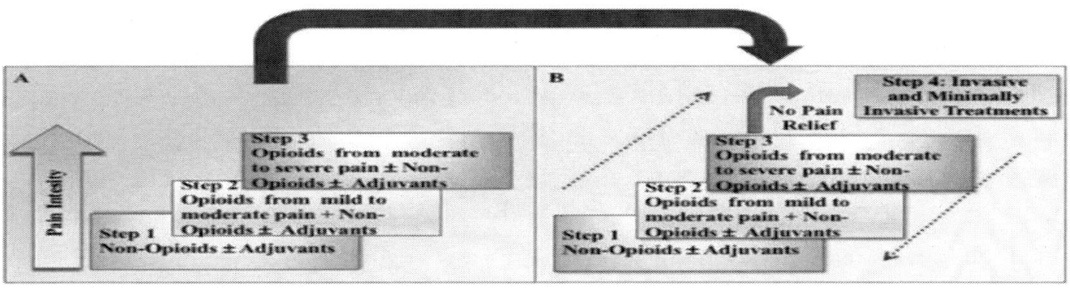


Transition from the original WHO three-step analgesic ladder (**A**) to the revised WHO fourth-step form (**B**). The additional step 4 is an "interventional" step and includes invasive and minimally invasive techniques. This updated WHO ladder provides a bidirectional approach.

Figure 3. The WHO analgesic ladder (Anekar, Aabha & Cascella, 2021).

Pain is a complex condition, so a multifaceted approach is required in the treatment. Analgesic therapy alone may not be sufficient, especially in musculoskeletal pain treatment. The patient should be led to non-drug treatment methods to prevent a new-onset pain from becoming chronic and to increase the patient's life quality.

Non-drug treatment methods include physical activity, patient education, physical therapy, traditional and complementary medicine practices such as hypnosis and acupuncture, and cognitive behavioral therapy. Walking, running, aerobics, swimming, cycling, and stretching and strengthening exercises can be recommended as physical activities. The most appropriate activity for the age and conditions of the patient should be preferred.

It has been shown that physical exercise, especially in musculoskeletal pain, increases the patient's functionality and decreases pain. Physical therapy is beneficial in reducing pain and enhancing functionality when applied within a treatment plan by experts. It has been observed that cognitive-behavioral therapy, in addition to medical treatment, has positive effects, especially in diseases such as fibromyalgia. Generally, these treatments alone are not sufficient for pain control. In addition to medical treatment, applying all non-drug treatment methods together raises treatment success and the patient's life quality (Bergman, 2007).

The patient's lifestyle should be understood. Risk factors such as smoking, obesity, and a sedentary life that may lead to pain or cause pain to become chronic should be intervened in patient education. The patient should be informed of conditions that may provoke pain, and it should be explained that drugs alone may not be sufficient in treating pain. The patient should be encouraged to do physical exercise. It should be explained that the most appropriate non-drug treatment methods will be beneficial in pain control in addition to medical treatment. The patient should be supported to quit smoking. The patient should be given counseling about proper nutrition behaviors in the presence of obesity.

Individuals with a coexisting psychiatric illness history, personality disorder, or substance abuse may show incoordination with patient education and pain management. These conditions also reduce the patient's ability to cope with pain. However, patients with chronic pain complaints are complex patients for doctors, even if they do not have a history of coexisting diseases. The concomitant psychiatric disease may make pain management more difficult for the physician (Jameson, 2019). Therefore, a multidisciplinary approach in pain management becomes more critical. Family physicians undertake an essential mission in treating pain by evaluating the patients from many aspects and guiding them whenever necessary with the biopsychosocial approach.

## Conclusion

All people experience pain at least once in their lifetime. Musculoskeletal pain is particularly one of the most common reasons for applying to polyclinics. The physiology of pain should be known to understand pain. As the health care providers who can be most easily reached, family physicians should evaluate musculoskeletal pain correctly. A personalized treatment should be administered, with consideration of the pain physiology to treat pain effectively. The patient's condition should be evaluated, the appropriate analgesics should be prescribed, and/or lifestyle changes should be recommended. If necessary, the patient should be referred to the relevant specialist. Chronic pain can be prevented by an appropriate intervention in the acute phase. So, secondary problems caused by pain can be prevented, and the patient's life quality can be raised. An individual with a high life quality takes part in society more effectively and efficiently.

## REFERENCES


Agaezi Onwuasoanya, D. (2016). Pain Management and Assessment for Healthcare Practitioners: Review Article. *Journal of Anesthesia & Pain Medicine*, *1*(2), 1–4. https://doi.org/10.33140/japm/01/02/00003.

Anekar, Aabha, A., & Cascella, M. (2021). *WHO Analgesic Ladder - StatPearls - NCBI Bookshelf*. Treasure Island (FL): StatPearls Publishing. https://www.ncbi.nlm.nih.gov/books/NBK554435/.

Apkarian, A. V., Bushnell, M. C., Treede, R. D., & Zubieta, J. K. (2005). Human braiEmechanisms of pain perception and regulation in health and disease. *European Journal of Pain*, *9*(4), 463. https://doi.org/10.1016/j.ejpain.2004.11.001.

Basbaum, A. I., Bautista, D. M., Scherrer, G., & Julius, D. (2009). Cellular and Molecular Mechanisms of Pain. *Cell*, *139*(2), 267–284. https://doi.org/10.1016/j.cell.2009.09.028.

Bergman, S. (2007). Management of musculoskeletal pain. *Best Practice and Research: Clinical Rheumatology*, *21*(1), 153–166. https://doi.org/10.1016/j.berh.2006.10.001

Breivik, H., Collett, B., Ventafridda, V., Cohen, R., & Gallacher, D. (2006). Survey of chronic pain in Europe: Prevalence, impact on daily life, and treatment. *European Journal of Pain*, *10*(4), 287. https://doi.org/10.1016/j.ejpain.2005.06.009.

Brown, D. A., & Passmore, G. M. (2009). Neural KCNQ (Kv7) channels. *British Journal of Pharmacology*, *156*(8), 1185–1195. https://doi.org/10.1111/j.1476-5381.2009.00111.x.

Bushnell, M. C., Čeko, M., & Low, L. A. (2013). Cognitive and emotional control of pain and its disruption in chronic pain. *Nature Reviews Neuroscience*, *14*(7), 502–511. https://doi.org/10.1038/nrn3516.

Coghill, R. C., Sang, C. N., Maisog, J. M., & Iadarola, M. J. (1999). Pain intensity processing within the human brain: A bilateral, distributed mechanism. *Journal of Neurophysiology*, *82*(4), 1934–1943. https://doi.org/10.1152/jn.1999.82.4.1934.

Deniz, S., Atim, A., Purtuloğlu, T., & Kurt, E. (2013). Results of the assessment of the council of multidisciplinary pain. *Agri*, *25*(3), 123–128. https://doi.org/10.5505/agri.2013.77045.

Garland, E. L., & Ph, D. (2013). Pain Processing in the Nervous System. *Prim Care*, *39*(3), 561–571. https://doi.org/10.1016/j.pop.2012.06.013.Pain.

Haefeli, M., & Elfering, A. (2006). Pain assessment. *European Spine Journal*, *15*(SUPPL. 1), 17–24. https://doi.org/10.1007/s00586-005-1044-x.

*IASP Terminology - IASP*. (n.d.). Retrieved May 15, 2021, from https://www.iasp-pain.org/Education/Content.aspx?ItemNumber=1698#Pain.

Jameson, R. N. (2019). The Doctor–Patient Relationship in Pain Management: Dealing with Difficult Clinician–Patient Interactions. In J. C. Ballantyne, S. M. Fishman, & J. P. Rathmell (Eds.), *Bonica's Management of Pain* (5th ed., pp. 1590–1614). Wolters Kluwer -- Medknow Publications.

Kopf, A., & Patel, N. B. (2010). Guide to Pain Management in Low-Resource Settings. *IASP Press*, 1–384. papers2://publication/uuid/C6AF8061-CDFC-4664-92EE-549338C9A317.

MacKichan, F., Wylde, V., & Dieppe, P. (2008). The Assessment of Musculoskeletal Pain in the Clinical Setting. *Rheumatic Disease Clinics of North America*, *34*(2), 311–330. https://doi.org/10.1016/j.rdc.2008.03.002.

Mccarberg, B. H., Nicholson, B. D., Todd, K. H., Palmer, T., & Penles, L. (2008). *The Impact of Pain on Quality of Life and the Unmet Needs of Pain Management : Results From Pain Sufferers and Physicians Participating in an Internet Survey*. *320*, 312–320.

Min, B. K. (2010). A thalamic reticular networking model of consciousness. *Theoretical Biology and Medical Modelling*, *7*(1), 1–13. https://doi.org/10.1186/1742-4682-7-10.

*Pain | Definition of Pain by Merriam-Webster*. (n.d.). Retrieved May 15, 2021, from https://www.merriam-webster.com/dictionary/pain.

Pınar, L. (2016). *Fundamentals of Nervous System and Muscle Physiology* (4th ed.). Akademisyen Kitabevi.

Tsang, A., Von Korff, M., Lee, S., Alonso, J., Karam, E., Angermeyer, M. C., Borges, G. L. G., Bromet, E. J., de Girolamo, G., de Graaf, R., Gureje, O., Lepine, J. P., Haro, J. M., Levinson, D., Oakley Browne, M. A., Posada-Villa, J., Seedat, S., & Watanabe, M. (2008). Common Chronic Pain Conditions in Developed and Developing Countries: Gender and Age Differences and Comorbidity With Depression-Anxiety Disorders. *Journal of Pain*, *9*(10), 883–891. https://doi.org/10.1016/j.jpain.2008.05.005.

Turk, D. C., Wilson, H. D., & Cahana, A. (2011). Pain 2 Treatment of chronic non-cancer pain. *The Lancet*, *377*(9784), 2226–2235. https://doi.org/10.1016/S0140-6736(11)60402-9.

Yam, M. F., Loh, Y. C., Tan, C. S., Adam, S. K., Manan, N. A., & Basir, R. (2018). General pathways of pain sensation and the major neurotransmitters involved in pain regulation. *International Journal of Molecular Sciences*, *19*(8). https://doi.org/10.3390/ijms19082164.

Zubrzycki, M., Liebold, A., Skrabal, C., Reinelt, H., Ziegler, M., Perdas, E., & Zubrzycka, M. (2018). Assessment and pathophysiology of pain in cardiac surgery. *Journal of Pain Research*, *11*, 1599–1611. https://doi.org/10.2147/JPR.S162067.

In: Musculoskeletal Pain (Common Clinical Presentations) ISBN: 978-1-68507-410-4
Editors: Mehmet Cenk Turgut and Serdar Toy 

*Chapter 2*

# Low Back Pain

***Cuma Uz*[*], *MD***
Department of Physical Therapy and Rehabilitation,
Kirikkale High Specialized Hospital, Kirikkale, Turkey

## Abstract

Low back pain is an important reason for hospital admissions. Low back pain affects the families and environment of patients by causing economic losses, decreases in work performance, need for medical care and psychological stress. We classify low back pain according to the duration of symptoms as acute, subacute and chronic. The diagnosis and treatment process is shaped according to this classification. We can collect the etiology of low back pain under three main headings. These are mechanical low back pain, non-mechanical low back pain and referred pain. Age, weight, occupational, sociocultural and psychosocial factors are important risk factors for low back pain. In the approach to the patient with low back pain, detailed anamnesis, detailed physical examination and imaging methods are used. Although the treatment varies according to the etiology, rest, medical treatments, exercise, physical therapy programs and surgical treatments are the primary approaches.

**Keywords:** low back pain, lumbar disc hernia, physical therapy

## Introduction

Low back pain is a significant health problem causing limitation in daily life activities and loss of labor. Low back pain is defined as the pain felt between the 12th rib and the inferior gluteal fold. Depending on the etiology, the pain may radiate to the thighs, legs, or feet.

[*] Corresponding Author's E-mail: cumauz12@gmail.com.

The prevalence of low back pain is over 70%, and its annual prevalence varies between 15 and 45% (Tulder et al., 2006). 63.2% of women and 33.8% of men have experienced back pain at least once in their lifetime (Altinel et al., 2008).

The years lived with disability caused by low back pain have increased by 54%, mainly due to population growth and aging, with the most significant increase in low-income and middle-income countries. Low back pain is the leading cause of disability nowadays (Hartvigsen et al., 2018). For these reasons, low back pain should be handled in a multidisciplinary manner, and measures to reduce the disability, labor loss, and burden on health expenditures and diagnosis and treatment strategies should be determined.

Low back pain is divided into acute, subacute, and chronic by the duration of symptoms. The condition in which the pain persists for six weeks or less is defined as acute low back pain. Low back pain is considered to be subacute if it lasts for 6-12 weeks and chronic if it lasts longer than 12 weeks (Parfenov and Golovachera, 2019). Diagnosis and treatment strategies differ according to whether low back pain is acute, subacute, or chronic.

## Low Back Pain (Lumbago)

Low back pain is a health problem with different underlying causes and negatively affects the life quality of affected individuals.

**Table 1. Low back pain classification**

| Mechanical Back Pain | Non-Mechanical Back Pain | Referred Pain |
|---|---|---|
| • Lumbar strain, sprain<br>• Spondylosis, spondylolisthesis<br>• Discogenic pain (disc herniation, radiculopathy<br>• Scoliosis, transitional vertebra, sacralization, lumbarization)<br>• Osteoporotic compression fractures<br>• Trauma<br>• Sacroiliac dysfunction<br>• Thoracolumbar junction syndrome<br>• Myofascial pain syndromes<br>• Coccydynia (tailbone pain)<br>• Posture disorder<br>• Failed back surgery | • Neoplasia (multiple myeloma, leukemia, lymphoma, spinal cord tumors, metastasis, renal tumors, primary vertebral tumors<br>• Infection (osteomyelitis, septic discitis, epidural abscess, shingles)<br>• Rheumatological (spondyloarthropathies, fibromyalgia, polymyalgia rheumatica)<br>• Metabolic bone diseases (osteoporosis, osteomalacia, Paget's disease, Scheuermann's disease) | • Gastrointestinal system diseases (cholecystitis, pancreatitis, peptic ulcer)<br>• Pelvic organ diseases (prostatitis,<br>• endometriosis, pelvic inflammatory disease)<br>• Renal diseases (nephrolithiasis, pyelonephritis, perinephric abscess)<br>• Aortic aneurysm |

According to the etiology, it can be classified as idiopathic, mechanical, rheumatological, metabolic, infectious, endocrine, neoplastic, neurological/psychiatric, and visceral-originated pains. It can also be classified as mechanical back pain, non-mechanical back pain, and referred back pain by symptom characteristics (Table 1).

## Low Back Pain Risk Factors

Age, gender, body weight, genetics, occupational factors, smoking, sociocultural level, and psychosocial factors play an essential role in developing low back pain (Ferreira et al., 2011).

Age: Degenerative changes in the lumbar spine increase with age. Therefore, age is a significant risk factor for low back pain.

Gender: Low back pain with occupational mechanical factor etiology is frequent in men. In the general population, low back pain is more common in women due to menstruation, pregnancy, childbirth, and postmenopausal osteoporosis (Wáng et al., 2016).

Genetic predisposition: Genetic factors that determine the building and destruction of the structural and biochemical content of the intervertebral disc cause a faster degenerative process (Kalichman and Hunter, 2008).

Obesity: In a meta-analysis including 33 studies, a strong association was found between being overweight/obese and seeking care for low back pain and chronic low back pain (Shiri et al., 2010).

Smoking: Long-term smoking has a significant relationship with chronic low back pain (Kwon et al., 2006).

Psychosocial factors: Psychosocial factors such as stress, depression, and anxiety are significant in developing chronic low back pain (Linton, 2005).

Occupational factors: Low back pain development is more common in occupations requiring physical strength and involving physical conditions such as manual handling, bending forward, and vibration (Hoogendoorn et al., 2000).

Education level: Some studies have found a relationship between low education and increased prevalence of low back pain. The duration of low back pain and the frequency of recurrence were higher in those with a low education level in a review (Dionne et al., 2001).

## Clinical Evaluation of Low Back Pain

A detailed anamnesis should be taken in a patient presenting with low back pain. The following should be questioned in the patient with low back pain: age, gender, occupation, onset time and type of pain, severity, localization, whether it radiates to the legs, what increases or decreases pain, night pain, urinary and stool incontinence, numbness, tingling and weakness, morning stiffness and duration. In addition, the presence of fever, sweating and shivering for the infection and the treatments applied, the response to painkillers and comorbid diseases should be questioned. Red flags in low back pain are the findings suggesting severe spinal pathologies requiring urgent intervention. Questioning these findings is essential for differential diagnosis.

Red flag findings: These are conditions suggesting malignancy, infection, and inflammatory rheumatic disease requiring detailed examination. The findings are as follows: being younger than 18 years old or older than 55 years, history of severe trauma, fever, chills, and night sweats, involuntary weight loss, immunosuppressive drugs usage, drug abuse, pain that does not decrease with rest, awakening from sleep at night, saddle anesthesia, urinary retention and/or lower limb weakness, and morning stiffness

Yellow flag findings are psychosocial factors that can be effective in low back pain. These factors include the belief that pain will lead to severe disability, avoidance of activities, belief in passive treatment rather than active treatment, low or negative mood, job dissatisfaction, an overprotective family, or lack of family support. Yellow flags should be identified and treated to prevent low back pain from becoming chronic (Bratton, 1999; Watson and Collett, 2003).

## Physical Examination

Physical examination starts with the measurement of vital signs in patients with low back pain. The patient's posture and gait should be observed when the patient enters the room. The increase/decrease in lordosis, the presence of scoliosis, skin lesion, and muscular atrophy/hypertrophy should be evaluated by inspection. On palpation, paravertebral spasm, myofascial trigger points, and painful spinous protrusions can be detected. Painful spinous processes may be significant for fracture, infection, and trauma. The lumbar spine range of motion should be evaluated. The normal lumbar spine range of motion is 40-60° in flexion, 20-35° in extension, 15-20° in lateral flexion, and 3-18° in rotations. Increasing pain with flexion indicates posterolateral localization, while pain in extension indicates central localization, and pain in ipsilateral bending indicates lateral herniation (Al Nezari et al., 2013). In physical examination, the sacroiliac and hip joint examination should also be performed.

## Neurological Examination

A manual muscle strength evaluation, deep tendon reflexes, pathological reflexes, and sensory examination are performed by neurological examination.

The L4, L5, and S1 roots are most commonly affected in lumbar spine disc pathologies. Sensory symptoms are seen in the anterior thigh in L1, L2, and L3 root compression. In the motor examination, the iliopsoas, sartorius, hip flexor and adductor muscles are evaluated. In L4 root compression, sensory loss extending from the medial of the leg to the medial of the foot, a decrease or loss of patella reflexes, and weakness in the quadriceps, and tibialis anterior muscles are observed. In L5 root compression, sensory impairment in the area on the lateral aspect of the leg extending to the medial of the foot dorsum and weakness in the extensor hallucis longus, gluteus medius, extensor digitorum longus, and brevis muscles are seen. The Achilles reflex is weak or missing in S1 root compression. Weakness is observed in the toe flexors, peroneus longus and brevis, triceps surae, and gluteus maximus muscles, together with sensory impairment in the area extending from the back of the leg to the foot lateral (Oğuz, 2011). Since the spinal cord conus ends at L1-L2 in lumbar radiculopathy, no upper motor neuron findings such as Babinski reflex, spasticity, and hyperreflexia are seen. If there are any, upper motor neuron abnormalities should be investigated.

Distinctions between an upper motor neuron (multiple sclerosis), nerve root (disc herniation), and peripheral nerve lesions (diabetes mellitus) are essential for the differential diagnosis of low back pain.

## Specialized Tests (Kosteljanetz, 1984; Windt, 2010)

### *SLR (Straight Leg Raise) Test*

This is positive in the compression of L4, L5, S1, S2, and S3 roots, especially L5 and S1 roots, forming the sciatic nerve. While the patient is lying in the supine position, the leg is lifted passively by holding the heel with the knee in extension, and it is evaluated whether the pain occurs in the waist and anatomical distribution area of the sciatic nerve. Pain between 30 and 70 degrees indicates sciatic nerve root compression. At the same time, pain above 70 degrees suggests facet joint and sacroiliac joint pain. The Bragard test is used to distinguish pain felt at the back of the leg during the SLR test from hamstring shortness. The test is started by performing the SLR test; then, the leg is lowered 10 cm at the point where the pain is felt, and the ankle is brought to dorsiflexion. The recurrence of pain radiating to the leg indicates compression of the sciatic nerve.

***Contralateral SLR Test***

When an SLR test is performed on the painless leg, the feeling of pain on the affected side suggests a large central herniation.

***Double Leg Raise Test***

The patient's legs lying in the prone position are raised to 30 degrees with the knees in extension, and the patient is asked to maintain the position. The presence of pain in the lower back indicates test positivity. This test suggests pathology in the posterior elements of the lumbar spine, such as facet syndrome or spondylolisthesis.

***Femoral Nerve Stretch Test***

The test evaluates irritation of the L2-L3 nerve roots forming the femoral nerve. The hip of the patient lying in the prone position is passively hyperextended with the knee in extension. Pain on the anterior surface of the leg indicates test positivity.

***Waddell's Test***

This identifies patients with functional or exaggerated findings and reveals psychosomatic disease. The presence of three of the five findings is clinically significant.

- Sensitivity by superficial touch,
- Pain sensation in movements that do not typically cause pain (e.g., low back pain with slight axial loading),
- Conflicting results in the same tests in different positions (e.g., no pain in the SLR test when repeatedly sitting),
- Regional sensory and motor disorders not conforming to neuroanatomical structures,
- Excessive reaction during physical examination (disproportionate reactions such as bouncing and retraction).

Laboratory and Radiological Evaluation in Low Back Pain: The use of laboratory tests in evaluating low back pain is limited, and it is preferred in distinguishing systemic diseases from mechanical diseases. Sedimentation and CRP (c-reactive protein) are tests that can be used to evaluate infection and inflammatory back pain. Laboratory examination may be helpful in systemic diseases and malignancies, especially in elderly patients. Clinical findings in patients presenting with nonspecific low back pain are not directly related to radiological findings. Imaging findings of people with and without low back pain may be similar. Spondylosis and degeneration can be found in 40-50% of patients without pain.

On the contrary, most patients with low back pain may not present imaging findings. Therefore, imaging is not recommended primarily in patients with nonspecific low back pain. However, if red flags related to fracture, cancer, infection, or cauda equina syndrome are present, imaging must be requested, and a detailed examination should be performed.

### *Plain Radiography*

Despite advanced diagnostic methods, anteroposterior and lateral radiographs of the lumbar region are the first imaging method to be performed. It helps to detect inflammatory, neoplastic, structural and degenerative spinal changes, fractures, dislocations, degenerative joint diseases, spondylolisthesis, and some bone diseases and vertebral tumors (Hansen et al., 2016). Oblique radiographs are used to visualize the neural foramina. Radiological findings of disc herniation are flattening in lordosis, scoliosis, and narrowing of the disc space. Narrowing of the disc space is detected in approximately one-third of the patients with low back pain. Spondylosis is detected in one-third of the patients.

### *Ultrasonography (USG)*

The most important indication of USG in patients with low back pain is determining the primary etiology in referred pain. Since the spinal canal is completely ossified in adults, USG use is limited to applications during surgery.

### *Computed Tomography (CT)*

CT may be required to diagnose degenerative diseases, obtain more information about bone morphology and structural/acquired vertebral anomalies, and demonstrate the presence or suspicion of fractures or foreign bodies. It has an important place in spinal trauma. In conclusion, CT's speed, resolution, and image reconstruction advantages and its ability to visualize both bone and soft tissue place this examination at the forefront of spinal examination (van Rijn et al., 2012).

### *Magnetic Resonance Imaging (MRI)*

MRI is preferred in degenerative spinal disease because it shows contrast resolution and internal disc structure. It has superior diagnostic ability in disc disease and imaging of a sequestered and ripped disc from its level. In the case of extradural neoplasia, infiltrative diseases, and myelopathy, it helps to diagnose with high sensitivity. Dehydration, annular tears, and herniations in the intervertebral disc are visualized on MRI with superior soft-tissue contrast. Evaluation of sequestered disc hernias and peridiscal degeneration and differentiation of hernias from other lesions is more straightforward with MRI (Hansen et al., 2016).

### *Electromyography (EMG)*

With inconsistent imaging and clinical findings, neurophysiological tests may be needed. Electrodiagnostic evaluation helps to reveal radiculopathy and determine the affected root level in patients with low back and leg pain. It can help to distinguish neuropathy from radiculopathy (Dillingham et al., 2002).

### *Radionuclide Imaging*

Radionuclide studies are most commonly used to screen metastases, detect primary spinal neoplasia or infection, and evaluate unexplained low back pain.

## Lumbar Strain/Sprain

This has an important place in the etiology of patients presenting with low back pain. Pain is often in the lumbosacral region and does not radiate to the lower extremity. Flexion and extension movements are painful, and pain increases with activity and decreases with rest. There is lumbar movement limitation and paravertebral muscle spasm on physical examination. Radicular and neurological findings are generally absent. Most patients recover completely within two weeks, 90% within two months, while in 10%, the condition becomes chronic (Jenkins, 2002).

## Lumbar Disc Hernia

Lumbar disc herniation is defined as the protrusion of the intervertebral disc material out of the intervertebral disc space. Radiculopathy occurs when the herniated disc compresses the spinal nerve root. It constitutes 4% of mechanical back pain.

The intervertebral disc consists of the gelatinous nucleus pulposus and the annulus fibrosus surrounding it. Tears occur in the annulus fibrosus fibers with inadequate hydration due to factors such as excessive and disproportionate overloading, aging, obesity, and smoking. The nucleus pulposus then becomes herniated from these tears.

The posterior longitudinal ligament (PLL), surrounding the intervertebral disc and vertebral bodies, has a thinner and weaker structure than the annulus fibrosus. Disc herniations are often posterolaterally localized, as the PLL fibers gradually become thinner from the midline towards the lateral and the remaining posterolateral part of the disc is empty (Loughenbury et al., 2006). When considering the entire spine, herniation is most common in the lumbar region. In the lumbar spine, herniation is most common at the levels of L4-L5 and L5-S1, the most mobile and load-bearing segments. The frequency of herniation is high at these levels due to higher load-bearing, a narrower central channel diameter, and a more mobile segment (McNamee et al., 2013).

## Risk Factors

Genetics, age, obesity, and jobs requiring heavy lifting are the main factors in developing lumbar disc herniation. Ages between 15 and 55 are the riskiest group for lumbar disc herniation (Demir et al., 2014). Heavy lifting, sudden rotational movements, and posture impairment cause the pressure increase on the intervertebral disc and form the basis for disc degeneration and herniation.

## History and Clinic

The most significant complaint of the patients is localized low back pain. The pain develops gradually, is widespread and stinging, increases with movement, decreases with rest, and is in the lower back and radiates to the leg by the anatomical distribution of the affected nerve root. It can start suddenly with an adverse movement like leaning forward or turning back and is aggravated by the slightest movement, leading to locking and back stiffness. Pain is enhanced by coughing, sneezing, sitting, standing, driving, and spine flexion due to increasing intradiscal pressure, and relieved by lying down, supporting lumbar lordosis, and extension movement.

The syndrome characterized by findings such as stool and urinary incontinence, perianal anesthesia, difficulty in walking, and loss of anal reflex is called cauda equina syndrome, caused by paralysis of the sacral roots due to large posterior herniation (Korse et al., 2017). Red flags should be determined to exclude severe underlying pathologies such as cancer, infection, and fracture in patients presenting with low back pain.

## Physical Examination

This should include inspection, palpation, a lumbar range of motion evaluation, sensory and motor examination, muscle strength evaluation, and provocative tests. The patient's gait should be evaluated during the inspection as antalgic gait can be seen in patients with disc herniation. Lumbar lordosis is mostly flattened. The paravertebral muscles of the patient should be palpated for spasm and trigger points. Valleix points should be palpated for radicular pain.

## Lumbar Range of Motion

The patient's flexion, extension, rotation, and lateral flexion should be measured with the aid of an inclinometer. Increasing pain in flexion indicates posterolateral localization, increasing pain in extension indicates central localization, and increasing pain with ipsilateral bending indicates lateral herniation (Al Nezari et al., 2013).

## Neurological Examination

This includes muscle strength, reflex, and sensory examination. Reflex examination compromises deep tendon, superficial, and pathological reflexes. In the reflex examination, patellar (L3-L4), medial hamstring (L5), and Achilles (S1) reflexes, and in the sensory examination, light touch, sense of heat, and pinpoint touch methods should be performed comparative to the other extremities (Al Nezari et al., 2013).

There are different types and degrees of disc herniation. Classification of disc herniation consistent with MRI findings is beneficial in evaluation. Pathology in disc herniation is classified as bulging, protrusion, extrusion, and sequestration of the annulus fibrosis (Figure 1).

## Bulging

This is the bulging and convexification of the disc material beyond normal limits. The annulus fibrosis is normal. It is asymptomatic unless spinal stenosis occurs or neural tissues are affected.

## Protrusion

This is posterior displacement of the disc material within the weakened and torn annulus fibrosis. The PLL is intact.

## Extrusion

This is displacement of the disc material due to completely torn annulus fibrosis. The PLL is torn.

**Sequestration**

The herniated disc is wholly separated from the disc as a free fragment and displaces cranially or caudally.

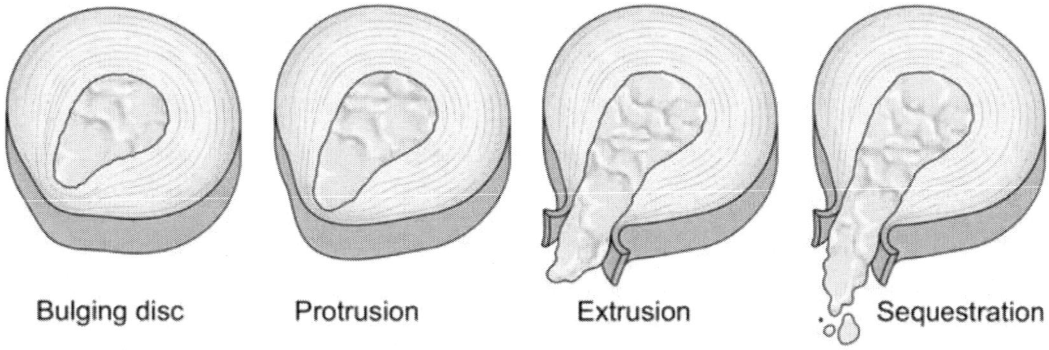


Figure 1. Classification of disc herniation (Cunha et al., 2018).

## LUMBAR SPONDYLOSIS

Lumbar spondylosis, in other words, spine osteoarthritis, is a clinical picture that occurs from degenerative changes in the intervertebral disc, corpus, intervertebral foramen, facet joints, lamina, and ligaments, often due to age and chronic mechanical stress. Radiographically, it is characterized by narrowed joint space, subchondral sclerosis, and cyst formation. Smoking, occupational factors, and genetics are responsible for the etiology. The frequency of degeneration increases with age, and a normal spine is rare after the age of 60. Instability due to spondylosis is also typical. Clinically, the main complaint is pain localized in the lower back, and when spinal stenosis develops due to spondylosis, the pain radiates to the gluteals and leg.

## FACET JOINT SYNDROME

Facet joint pain often occurs from the degeneration of the facet joints. It is clinically characterized by pain in the lumbosacral region. The pain can radiate to the legs but not below the knees – pain increases, especially with rest, extension, and rotational movements. Palpation of the facet joints is painful, and neurogenic claudication can be seen. While the straight leg raising test is negative, the double leg raising test is positive. Neurological examination is often regular. Lumbar bidirectional radiographs are auxiliary in diagnosis (Perolat et al., 2018).

## Spinal Stenosis

Lumbar spinal stenosis is caused by the compression of neural elements from any narrowing in the spinal canal, nerve root canal, or intervertebral foramen. It is divided into central and lateral according to anatomical location and primary and secondary according to etiology. Central stenosis develops from the narrowed sagittal and/or coronal diameter of the spinal canal and is usually at the intervertebral disc level. The canal diameter can be narrowed due to facet joint hypertrophy, ligamentum flavum thickening, intervertebral disc bulging, or spondylolisthesis. Lateral canal stenosis is a clinical picture that occurs with facet joint hypertrophy of the lateral canal, a decrease in disc height, posterolateral disc protrusion, or narrowing due to spondylolisthesis. It is localized in the region from which the nerve root sheath separates from the dural sac and ends at the lateral of the intervertebral foramen where the spinal nerve joins the lumbosacral plexus (Şendur, 2011). Although the anteroposterior diameter of the lumbar canal is stated differently in different sources, a diameter of 17-23 mm is generally accepted as normal. In symptomatic people, this diameter is as low as 10-15 mm. The mid-sagittal diameter is less than 13 mm in relative stenosis and <10 mm in absolute stenosis. The anteroposterior diameter is <3 mm in lateral canal stenosis.

Spinal stenosis progresses with symptoms decreasing and increasing according to posture, loading, and even loading time. Patients are usually over the age of 50, as the underlying causes are primarily degenerative. Patients complain of low back pain that has been present for a long time and has recently increased. Leg pain can be unilateral or bilateral and can radiate from the thigh to the calf or foot. With the flexion of the waist, the spinal canal's anteroposterior diameter increases due to the separation of the lamina and the decrease in the ligamentum flavum thickness, and the symptoms are relieved. Therefore, patients tend to stand in a forward-bent posture. Symptoms are intensified in extension and under load. In physical examination, although flexion is usually painless and regular, extension is limited and painful. In lateral canal stenosis, the patient usually complains of single-leg pain, and leg pain is prominent with no low back pain (Şendur, 2011).

## Lumbar Myofascial Pain Syndrome

Myofascial pain syndrome is characterized by intramuscular trigger points that are sensitive on palpation. It often causes acute pain but can also cause chronic recurrent pain. Although any muscle can be affected, the multifidus, quadratus lumborum, erector spinae, and psoas muscles, and interspinous and supraspinous ligaments are most commonly affected. Depending on the affected muscle, flexion, lateral flexion, and rotations are painful, whereas the pain decreases in extension. The diagnosis is usually made clinically, and local injections are helpful in treatment.

## SPONDYLOLYSIS – SPONDYLOLISTHESIS

The defect occurring in the pars interarticularis of the vertebra is called spondylolysis. Spondylolisthesis is the displacement of all or part of a vertebra over the underlying vertebra and consists of 5 types (Niggemann et al., 2012). The backward sliding or displacement of one vertebra over the other is called retrolisthesis.

Type 1 – Dysplastic spondylolisthesis is characterized by the forward subluxation of the lumbosacral joint due to dysplasia of the sacral vertebra.

Type 2 – Isthmic or spondylotic spondylolisthesis is the most common type. It is often acquired and develops after spondylolysis or stress fracture in the pars interarticularis.

Type 3 – Degenerative spondylolisthesis is not a pars interarticularis defect and develops due to facet joint degeneration.

Type 4 – Traumatic spondylolisthesis develops due to acute fracture in the posterior structures of the vertebra.

Type 5 – Pathological spondylolisthesis is seen when the bone structure is weakened by infection, malignancy, or osteoporosis.

Spondylolisthesis is graded by the Meyerding staging method by the vertebral shift amount (Figure 2).

Spondylolisthesis causes low back pain that decreases with rest and increases with activity. It is common in the young population. Lumbar lordosis increases, and a step-off sign is detected in palpation. If there is no spinal stenosis, radicular and neurological findings are not observed. The extension is painful. Lumbosacral corsets with steel baleen, exercise, physical therapy, and injections are used in the treatment due to the risk of instability. Surgical treatment is considered in patients developing neurological deficits and not responding to conservative treatment.

Failed back surgery includes spinal stenosis, degenerative changes, pseudoarthrosis, recurrent disc herniation, and vertebral instability due to deficient lumbar surgical methods.

Inflammatory low back pain is often seen under the age of 40, has an insidious onset, decreases with exercise, and increases with rest. Restriction of the spine movements and chest expansion, pain radiating to the hip and thigh, peripheral arthritis, tenderness in enthesitis areas, and dactylitis can be detected on the physical examination. In addition, extra-articular involvement such as inflammatory bowel disease, psoriatic skin rash, and uveitis may accompany the clinical picture (Erol et al., 2018).

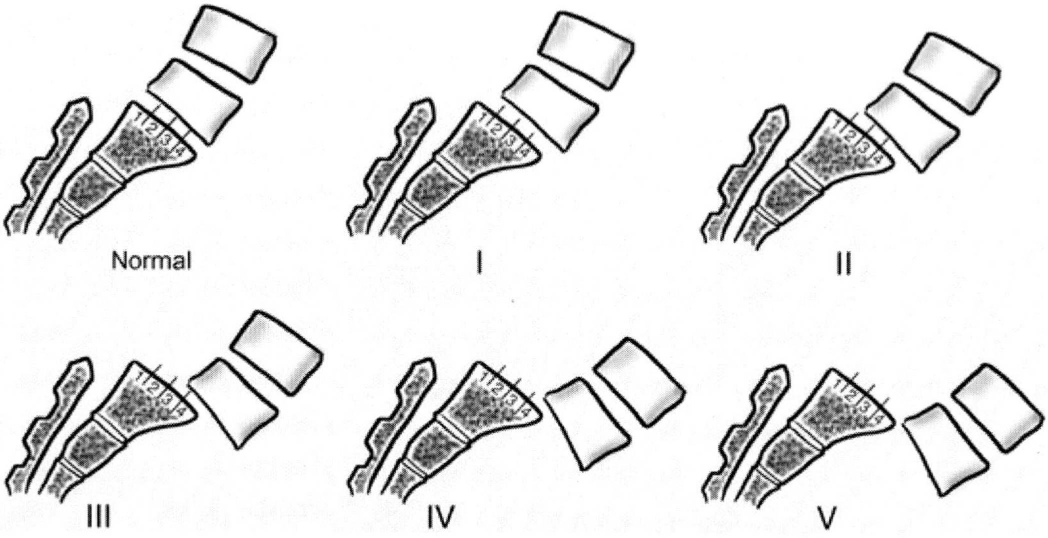


Figure 2. The Meyerding classification of spondylolisthesis (Lasanianos, 2015).

Findings suggesting low back pain associated with malignancy are as follows;

- Lack of typical features of mechanical back pain,
- Continuous and non-decreasing pain in atypical areas or more than one area,
- Pain unrelated to movement and posture,
- Widespread bone pain,
- Systemic and constitutional symptoms,
- Being over the age of 55 and not having previous similar pain attacks,
- High sedimentation rate.

In the presence of these findings, a further examination must be required.

## Treatment in Low Back Pain

Half of the patients with acute low back pain recover without treatment in the first two weeks, while 40% recover in 4-12 weeks with treatment. In the remaining 10% of patients, back pain becomes chronic. Low back pain treatment aims to relieve pain and prevent recurrence of pain and chronicity.

## Education

The first step of treatment in pain management is to explain the natural course of the symptoms to the patient and give information about the treatment process. Patient education content should include the course of the disease, the factors that increase pain, the treatment process, and the expected recovery duration. Patients should be informed about not lifting anything heavy, avoiding shearing movements, and not sitting and standing for a long time (Taşçı et al., 2021).

## Bed Rest

There are different opinions about bed rest in the literature. In current treatment guidelines, patients with acute low back pain are recommended to have bed rest not exceeding four days. Long-term bed rest is not recommended as it may lead to the weakening of the lumbar region muscles.

## Exercise

This is given to expand the range of motion, strengthen lumbar region muscles, stretch tense structures, or strengthen patients physically and mentally. Flexion, extension, stretching, aerobic exercises, and a dynamic lumbar stabilization program are suggested (Meray et al., 2015; Akuthota et al., 2008). The NICE guideline recommends exercises such as stretching, yoga, and aerobics as first-line treatments for patients with acute low back pain. In addition, patients should be encouraged to continue their normal daily activities.

Posture and lumbar protection training are the beginning of rehabilitation in patients with acute low back pain. In patients with acute low back pain, abdominal contraction exercises, lower extremity stretching, and strengthening exercises should be performed without increasing intrathecal pressure by avoiding waist flexion exercises.

In the subacute period, core stabilization exercises are essential in forming static and dynamic lumbar recovery. Core stabilization exercises increase neuromuscular control, strength, and endurance of the multifidus, transversus abdominis, and pelvic floor muscles, stabilizing the lumbar region. As the first step in core stabilization exercises, exercises for ensuring normal muscle mobility and length should be performed. After that, lumbopelvic stability exercises should be added to the training program. Then, functional exercises increasing balance coordination at standing should be initiated (Meray et al., 2015; Akuthota et al., 2008).

In the first phase of core stabilization training, it is essential to activate the transversus abdominis and the external and internal oblique muscles and initiate abdominal corset application. The abdominal corset application should be continued throughout the exercise, and rhythmic diaphragmatic breathing should be performed with expiration during the abdominal muscle contraction and inspiration during the abdominal muscle relaxation. Stretching and strengthening the lumbar extensors and hamstring muscles should not be omitted in patients undergoing core stabilization and abdominal flexor strengthening. After the exercises in the lying position are completed, the exercises during sitting, standing, and walking should be started (Meray et al., 2015; Akuthota et al., 2008). In the chronic period, in addition to core stabilization exercises, walking, running, cycling, aerobic exercises such as gymnastics (calisthenic), aquatic exercises, Pilates, Yoga, and Tai Chi exercises could be done.

Pilates is mind-body exercises targeting core stabilization, endurance, flexibility, posture, breathing techniques, and muscle control. Pilates is thought to be effective in reducing pain and disability in patients with low back pain. There are also publications stating that Tai Chi and Yoga are effective on pain and disability in patients with low back pain. Since aerobic exercises effectively improve physical and psychological functions and decrease pain intensity, they can be recommended, especially in patients with chronic low back pain (Meray et al., 2015). Therapeutic massage in addition to exercise has been found to affect pain and functional recovery.

## Pharmacological Treatment

Acetaminophen is the drug of choice in low back pain guidelines due to its low risk of side effects and effectiveness. However, in some guidelines, 4-week treatment was not superior to placebo (Qaseem, 2017). Nonsteroidal anti-inflammatory drugs (NSAIDs) could be initiated in patients not responding to acetaminophen treatment. There is no difference in the efficacy of different NSAI drugs. The most common side effects of NSAIDs are gastrointestinal complaints. Studies have shown that the risk of ulcers and complications increases 4-10 times in nonspecific NSAID users compared to non-users. Since gastrointestinal, renal, and cardiac side effects are dose-dependent, the use of NSAI drugs at the lowest effective dose and for the shortest duration should be preferred (Garcia and Barreales 2007).

In the case of an inadequate response to NSAIDs, a weak opioid addition to the treatment is recommended. Despite their strong analgesic effects, they should be used cautiously due to side effects such as respiratory depression, constipation, and sedation (Bratton, 1999).

Myorelaxants can be used in patients who are thought to have low back pain of myofascial origin. They have addictive potential and can induce drowsiness. There is insufficient evidence regarding the long-term use of myorelaxants in pain treatment (Bhatia et al., 2020; Foster et al., 2018).

Gabapentin and pregabalin are used in the treatment of neuropathic pain accompanied by radicular pain. Patient selection is important because of their side effects, such as confusion, dizziness, and addictive potential. Treatment should always be started at a low dose, and then the dose could be increased according to patient compliance. The onset of effect occurs after two weeks, and the treatment should be discontinued by tapering the dose in patients with an inadequate response in the 4th week (Bhatia et al., 2020).

Duloxetine is frequently used among antidepressant drugs, especially in chronic low back pain with a neuropathic component. Studies have shown that duloxetine is superior to placebo in controlling pain and increasing functionality in patients with chronic low back pain. Treatment should be started with 30 mg and increased to 60 mg after two weeks. In patients with an inadequate response at the end of the 4th week, the treatment should be discontinued by dose tapering (Weng et al., 2020).

## Physical Therapy Modalities

Various physical therapy modalities commonly used to treat low back pain cause early mobilization by improving symptoms such as pain and spasm. For this purpose, therapeutic hot, cold, and deep heaters, low and medium frequency currents, transcutaneous electrical nerve stimulation (TENS), laser, acupuncture, manipulation and massage, balneotherapy, magnetic field therapy, biofeedback, cognitive behavioral therapy, mindfulness-based stress reduction, and yoga can be used (Yurdakul et al., 2019). These modalities should be applied with the correct technique considering contraindications.

## Back School

This is an essential part of the rehabilitation of patients with low back pain. The main objectives of the back school are to inform people about low back pain, teach them to use the correct body mechanics during daily life and work, improve their ability to cope with back problems and their quality of life by increasing self-confidence, and reduce recurrences. Some reviews about the effectiveness of back school on chronic low back pain stated that it has a moderate effect on short-term pain and functional status. There was moderate evidence that it is no different to other treatments in the long term. A review of the current guidelines recommended patient education most frequently in nonspecific acute low back pain (Tulder et al., 2000).

## Interventional Methods

Intervertebral disc stimulation, medial bundle branch block, and facet and sacroiliac joint injections could be performed for diagnostic purposes. Therapeutic epidural steroid injections, on the other hand, increase the physical activity level of the patient by helping the healing of intervertebral disc and spinal root lesions. Peripheral nerve blocks, epidural steroid and local anesthetic injections, sympathetic blocks, radiofrequency applications, peripheral nerve stimulation, spinal cord stimulation, intrathecal drug applications, and cerebral and cortical neurostimulation are among the other methods used. Although these treatment methods are not therapeutic alone, they could be effective in the short-medium term when the correct procedure is applied to the appropriate patient at the right time (Tecer and Taşkaynatan, 2017).

## Surgical Treatment

The primary purpose of surgical treatment is to remove the compression on neural structures in pathologies such as lumbar disc herniation, in which neurological losses are prominent with radicular pain due to nerve root compression. Surgical intervention should be considered when progressive and neurological deficits and relapses develop despite conservative treatment. Cauda equina syndrome is the only emergency surgery indication in lumbar disc herniation (LDH). The patient should be operated on within the first 48 hours after symptom onset. Otherwise, there is a risk of developing paraplegia. Surgical indication exists relatively in the following conditions; sciatica with large disc herniation unresponsive to analgesics; sciatica lasting more than 4-6 weeks and moderate loss of muscle strength (>3/5); radicular pain lasting longer than 6-12 weeks and unresponsive to conservative treatments; and persistent radicular pain accompanied by spinal canal stenosis (McAfee, 2004).

# CONCLUSION

Low back pain is a common symptom in our daily clinical practice causing severe disability in patients. It has an important place in labor loss and health expenses. The primary purpose of the approach to low back pain is to correctly identify and treat the factors causing low back pain and prevent the pain from becoming chronic. It should be kept in mind that there may be reasons other than the lumbar region in the etiology of low back pain, so the approach should be multidisciplinary.

## REFERENCES


Akuthota, V., Ferreiro, A., Moore, T., & Fredericson, M. (2008). Core stability exercise principles. *Current sports medicine reports*, *7*(1), 39–44.

Al Nezari, N. H., Schneiders, A. G., Hendrick, P. A. (2013). Neurological examination of the peripheral nervous system to diagnose lumbar spinal disc herniation with suspected radiculopathy: a systematic review and meta-analysis. *The spine journal: official journal of the North American Spine Society*, *13*(6), 657–674.

Altinel, L., Köse, K. C., Ergan, V., Işik, C., Aksoy, Y., Ozdemir, A., Toprak, D., & Doğan, N. (2008). Afyonkarahisar ilinde erişkinlerde bel ağrisi sikliği ve etkileyen faktörler [The prevalence of low back pain and risk factors among adult population in Afyon region, Turkey]. *Acta orthopaedica et traumatologica turcica*, *42*(5),328–333.

Bhatia, A., Engle, A., & Cohen, S. P. (2020). Current and future pharmacological agents for the treatment of back pain. *Expert opinion on pharmacotherapy*, *21*(8), 857–861.

Bratton R. L. (1999). Assessment and management of acute low back pain. *American family physician*, *60*(8), 2299–2308.

Cunha, C., Silva, A. J., Pereira, P., Vaz, R., Gonçalves, R. M., & Barbosa, M. A. (2018). The inflammatory response in the regression of lumbar disc herniation. *Arthritis research & therapy*, *20*(1), 251.

Demir, S., Dulgeroglu, D., & Cakci, A. (2014). Effects of dynamic lumbar stabilization exercises following lumbar microdiscectomy on pain, mobility and return to work. Randomized controlled trial. *European journal of physical and rehabilitation medicine*, *50*(6), 627–640.

Dillingham, T. R., Lauder, T. D., Andary, M., Kumar, S., Pezzin, L. E., Stephens, R. T., & Shannon, S. (2000). Identifying lumbosacral radiculopathies: an optimal electromyographic screen. *American journal of physical medicine & rehabilitation*, *79*(6), 496–503.

Dionne, C. E., Von Korff, M., Koepsell, T. D., Deyo, R. A., Barlow, W. E., & Checkoway, H. (2001). Formal education and back pain: a review. *Journal of epidemiology and community health*, *55*(7), 455–468.

Erol, K., Gok, K., Cengiz, G., Kilic, G., Kilic, E., & Ozgocmen, S. (2018). Extra-articular manifestations and burden of disease in patients with radiographic and non-radiographic axial spondyloarthritis. Extra-articular manifestations and burden of disease in patients with radiographic and non-radiographic axial spondyloarthritis. *Acta reumatologica portuguesa*, *43*(1), 32–39.

Ferreira, G. D., Silva, M. C., Rombaldi, A. J., Wrege, E. D., Siqueira, F. V., & Hallal, P. C. (2011). Prevalence and associated factors of back pain in adults from southern Brazil: a population-based study. *Rev Bras Fisioter*, 15(1): p. 31-6.

Foster, N. E., Anema, J. R., Cherkin, D., Chou, R., Cohen, S. P., Gross, D. P., Ferreira, P. H., Fritz, J. M., Koes, B. W., Peul, W., Turner, J. A., Maher, C. G., & Lancet Low

Back Pain Series Working Group (2018). Prevention and treatment of low back pain: evidence, challenges, and promising directions. *Lancet (London, England)*, *391*(10137), 2368–2383.

García Rodríguez, L. A., & Barreales Tolosa, L. (2007). Risk of upper gastrointestinal complications among users of traditional NSAIDs and COXIBs in the general population. *Gastroenterology*, *132*(2), 498–506.

Hansen, B. B., Hansen, P., Carrino, J. A., Fournier, G., Rasti, Z., & Boesen, M. (2016). Imaging in mechanical back pain: Anything new?. *Best practice & research. Clinical rheumatology*, *30*(4), 766–785.

Hartvigsen, J., Hancock, M. J., Kongsted, A., Louw, Q., Ferreira, M. L., Genevay, S., Hoy, D., Karppinen, J., Pransky, G., Sieper, J., Smeets, R. J., Underwood, M., & Lancet Low Back Pain Series Working Group (2018). What low back pain is and why we need to pay attention. *Lancet (London, England)*, *391*(10137), 2356–2367.

Hoogendoorn, W. E., van Poppel, M. N., Bongers, P. M., Koes, B. W., & Bouter, L. M. (2000). Systematic review of psychosocial factors at work and private life as risk factors for back pain. *Spine*, *25*(16), 2114–2125.

Jenkins H. (2002). Classification of low back pain. *Australas Chiropr Osteopathy*, 10(2):91-7.

Kalichman, L., & Hunter, D. J. (2008). The genetics of intervertebral disc degeneration. Familial predisposition and heritability estimation. *Joint bone spine*, *75*(4), 383–387.

Korse, N. S., Pijpers, J. A., van Zwet, E., Elzevier, H. W., & Vleggeert-Lankamp, C. (2017). Cauda Equina Syndrome: presentation, outcome, and predictors with focus on micturition, defecation, and sexual dysfunction. *European spine journal: official publication of the European Spine Society, the European Spinal Deformity Society, and the European Section of the Cervical Spine Research Society*, *26*(3), 894–904.

Kosteljanetz, M., Espersen, J. O., Halaburt, H., & Miletic, T. (1984). Predictive value of clinical and surgical findings in patients with lumbago-sciatica. A prospective study (Part I). *Acta neurochirurgica*, *73*(1-2), 67–76.

Kwon, M. A., Shim, W. S., Kim, M. H., Gwak, M. S., Hahm, T. S., Kim, G. S., Kim, C. S., Choi, Y. H., Park, J. H., Cho, H. S., & Kim, T. H. (2006). A correlation between low back pain and associated factors: a study involving 772 patients who had undergone general physical examination. *Journal of Korean medical science*, *21*(6), 1086–1091.

Lasanianos N. G., Triantafyllopoulos G. K., Pneumaticos S. G. (2015). Spondylolisthesis Grades. In: Lasanianos N., Kanakaris N., Giannoudis P. (eds) *Trauma and Orthopaedic Classifications*. Springer, London, pp 239-242.

Linton S. J. (2005). Do psychological factors increase the risk for back pain in the general population in both a cross-sectional and prospective analysis?. *European journal of pain (London, England)*, *9*(4), 355–361.

Loughenbury, P. R., Wadhwani, S., & Soames, R. W. (2006). The posterior longitudinal ligament and peridural (epidural) membrane. *Clinical anatomy (New York, N.Y.)*, *19*(6), 487–492.

McAfee P. C. (2004). The indications for lumbar and cervical disc replacement. *The spine journal: official journal of the North American Spine Society*, *4*(6 Suppl), 177S–181S.

McNamee, J., Flynn, P., O'Leary, S., Love, M., & Kelly, B. (2013). Imaging in cauda equina syndrome--a pictorial review. *The Ulster medical journal*, *82*(2), 100–108.

Meray J., Tecer D. (2015). Lomber Diskopatilerde Egzersizler ve Korunma [Exercise in Lumbar Disc Herniation and Prevention] *Turkiye Klinikleri Journal of Physical Medicine Rehabilitation Special Topics*, 8(4):50-56.

Niggemann, P., Kuchta, J., Grosskurth, D., Beyer, H. K., Hoeffer, J., & Delank, K. S. (2012). Spondylolysis and isthmic spondylolisthesis: impact of vertebral hypoplasia on the use of the Meyerding classification. *The British journal of radiology*, *85*(1012), 358–362.

Oğuz H. (2011). Bel Ağrılarında Klinik Değerlendirme. [Clinical Evaluation of Low Back Pain] *Turkiye Klinikleri Journal of Physical Medicine Rehabilitation Special Topics*, 4(1):12-16.

Parfenov, V. A., & Golovacheva, V. A. (2019). *Terapevticheskii arkhiv*, *91*(8), 155–159.

Perolat, R., Kastler, A., Nicot, B., Pellat, J. M., Tahon, F., Attye, A., Heck, O., Boubagra, K., Grand, S., & Krainik, A. (2018). Facet joint syndrome: from diagnosis to interventional management. *Insights into imaging*, *9*(5), 773–789.

Qaseem, A., Wilt, T. J., McLean, R. M., Forciea, M. A., & Clinical Guidelines Committee of the American College of Physicians (2017). Noninvasive Treatments for Acute, Subacute, and Chronic Low Back Pain: A Clinical Practice Guideline from the American College of Physicians. *Annals of internal medicine*, *166*(7), 514–530.

Şendur, Ö. F. (2011). Lomber Spinal Stenoz [Lumbar Spinal Stenosis] *Turkiye Klinikleri J PM&R-Special Topics,* 4(1):44-52

Shiri, R., Karppinen, J., Leino-Arjas, P., Solovieva, S., & Viikari-Juntura, E. (2010). The association between obesity and low back pain: a meta-analysis. *American journal of epidemiology*, *171*(2), 135–154.

Taşçı Bozbaş G., Gürer G. (2021). Akut bel ağrılarında tanı ve tedavi yaklaşımı.[Approach to Diagnosis and Treatment in Acute Low Back Pain] Tuncer T, Çubukçu Fırat S, Kaçar C, Sezer İ, editörler. Bel Ağrıları. 1. Baskı. Ankara: *Türkiye Klinikleri*, p.86-91.

Tecer D., Taşkaynatan M. A. (2017). Spinal Ağrılarda Algoritmik Yaklaşım [Algorithmic Approach in Spinal Pain]. *Turkiye Klinikleri Journal of Neurology Special Topics*, 10(4):395-399.

van der Windt, D. A., Simons, E., Riphagen, I. I., Ammendolia, C., Verhagen, A. P., Laslett, M., Devillé, W., Deyo, R. A., Bouter, L. M., de Vet, H. C., & Aertgeerts, B.

(2010). Physical examination for lumbar radiculopathy due to disc herniation in patients with low-back pain. *The Cochrane database of systematic reviews*, (2), CD007431.

van Rijn, R. M., Wassenaar, M., Verhagen, A. P., Ostelo, R. W., Ginai, A. Z., de Boer, M. R., van Tulder, M. W., & Koes, B. W. (2012). Computed tomography for the diagnosis of lumbar spinal pathology in adult patients with low back pain or sciatica: a diagnostic systematic review. *European spine journal: official publication of the European Spine Society, the European Spinal Deformity Society, and the European Section of the Cervical Spine Research Society*, *21*(2), 228–239.

van Tulder M. W., Koes B. W., Assendelft W. J., Buter L. M. (2000). Chronic low back pain: exercise therapy, multidisciplinary programs, NSAID's, back schools and behavioral therapy effective; traction not effective; results of systematic reviews. *Ned Tijdschr Geneeskd*, 144:1489-94.

van Tulder, M., Becker, A., Bekkering, T., Breen, A., del Real, M. T., Hutchinson, A., Koes, B., Laerum, E., Malmivaara, A., & COST B13 Working Group on Guidelines for the Management of Acute Low Back Pain in Primary Care (2006). Chapter 3. European guidelines for the management of acute nonspecific low back pain in primary care. *European spine journal: official publication of the European Spine Society, the European Spinal Deformity Society, and the European Section of the Cervical Spine Research Society*, *15 Suppl 2*(Suppl 2), S169–S191. https://doi.org/10.1007/s00586-006-1071-2.

Wáng, Y. X., Wáng, J. Q., & Káplár, Z. (2016). Increased low back pain prevalence in females than in males after menopause age: evidences based on synthetic literature review. *Quantitative imaging in medicine and surgery*, *6*(2), 199–206.

Watson P. J., Collett B. (2003). Chronic low back pain: Patient had chronic rather than acute pain. *BMJ*, *327*(7406), 107.

Weng, C., Xu, J., Wang, Q., Lu, W., & Liu, Z. (2020). Efficacy and safety of duloxetine in osteoarthritis or chronic low back pain: a Systematic review and meta-analysis. *Osteoarthritis and cartilage*, *28*(6), 721–734.

Yurdakul, O. V., Beydoğan, E., & Yılmaz Yalçınkaya, E. (2019). Effects of physical therapy agents on pain, disability, quality of life, and lumbar paravertebral muscle stiffness via elastography in patients with chronic low back pain. *Turkish journal of physical medicine and rehabilitation*, *65*(1), 30–39.

In: Musculoskeletal Pain (Common Clinical Presentations) ISBN: 978-1-68507-410-4
Editors: Mehmet Cenk Turgut and Serdar Toy 

*Chapter 3*

# CERVICAL PAIN

***Gökhan Çağlayan*, MD***
Department of Rheumatology,
Giresun University Training and Research Hospital, Giresun, Turkey

## ABSTRACT

Cervical pain is one of the most common musculoskeletal pain syndromes. Its prevalence is similar to low back pain and it may lead to disability. Intervertebral discs, zygapophyseal joints, cervical nerve roots and referred pain are causes of cervical pain. Neck pain is acute, subacute or chronic; nociceptive or neuropathic. Red flags are important and need to be investigated. Rheumatological diseases such as spondyloarthropathies and rheumatoid arthritis are important besides cervical sprains, strains and myofascial pain. Spondylosis gains importance with aging. Disc hernias should be kept in mind for radicular pain and myelopathy. Taking history and physical examination are two cornerstones for reaching a diagnosis. Radiological imaging and laboratory tests are used when needed. Nonsteroidal anti-inflammatory drugs, rest or exercises, physical therapy modalities or cervical collars are first treatment options. For resistant cases therapeutic injections or cervical spine interventions are considered.

## INTRODUCTION

The neck is the anatomical region between the head and trunk. It has important conduits for vascular and neural tissues between the brain and other parts of the body. Most of them are provided by the cervical spine which combines strength and a wide range of movement. Cervical vertebrae supply strength to the neck region and have

* Corresponding Author's E-mail: gokhancaglayan@yahoo.com.tr.

structures for cervical movements. These complex articular system elements are intervertebral discs, zygapophyseal (facet, apophyseal) joints at the posterior lower parts, looser synovial joints at the upper parts and uncovertebral joints (Luschka joints). The discs permit rotatory movements. Zygapophyseal joint movements involve gliding which permits flexion and extension and rotation. Patients with neck pain have varied limitations for a cervical range of movement which is controlled by complex neuromuscular activity (Barnsley, 2018).

Neck pain may originate from local structures of the cervical spine or distant parts that refer pain to the neck (referred pain). Most chronic cases are musculoskeletal in origin but others must be excluded by history, physical examination and laboratory or radiological investigations if necessary. “Red flags” or “alerting features” are important to ask the patient. These are weight loss, fever, malignancy in the history, and neurological deficits. Cervical nerve root and cervical cord compression are two important issues related to the neck region.

## EPIDEMIOLOGY

### Incidence and Prevalence

Cervical pain is less common than low back pain but it is the fourth reason for global disability. 1 in 20 people have cervical pain at any time. One-year incidence is between 10% and 21% and mean one-year prevalence is 25.8% according to a comprehensive review (Barnsley, 2018).

### Risk Factors

Trauma especially whiplash injury, occupation especially manual working with a heavy workload, level of education, and depression are important risk factors for chronic or recurrent mechanical neck pain. Others are high body mass index and metabolic syndrome. Increased flexibility in adolescence is good for future neck health. Some degree of genetic component for neck pain has been shown in twin studies (Barnsley, 2018).

### Classification of Cervical Pain

Neck pain is classified according to duration; acute for less than 6 weeks, subacute between 6 weeks and 3 months, and chronic for more than 3 months. It is classified according to the mechanism, as mechanical, neuropathic or referred pain and according to type; nociceptive and neuropathic pain. Mixed neuropathic-nociceptive pain may be seen with degenerative discs and failed neck surgery (Cohen, 2015). Differentiating types of pain affect treatment choices.

## Pathogenesis of Neck Pain

The exact cause of neck pain is difficult to find generally. In the acute pain entrapment of menisci in the zygapophyseal joints, inflammation is suggested to be the cause. Discal annular tears and trauma are other sources of pain. They may result in premature osteoarthritis. Adhesion, capsulitis and synovitis in zygapophyseal joints may be causes for chronic neck pain. The biopsychosocial model is important in which psychological and social factors also play a role (Barnsley, 2018).

There are seven cervical vertebrae and eight cervical spinal nerves. Uncovertebral (Luschka) joints are located in the lower cervical vertebral (C3-C7) uncinate processes which look like synovial joints. They are close to cervical spinal nerve roots. These joints are prone to osteoarthritic changes which cause constriction in the intervertebral foramens.

In the center of the intervertebral discs there is gelatin-like nucleus pulposus. The intervertebral discs are thicker at the anterior parts that contribute to normal cervical lordosis. Damage of the normal cervical anatomy, by degenerative and traumatic factors, causes some cervical vertebral diseases. In the neck region, the pain focus is on nerves, intervertebral discs, facet joints, posterior longitudinal ligaments and cervical muscles (DePalma and Slipman, 2010).

Pain from cervical facet joints extends to some anatomic regions: C2-3 extends to the occipital region; C3-4, C4-5 in the posterior part of the neck; C5-6 to the supraspinatus fossa of the scapula and C6-7 to the scapular region (DePalma and Slipman, 2010). Intervertebral discs cause bilateral vertebral pain in 34% to 50% of patients (Grubb and Kelly, 2010). Cervical radicular pain is different because it is actually upper extremity pain; arm, forearm or hands. Pain in the scapular region or trapezius muscles may originate from the C4 or C5 nerve root. C5 nerve root pain radiates to the arm; C6, C7 and C8 nerve root pains radiate to the forearm and hand. Nerve injuries through the intervertebral foramina may originate from these 3 structures; intervertebral discs which are most common, facet joints or uncovertebral joints. The second most common reason for cervical radiculopathies is cervical spondylosis that sometimes accompanies cervical myelopathy. In some radiculopathies there is only myotomal weakness without any pain (Liversedge et al., 1953). Hypotheses for pain mechanisms in cervical radiculopathies are inflammation in nerve roots (Bogduk, 2003), increased discharge in the dorsal root ganglion, mechanosensitivity or chemosensitivity in the nerve root, and direct pressure to axons or the dorsal root ganglia (Howe et al., 1977). Some other causes of cervical radiculopathy are tumors (Vargo and Flood, 1990), trauma (Poindexter and Johnson, 1984) and sarcoidosis (Atkinson, 1987).

Diseases affecting the neck region are classified as mechanical disorders (cervical sprain, cervical strain, herniation of the nucleus pulposus, cervical spondylosis, cervical stenosis, osteoarthritis), rheumatologic diseases (ankylosing spondylitis, psoriatic arthritis, rheumatoid arthritis, polymyalgia rheumatica, diffuse idiopathic skeletal hyperostosis, reactive arthritis, enteropathic arthritis, fibrositis, fibromyalgia), endocrinologic and metabolic diseases (osteoporosis, Paget's disease, osteomalacia, parathyroid disease), infectious diseases (osteomyelitis, discitis, epidural, intradural or subdural abscesses), benign tumors (osteochondroma, osteoid osteoma, osteoblastoma, hemangioma), malignant tumors (multiple myeloma, chondrosarcoma, Ewing's tumor, lymphoma, metastatic tumors), syringomyelia and arteriovenous malformation (DePalma and Slipman, 2010).

Non-musculoskeletal-related sources of cervical pain are laryngitis, pharyngitis, tracheitis, thyroiditis, lymphadenitis, carotidynia, angina, myocardial infarction, and pericarditis (Barnsley, 2018).

Disc herniations are classified as protrusion, extrusion and sequestration.

Disc degeneration starts with fissures in the peripheral annulus by the effect of microtrauma and insufficient nourishment of the discs. Both biomechanic and biochemical changes occur (Saal, 1995). In spinal stenosis pain increases with extension due to reduced spinal canal area however in discogenic pain forward flexion worsens pain (Cohen, 2015).

## Common Clinical Diagnoses

### Cervical Strain and Sprain

Cervical strain is the overloading injury of musculotendinous structures in the cervical spine. Cervical sprain is the injury of the cervical ligaments. Cervical muscular strains are more common where the upper trapezius and sternocleidomastoid muscles are injured (Press et al., 1996). Acute, relapsing or chronic injuries are the cause of about 85% of neck problems (Jackson, 1982). These injuries are observed in motor vehicle accidents and sport injuries. In whiplash (acceleration and deceleration) injuries there may be muscle rupture or hemorrhage, and anterior longitudinal ligament ruptures.

Physical examination findings are local tenderness in the paracervical muscles and a decrease in the cervical range of motion.

Nonsteroidal anti-inflammatory drugs (NSAIDs) are used for first line drugs for pain treatment. Muscle relaxants such as cyclobenzaprine may be used for acute neck pain. A soft collar is generally used for the first 72 hours. Physical modalities such as cold or heat, and electrical stimulation may be used. Exercises should be started after a decrease in pain.

## Cervical Radiculopathy and Radicular Pain

Cervical radiculopathy is a disorder of the nerve root. The most common cause is cervical intervertebral disc herniations, and the second is cervical spondylosis. There is usually unilateral arm and neck pain or both. Physical examination findings are a decrease in myotomal strength, paresthesias, sensory deficits and a decrease or loss in deep tendon reflexes. The C7 root (C6-7 herniation) is the most commonly affected nerve root, the C6 root (C5-6 herniation) and C8 root (C7-T1 herniation) are others (Iyer and Kim, 2016). Cervical and lumbar disc herniations may occur with the sudden exertion of heavy lifting. There is mechanical compression and inflammation (Theodore, 2020). The Valsalva maneuver increases pain. Radicular pain from C5-7 is felt in the scapula medial border; C5-6 in the upper trapezius, anterior chest wall, deltoid region, and lateral arm; C6-7 in the anterolateral forearm; C7-T1 in the anterolateral and posterior of the forearm and the posteromedial arm; and C6-T1 in the fingers. Muscle weakness or atrophy due to C5 or C6 radiculopathy is observed in the supra or infrascapular fossa or deltoid; from C7 in the triceps muscle; and C8 in the thenar or first dorsal interosseous regions. True neurological weakness should be distinguished from pain induced weakness. Deep tendon reflexes are examined as the biceps reflex for C5-C6 nerve roots, the brachioradialis reflex for the C6 nerve root and the triceps reflex for the C7 nerve root.

There are maneuvers that provoke radiculopathy. The Spurling test is cervical extension, lateral flexion, and axial rotation to the same side. Its mechanism depends on the narrowing of the neural foramen and production of the symptoms (Iyer and Kim, 2016). It has low sensitivity (30%) but high specificity (94%) according to a study (Tong et al., 2002). According to a systematic review, when rotation and extension are combined, the Spurling test becomes the most sensitive (30-100%) and specific (75-100%) test among other provocative tests like the Valsalva maneuver and neck distraction (Rubinstein et al., 2007). The Lhermitte sign is the sensation of an electric-like shock in the neck and upper extremities with passive neck flexion. It may be positive in multiple sclerosis, cervical tumor or spondylosis.

If there is exertional pain only in the arm, thoracic outlet syndrome should also be investigated. In a study with patients with shoulder and neck pain, a detailed history, physical examination and imaging studies are emphasized for a differential diagnosis of cervical radiculopathy/cervical foraminal stenosis from rotator cuff pathologies (Wu et al., 2018).

Cervical X-rays are generally the first radiological study especially for traumatic injuries, rheumatologic diseases (rheumatoid arthritis, ankylosing spondylitis), spondylolisthesis, scoliosis and degenerative disease. Routinely, anteroposterior and lateral views of the cervical spine are used. Oblique radiographs of the cervical spine are better for neural foramens.

Magnetic resonance imaging (MRI) is the best and most sensitive technique for radiculopathy. It depicts discs, muscles, ligaments, bone and nerves. MRI is recommended in patients with red flag signs, patients with a history of cancer and progressive neurologic deficits, for determining a fracture and for preprocedural and presurgical assessment (Popescu and Lee, 2020) Computerized tomography may be an option for bone tumors and fractures.

Electrodiagnostic tests (nerve conduction studies and electromyography) are useful for the functions of nerve roots, the cervical plexus and peripheral nerves. It enables the differentiation of nerve root impingement from peripheral entrapment syndromes (e.g., carpal and cubital tunnel syndromes). A patient may have both cervical radiculopathy and peripheral nerve entrapment, called the "double crush" phenomenon.

Treatment of cervical radiculopathy is done according to symptoms. Nonsteroidal anti- inflammatory drugs are first line drugs for nociceptive pain. Muscle relaxants may be added. For neuropathic pain, antiepileptic drugs especially gabapentin and pregabalin and tricyclic antidepressants (e.g., amitriptyline) may be used. Patient education and activity modification are important. Patients should be advised on the right posture and ergonomics. Soft collars for the short term may be suggested. Physical modalities such as heat, ultrasound, transcutaneous electrical nerve stimulation (TENS) and cervical traction may be suggested for proper patients. Traction is contraindicated in myelopathy. Range of movement, posture and isometric strengthening exercises should be started respectively.

Algologic diagnostic and treatment methods are suggested for patients who are resistant to conservative treatments. These are epidural corticosteroid and/or local anesthetic injections, and diagnostic and selective therapeutic nerve blocks by using fluoroscopy or ultrasonography (Chang et al., 2018).

Intractable pain (resistant to conservative management), neurological deficits and myelopathy are surgery indications. Percutaneous disc decompression, anterior cervical discectomy and fusion, cervical disc arthroplasty; and posterior decompression (foraminotomy) are surgical methods (Iyer and Kim, 2016). In a study about outcome predictors of anterior cervical decompression and fusion, a nonsmoking status is associated with better long-term results (Peolsson, A., and Peolsson, M., 2008).

## Cervical Facet Joint Pain

This may be traumatic (e.g., whiplash injuries) or spondylotic. The neck is examined for paraspinal tenderness on palpation. Headache may be present. Treatment after the above-mentioned conservative methods includes diagnostic or therapeutic facet joint blocks (injections) and radiofrequency ablation (other names are medial branch ablation, percutaneous radiofrequency neurotomy) (Cohen, S. P., Hooten, W. M., 2017).

## Cervical Internal Disc Derangement

Internal disc derangement is damage to the internal structure of the disc not the outer part so it occurs without nerve root compression. It may start with trauma and may get chronicity. A decreased fluid level of the disc, loss of disc height, annular fissure, osteophytosis, and end plate changes are signs of disc degeneration (Depalma and Slipman, 2010). Transforaminal epidural steroid injections may be tried after conservative treatments.

## Cervical Spondylosis

This is osteoarthritis of the cervical spine with disc degeneration, and osteophyte formation in the apophyseal and uncovertebral joints. Diffuse cervical pain may radiate to the occipital area, shoulders or interscapular area. Physical examination reveals midline tenderness and limited motion with extension and lateral flexion. Cervical X-rays show intervertebral narrowing and facet joint sclerosis (Borenstein, 2013). Treatment is acetaminophen, NSAIDs, exercises for neck flexibility, physical modalities or local injections. Topical NSAIDs may be more suitable than oral NSAIDs for older patients. Isometric exercises are recommended for chronic neck pain. Smoking and obesity are risk factors for cervical spondylosis (Kadow et al., 2015).

## Cervical Myelopathy

This occurs secondary to compression of the spinal cord or nerve roots. The most common reason is cervical spondylotic myelopathy, which is often seen, in older people. The usual cause is a decrease of volume of the spinal canal by compression with an osteophyte and degenerative disc. Other causes are disc herniation, multiple sclerosis, vasculitis, spine tumors, syringomyelia, motor neuron disease, trauma (spinal cord injury) and myelitis (Yu et al., 1987; Cohen 2015). Symptoms are numbness and paresthesias at the distal part of the extremities, weakness especially in the lower extremities, cervical axial pain, and walking disturbance. Bladder dysfunction, and urinary or rectal incontinence may occur in severe cases. Physical examination findings are upper motor neuron findings (Hoffman sign, hyperreflexia (increased deep tendon reflexes), Babinski sign, spasticity, clonus), atrophy in intrinsic hand muscles, ataxia and Romberg's sign (Theodore, 2020). MRI findings are spinal cord compression, myelomalacia, atrophy, and signal changes in the spinal cord (Depalma and Slipman, 2010). Surgery is indicated in patients with severe or progressive symptoms or failure of conservative treatments. Decompression surgeries such as anterior cervical discectomy, fusion, corpectomy, laminectomy, and laminoplasty are surgical methods.

## Cervicogenic Headache

Its prevalence is between 0.4% and 2.5% in the general population (Sjaastad and Fredriksen, 2000). It is one of the most common reasons for headache. It may originate from different cervical spinal structures.

## Whiplash Syndrome

This refers to symptoms related to whiplash injury which means hyperflexion then hyperextension of the neck during an accident (Barnsely et al., 1998). It is an acceleration-deceleration injury to the soft tissue structures of the cervical region. There is no direct trauma to the head or neck. It is generally due to a motor vehicle accident, but diving, falls, and sports injuries are also causes. Symptoms of stiffness and pain with motion generally start 12-24 hours after the accident. Neck pain with palpation, paracervical muscle contraction, and a decreased range of motion are examination findings. Severe whiplash can damage the sympathetic ganglia and results in Horner syndrome (Borenstein, 2013). A soft collar for the short term, rest, NSAIDs, and muscle relaxants are suggested. Most patients recover within the first weeks or first three months but some of them have chronic neck pain.

## Other Situations

When there is suspicion for infection or tumor, blood tests such as complete blood count, erythrocyte sedimentation rate, and C-reactive protein are ordered. The alkaline phosphatase test is useful for Paget disease. The isotope scan (bone scanning with technetium) is the first investigation method for the detection of metastases and useful for detecting bone infections.

In rheumatoid arthritis, the cervical spine may be affected especially in severe, erosive and seropositive disease. The most common situation is atlantoaxial subluxation. Separation of the anterior aspect of the odontoid process from the posterior inferior tubercle of the atlas is seen by using lateral X-rays, and a distance of more than 3 mm in women and more than 2.5 mm in men is pathologic (Komusi et al., 1985). Vertical subluxation of the odontoid may occur in some rheumatoid arthritis patients (Lipetz, J.S., and Lipetz, D.I., 2010). In patients with spondyloarthropathies or rheumatoid arthritis, early morning stiffness of the cervical spine is a common complaint which may last for hours in the morning. Patients with ankylosing spondylitis may have a decreased cervical range of movement. Patients with polymyalgia rheumatica have neck, shoulder and thigh pain. They are usually over 50 years of age and have early morning neck and shoulder stiffness with an increased erythrocyte sedimentation rate. Fibromyalgia is a chronic and widespread pain syndrome generally with tender points and other problems like fatigue and sleep or memory problems.

Rigid cervical collars can be used in patients with suspected instability. They restrict flexion and extension motions.

Spinal manipulation may have short-term benefits. It is contraindicated in cervical instability.

Myofascial pain is common in the neck region. Palpable trigger points in muscles which are taut muscle bands are important in physical examination. Posture exercises, analgesic medications, physical therapy, and trigger point injections are options for treatment. In a study comparing trigger point injection types lidocaine injection was found to be more practical than dry needling and more cost effective than Botulinum toxin-A injection (Kamanli et al., 2005).

## CONCLUSION

Neck pain is one of the most common musculoskeletal problems which is a big personal and social burden with disability. History taking and physical examination are two important key factors during the approach to cervical pain. Laboratory tests, imaging methods and electromyography are used when necessary. Pain treatment is recommended to begin with conservative methods and the stepped approach. The right posture, staying physically active and preventing cervical injuries should be emphasized.

## References

Atkinson R, Ghelman B, Tsairis P, et al., (1987) Sarcoidosis presenting as cervical radiculopathy. A case report and literature review. *Spine*, 7, 412-416.

Barnsely L, Lord S, Bogduk N. (1998) The pathophysiology of whiplash. *Spine State Art Rev.,* 12(2), 209-242.

Barnsley L. (2018) Neck pain. In: *Rheumatology*. Ed. Hochberg M. pp: 621-631.

Bogduk N. (2003) The anatomy and pathophysiology of neck pain. *Phys. Med. Rehabil. Clin. North Am.*, 14, 455-472.

Borenstein D. (2013) Approach to the patient with neck pain. In: *Current Diagnosis and Treatment Rheumatology*. Ed. Imboden J B, Hellmann D B, Stone J H.3th ed. Lange.pp: 79-85.

Chang K V, Wu W T, Özçakar L. (2018) Ultrasound-guided interventions of the cervical spine and nerves. *Phys. Med. Rehabil Clin. N. Am.*, 29(1), 93-103.

Cohen S P. (2015) Epidemiology, diagnosis and treatment of neck pain. *Mayo Clin. Proc.*, 90(2), 284-299.

Cohen S P, Hooten W M. (2017) Advances in the diagnosis and management of neck pain. *BMJ,* 358, j3221.

DePalma M J, Slipman C W. (2010) Treatment of common neck problems. In: *Physical Medicine and Rehabilitation*. Ed. Braddom R L. 3th edition.

Grubb S A, Kelly C K. (2000). Cervical discography: clinical implications from 12 years of experience. *Spine*, 25, 1382-1389.

Howe J F, Loeser J D, Calvin W H. (1977) Mechanosensitivity of dorsal root ganglia and chronically injured axons: a physiological basis for the radicular pain of nerve root compression. *Pain,* 3, 25-41.

Iyer S, Kim HJ. (2016). Cervical radiculopathy. *Curr. Rev. Musculoskelet. Med.*, 9, 272-280.

Jackson R. (1982). Cervical trauma: not just another pain in the neck. *Geriatrics*, 37,123.

Kadow T, Sowa G, Vo N, et al., (2015). Molecular basis of intervertebral disc degeneration and herniations: what are the important questions? *Clin. Orthop. Relat. Res.,* 473, 1903-1912.

Kamanli A, Kaya A, Ardicoglu O, et al., (2005) Comparison of lidocaine injection, botulinum toxin injection and dry needling to trigger points in myofascial pain syndrome. *Rheumatol. Int.,* 25(8), 604-611.

Komusi T, Munro T, Harth M. (1985) Radiologic view: the rheumatoid cervical spine. *Semin. Arthritis Rheum.*14,187-195.

Lipetz J S, Lipetz D I (2010). Disorders of the cervical spine. In: *DeLisa's Physical Medicine and Rehabilitation*. Ed. Frontera WR. Fifth edition. pp: 811-836.

Liversedge L A, Hutchinson E C, Lyons J B. (1953). Cervical spondylosis simulating motor neuron disease. *Lancet,* 2, 652-659.

Peolsson A, Peolsson M. (2008) Predictive factors for long-term outcome of anterior cervical decompression and fusion: a multivariate data analysis. *Eur. Spine J.,* 17(3), 406-414.

Poindexter DP, Johnson EW. (1984) Football shoulder and neck injury: a study of the 'stinger'. *Arch Phys Med Rehabil*, 65, 601-602.

Popescu A, Lee H. (2020) Neck pain and lower back pain. *Med. Clin. N. Am.*, 104, 279-292.

Press J M, Herring S A, Kibler WB. (1996) Rehabilitation of musculoskeletal disorders. In: *The textbook of military medicine.* Borden Institute: Office of the Surgeon General.

Rubinstein S M, Pool J J, van Tulder M W, et al., (2007) A systematic review of the diagnostic accuracy of provocative tests of the neck for diagnosing cervical radiculopathy. *Eur. Spine J.*, 16, 307-319.

Saal J. (1995). The role of inflammation in lumbar pain. *Spine*, 20, 1821-1827.

Sjaastad O, Fredriksen T. (2000) Cervicogenic headache: criteria, classification and epidemiology. *Clin. Exp. Rheumatol.,* 18(2 suppl 19), S3-6.

Vargo M M, Flood K M. (1990) Pancoast tumor presenting as cervical radiculopathy. *Arch. Phys. Med. Rehabil.* 71, 606-609.

Theodore N. (2020) Degenerative cervical spondylosis. *N. Engl. J. Med.*, 383,159-168.

Tong H C, Haig A J, Yamakawa K. (2002) The Spurling test and cervical radiculopathy. *Spine* (Phila Pa 1976), 27, 156-159.

Wu W T, Chang K V, Han D S, et al., (2018) Cross-talk between shoulder and neck pain: an imaging study of association between rotator cuff tendon tears and cervical foraminal stenosis. *Medicine*, 97, 36.

Yu Y L, Woo E, Huang C Y. (1987). Cervical spondylotic myelopathy and radiculopathy. *Acta Neurol. Scand.*, 75, 367-373.

In: Musculoskeletal Pain (Common Clinical Presentations) ISBN: 978-1-68507-410-4
Editors: Mehmet Cenk Turgut and Serdar Toy 

*Chapter 4*

# MUSCULOSKELETAL CHEST PAIN

***Mevlana Omeroglu**, MD***
Department of Emergency Medicine, Ataturk University,
Erzurum, Turkey

## ABSTRACT

Chest pain is the second most common cause of emergency admissions. Patients can describe discomfort in the chest as related to the heart, lungs, great vessels, esophagus, stomach and mediastinum, and abdominal organs. For emergency doctors, the patient examination is crucial in terms of clinical and vital findings, and defining and eliminating life-critical etiologies. Musculoskeletal chest pain (MSCP) forms 25% of admitting emergencies with a chest pain complaint. Though MSCP was observed in approximately 30-45% of patients who performed a percutaneous coronary intervention without any pathology, it should be known that the MSCP finding is not a reason to eliminate coronary disease (Brunse et al., 2010; E. Wolf, 1976). Diagnosing, differential diagnosis and treatment of isolated musculoskeletal chest pain (MSCP) will be discussed in this section of the book.

## INTRODUCTION

A patient describing a chest pain complaint is a situation where diagnosis and intervention should occur if necessary. First, it should be evaluated in terms of cardiopulmonary etiologies and acute coronary syndrome, acute aortic dissection, pulmonary embolism, tension pneumothorax, and pericardial tamponade, and esophageal rupture that may cause mediastinitis diagnoses should be eliminated. The presence of

* Corresponding Author's E-mail: mevlana.gul@atauni.edu.tr.

symptoms such as pain caused by effort, creeping pain to the neck, jaw and arms, weakness, fever, and cough is thought to be non-musculoskeletal etiology. It should be noted that musculoskeletal chest pain is a diagnosis of exclusion.

The patient's age, gender, family history, cardiac risk factors and comorbidity should be noted when starting the examination. MSCP occurs frequently in women. It can last for hours or even days. It is a sharp pain located in the xiphoid, parasternal area, middle of the sternum and floating rib. Pain can increase with movement, deep breathing, and movements of the arms. The localization of pain is sometimes not determinant in the differential diagnosis. Pain that increases with effort, creeping pain to the arm and neck, numbness, fever, chills, weakness, cough, shortness of breath, and localized pain in atypical areas such as the axilla indicate non-MSCP etiologies.

## Isolated MSCP Types

- Muscle strains. These are caused by the contraction of intercostal muscles. There is tenderness on palpation of the affected muscles. Especially with deep breathing, the pain will increase because the tension of the muscles increases.
- Costochondritis and Costochondral junction syndrome (Tietze syndrome). This is a pain syndrome involving one or more costochondral joints. Swelling on the joint is not expected in costochondritis. Tietze syndrome has nonsuppurative swelling. Generally, there is involvement in the second and third costochondral areas. It is frequently observed in young adults. It is rare. It may be developed secondary to upper respiratory tract infections or severe cough. Both clinics have pain and tenderness on palpation.
- Posterior Chest wall syndrome. This is caused by dysfunction of the costovertebral joints and/or thoracic vertebrae disc herniations. It can also occur after a throwing motion of the upper extremity. It is characterized by pain that creeps unilaterally across the band-shaped dermatome. Pain increases with coughing or deep inspirium.
- Lower rib pain syndrome. This is also called clicking-slipping rib syndrome, rib type syndrome, and 12th rib syndrome. Pain can be spreading or local. Pain increases with palpation of the costal margin. It can develop as a result of traumas such as bending over or heavy lifting.
- Osteoarthritis. Though osteoarthritis of the sternoclavicular joint is not common, it may be the cause of localized chest pain.
- Xiphoidalgia. This is characterized by pain of the xiphoid process, and it is not common. It may develop as a result of trauma, heavy activity and cough. Pain may increase by bending, stretching and eating large portions.

- Spontaneous sternoclavicular subluxation. This is observed in middle-aged women. It develops especially after repetitive moderate and heavy activity with a dominant extremity. Subluxation usually occurs in the superior and/or anterior directions. Sclerosis in the medial clavicle can be observed in radiography.
- Sternalis Syndrome. This is characterized by pain in the sternal body. After the palpation, bilateral creeping pain occurs.

## PHYSICAL EXAMINATION

A physical examination is for detecting abnormalities in the heart, lungs and abdomen. Inspection of the chest wall is crucial in terms of diagnosis, especially of herpes zoster, psoriasis, palmoplantar pustulosis, acne, furuncle, carbuncle, and hidradenitis suppurativa. Photophobia, eye pain and red eye may also help to evaluate underlying rheumatological diseases.

The musculoskeletal examination begins with evaluating the cervical area and shoulder range of motion. In the examination of the lumbar region, a limitation in flexion suggests spondyloarthropathies. Discomfort in the external rotation of the hip or compression of the anterior iliac wings leads to sacroiliitis. Chest pain caused by movements in the thoracic region supports MSCP (Yelland, 2001). Costovertebral joint movements are evaluated with chest expansion. Chest expansion is measured at the fourth intercostal space, just below the breast in females. When the patient takes a deep inspiration after a strong expiration, normal expansion is 5 cm and above; less than 2.5 cm, is abnormal.

### Examination of the Ribs and Chest Wall

The most important diagnostic feature is constant pain. The examination begins with locating the localized pain region. The sternoclavicular, acromioclavicular, upper costochondral, manubriosternal and xiphosternal joints and the xiphoid process should be palpated. In addition to direct palpation, there is diagnostic value in some movements increasing the pain.

- Crowing rooster maneuver; This is performed by the clinician standing behind the patient and pulling the upper arms back and slightly upward while the neck is in extension and rotation.

- Horizontal arm flexion maneuver; Extended traction is performed on the flexed arm in the horizontal direction from the front of the chest while the neck is in extension and rotation.
- Hooking Maneuver; This is performed by pulling the lower edge of the anterior rib forward with the fingers. It helps to diagnose clicking rib syndrome.

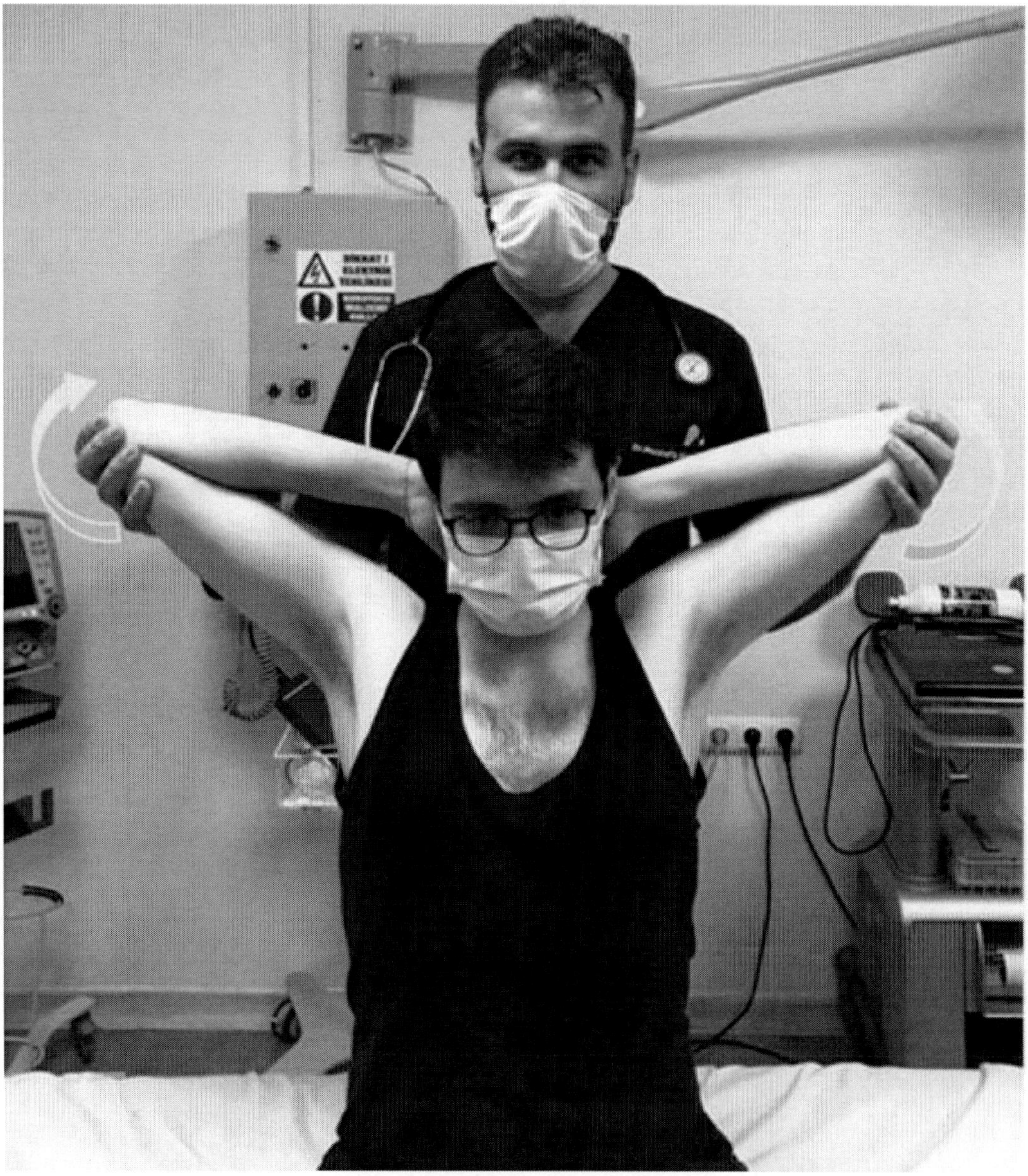

Figure 1. Crowing rooster maneuver.

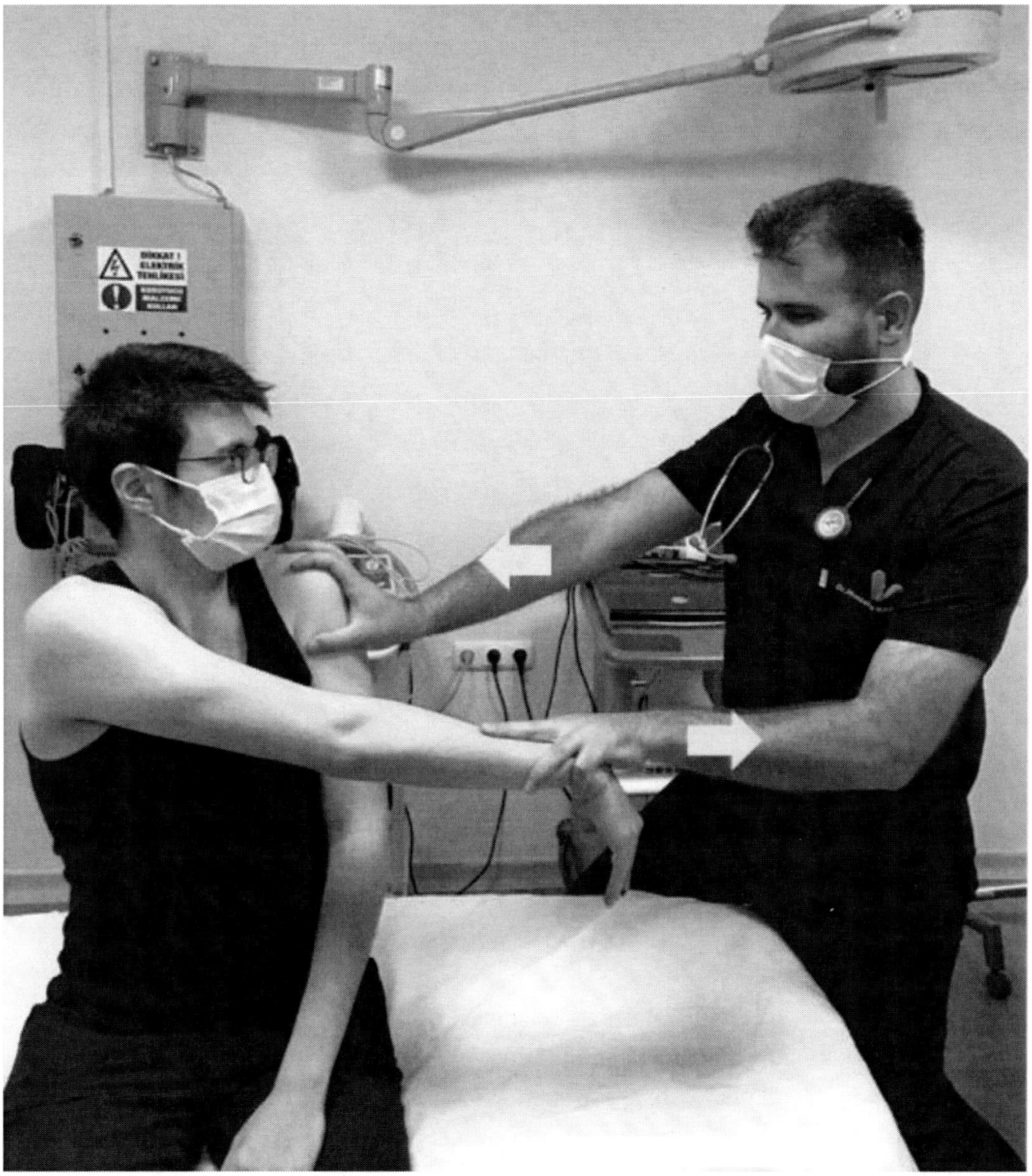

Figure 2. Horizontal arm flexion.

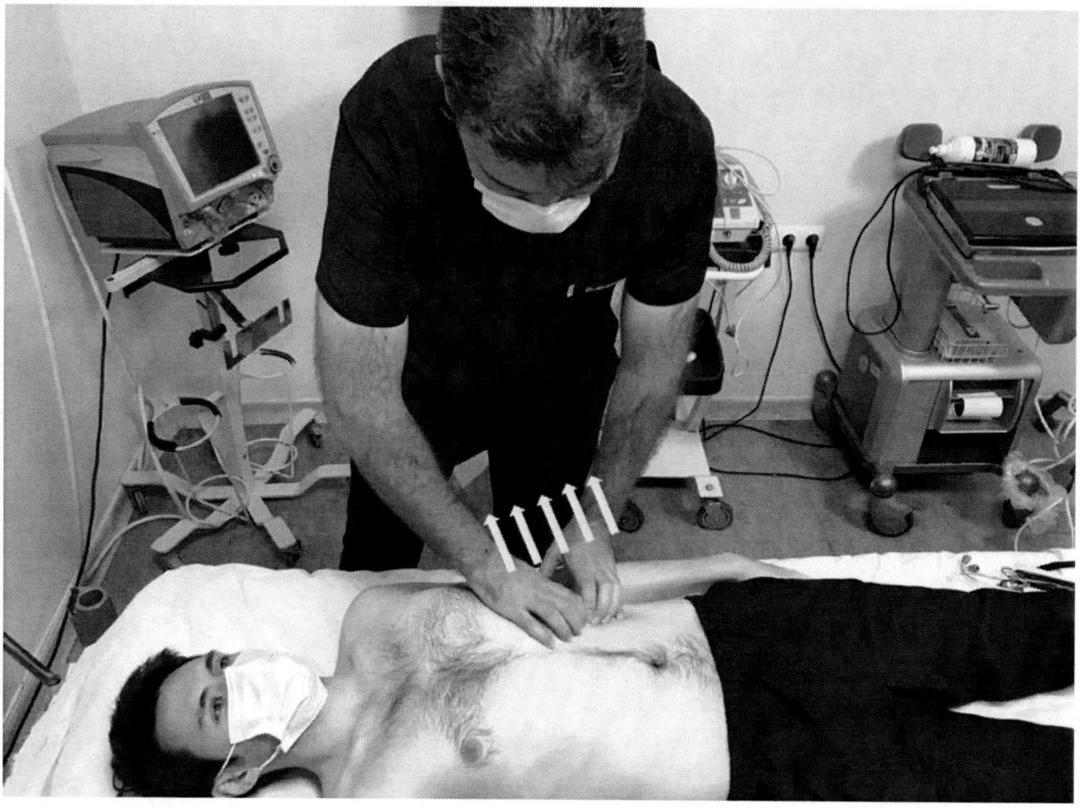

Figure 3. Hooking maneuver.

## Diagnosis

The selection of tests that help us to make a diagnosis or support our diagnosis depends on the patient's physical examination and anamnesis. While no examination is required in young patients with short-term pain and normal physical examination, in elderly patients, visceral pain should be eliminated if there is persistent pain, fever, cough, weight loss and additional disease. There are four main aims in the examination; to eliminate the causes of cardiac, pulmonary and abdominal pain, to detect those related with painful rheumatic diseases, and to locate the pain and define the adjacent anatomical region.

- Complete blood count, routine biochemistry, urinalysis, chest graph and electrocardiogram should be analyzed, and if there are coronary risk factors (age, gender, smoking, family history, diabetes, hypertension, etc.), a complete cardiac exclusion should be performed even in atypical chest pain.
- In unexplained sternoclavicular arthritis, the rheumatoid factor should be analyzed to eliminate atypical monoarticular rheumatoid arthritis.

- Spondyloarthropathies should be considered in patients with sacroiliac joint tenderness, lumbar and back stiffness, chest expansion and limitation in lumbar flexion and human leukocyte antigen (HLA) – B27 levels should be seen when narrowing, irregularity and sclerosis in the sacroiliac joint are observed.
- If there is distinct swelling and erythema in an isolated single joint (sternoclavicular), aspiration and a cell count of the joint fluid should be performed. In the case of a negative result, if there is a high suspicion of infection, aspiration should be repeated and cultures of atypical organisms such as mycoplasma and fungus should be performed. Primary or metastatic malignancies should also be considered.
- Conventional x-ray; consecutive and divergent radiographs can be taken to show fractures and primary or metastatic tumors.
- Scintigraphy is very useful with an increased uptake in inflammatory processes with spreading pain, such as ankylosing spondylitis and SAPHO (synovitis, acne, pustulosis, hyperostosis, osteitis) syndrome, post-traumatic pain and tumors. It can also show bone infarcts that may occur in sickle cell anemia.
- While examining pulmonary embolism, aortic dissection, and coronary artery pathologies by both CT and MRG in the musculoskeletal structure of the chest wall, pleural lesions and etiologies related to the vertebral column can be examined. It even enables us to evaluate the infection-malignancy distinction of the lesion in the soft tissue, the regular-irregular edges of the lesion, and the liquid-solid content.
- Both imaging methods should be used for the better detection of the degree of adjacent soft tissue involvement in patients with sternoclavicular joint infection and tenderness.
- Ultrasound can be used to indicate the presence of synovitis, increased blood flow, erosions and osteophytes in arthritis evaluation.

## Differential Diagnosis

- Fibromyalgia. This is a common pain syndrome characterized by diffuse musculoskeletal pain with weakness, sleep disorder, depression, anxiety, and cognitive disorder. Pain is most common in the neck, shoulders, waist and hips. 85% of diagnosed fibromyalgia patients describe a costochondral tenderness (Almansa, 2010). 3% of all emergency service admissions and 8% of patients admitting with chest pain are diagnosed with fibromyalgia (Disla, Rhim, Reddy, Karten, & Taranta, 1994).

- Rheumatoid arthritis. Chest pain is not a common clinic in rheumatoid arthritis, but it can be the first symptom of the disease. While symptomatic sternoclavicular joint involvement occurs in 19% of diagnosed patients, imaging findings such as synovitis, erosion, osteophyte, and synovial hyperperfusion are also found in 30% of these patients (Rodriguez-Henriquez et al., 2013).
- Ankylosing spondylitis. The involvement of the thoracic vertebrae and all structures related to this column can be observed. The involvement of the sternum, costosternal joints and sternoclavicular joints, which may result in chest expansion limitation, is also common and a diagnostic finding (Ramonda et al., 2012). Anterior chest involvement is seen in 5-20% of the patients, with 18% of these patients having sternoclavicular, and 51% having manubriosternal joint involvement as radiographic findings (Jurik, 1992).
- Psoriasis arthritis. About 10-25% of patients with diagnosed psoriasis may be observed as axial and/or peripheral arthritis. The involvement of the chest wall is rare; however, the involvement of the manubriosternal and sternoclavicular joints can result in radiological findings (Jurik, 1992).
- SAPHO syndrome. SAPHO syndrome is characterized by the presence of synovitis, acne, pustulosis, hyperostosis and osteitis. For diagnosis, infection, malignancy and other rheumatological etiologies should be eliminated. It is a rare disease and frequently observed in those of 30-50 years. Involvement of the chest wall, sacroiliac joint and vertebral column is accompanied by common active neutrophilic dermatosis (Hayem et al., 1999). Dermatological involvement occurs as palmoplantar pustulosis in 60% of patients (Nguyen et al., 2012).

The involvement of the chest wall is observed in 65-90% of patients and characteristic; the costoclavicular ligament is affected as well as the sternocostal and sternoclavicular joints. The "bull's head" appearance is specific.

- Systemic lupus erythematosus. The cause of chest pain in lupus is the muscle and joint involvement. There is increased pain with breathing. Inflammation of the pleura, pleural effusion or rarely observed fibrothorax, which is caused by visceral pleural thickening that limits chest expansion, may also cause chest pain in this patient group.
- Infectious arthritis. This is rare and commonly causes sternoclavicular joint involvement. It can be related to the usage of intravenous drugs, diabetes, rheumatoid arthritis and distant infection (Murga, Copeland, Hargrove, Wallen, & Zaheer, 2017).
- Repetitive Polychondritis. This is rare and characterized by the involvement of cartilage tissue in the respiratory tract, nose and ear. 25% of patients have costochondral and manubriosternal involvement (Chopra, 2013).

- Failure or Stress fractures. Rheumatic diseases that have had osteoporosis, osteomalacia and glucocorticoid therapy pose a risk for this. Stress fractures can occur after repetitive athletic activities in athletes with good bone mineralization.
- Malignancy. Primary malignancies of the chest wall can cause bone and soft tissue sarcoma and multiple myeloma chest pain. Especially breast and lung metastases that spread through hematogenous and adjacent, should also be considered.
- Sickle cell disease. Sickle cell crisis that leads to bone and pulmonary infarction can cause chest pain.

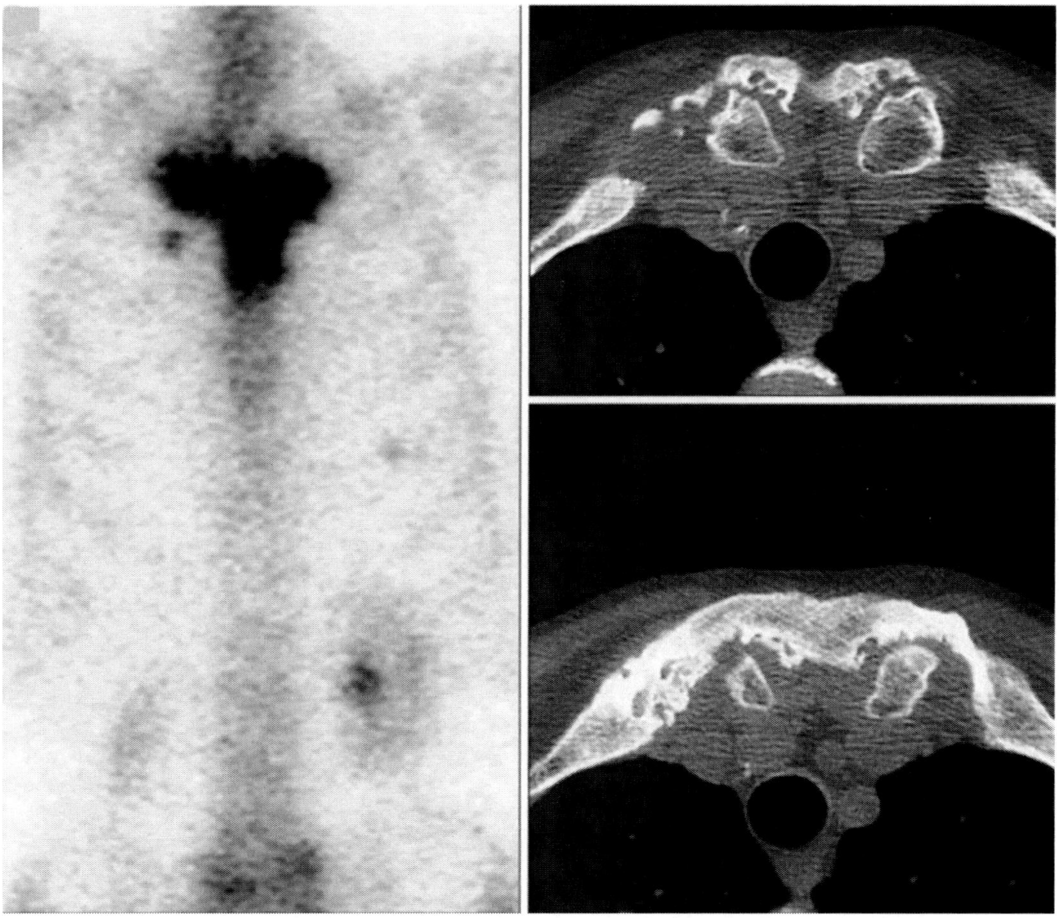

Figure 4. Appearance of scintigraphic and axial CT "Bull's Head" (Depasquale et al., 2012).

## TREATMENT

Isolated musculoskeletal chest pain may last for days, weeks or even months, depending on the underlying etiology. It should also be noted that pain lasting longer than

3 months may be related to chronic pain syndrome. The diagnosis should be confirmed and ensure that a life-threatening etiology is not missed before starting the treatment.

The first step of the treatment involves non-pharmacological approaches such as informing the patient about the disease and the treatment process, activity modification or restriction, and hot and cold application. The general approach is heat application for 20 minutes several times a day, at least 8 hours apart, in patients with muscle strain related to non-traumatic pain or overuse. Heat application in the first 48 hours is not recommended in traumatic patients because it may increase inflammation. A 20-minute cold application over 48 hours can be applied with intervals of 2-2.5 hours in patients with localized swelling. It should be noted that the patient should be at room temperature except for the application.

In addition to non-pharmacological approaches, analgesics are the basis of treatment. In the choice of drugs, the patient's age and comorbidity should be considered.

- Paracetamol or low-dose NSAIDs can be preferred for mild pain and situations that do not restrict light activities. In some patients, topical treatment may also be added.
    - Paracetamol can be safely prescribed in divided doses up to 3 grams per day.
    - NSAIDs can be preferred in a patient with paracetamol resistance. They can be used especially in patients for whom an anti-inflammatory effect is required, as the lowest dose results in the shortest time.
        - Naprosyn sodium 220 mg, 1-2 times/day
        - Ibuprofen 200 mg 2-3 tablets, 3-4 times/day
    - In topical treatment, analgesic and anti-inflammatory preparations are used for 2 weeks, but if they do not provide recovery or relief, their prescription is discontinued.
        - Creams with Capsaicin or salicylate content, 3-4 times/day
        - Diclofenac gel or ethyl chloride spray, 1-2 times/day
        - Lidocaine gel.
- In moderate pain, high-dose NSAIDs are prescribed in a situation that does not restrict light or moderate activities.
    - Naprosyn 375-500 mg, 2 times/day
    - Ibuprofen 400-800 mg 3-4 times/day
- In the case of an inadequate response to drugs;
    - Paracetamol 500 mg, 1-2 tablets every 3-4 hours at the most can be added to the treatment. 3000 mg per day should not be exceeded.

When prescribing NSAIDs, gastritis prophylaxis should be added to the treatment to minimize gastrointestinal side effects.

- In severe pain, it should be confirmed that there is no underlying rib fracture pathology in situations that restrict daily life activities.

Local injections, nerve blocks, and lidocaine injection combined with glucocorticoid and botulinum toxin injection are other treatment options in patients with pain lasting up to six weeks.

Tricyclic antidepressants, selective serotonin and norepinephrine reuptake inhibitors, and anti-convulsants such as gabapentin or pregabalin can be used in the treatment of patients with suspected fibromyalgia (Wang et al., 2012).

Though opiate usage is not recommended in the selected patient group for whom pain cannot be relieved by any method, low dose Tramadol 200 mg/day for 3 days can be added to the treatment.

In patients under 65 years of age who do not benefit from all the methods applied, centrally acting muscle relaxants such as cyclobenzaprine and methocarbamol can be added to the treatment.

- Cyclobenzaprine is biochemically more effective than other relaxants because of its similarity to the tricyclic antidepressant. It is taken before bed because of its excessive sedation and is not recommended for patients over 65 years of age due to having anticholinergic effects. It is started with an oral dose of 10 mg daily, and the dose can be increased up to a maximum of 30 mg (David G. Borenstein & Korn, 2003).
- Methocarbamol; 750-1500 mg can be taken three times a day.

Consultation with a rheumatologist, psychiatrist, or algologist may be required in cases of prolonged pain, and the indication of intercostal nerve block, glucocorticoid injection, and the diagnosis are unclear.

## Conclusion

The first step in diagnosing suspected musculoskeletal chest pain is to ensure that the patient is not experiencing chest pain due to a potentially life-threatening condition such as myocardial ischemia or infarction, pulmonary embolism, aortic dissection, or pneumothorax.

The first approach in the treatment of musculoskeletal chest pain includes general non-pharmacological interventions and the use of short-term analgesic drugs. Most of these patients improve within a few weeks or months.

The treatment process can be shortened by adding stretching exercises to the treatment of patients with costochondritis. Patients with spontaneous subluxation of the sternoclavicular joint may be referred to physical therapy for shoulder and scapular strengthening exercises.

Patients with isolated musculoskeletal pain due to posterior chest wall syndromes, sternoclavicular osteoarthritis, costochondritis, costochondral junction (Tietze) syndrome, or xiphoidalgia with symptoms that cannot be adequately controlled with initial therapy may benefit from local nerve blocks or glucocorticoid injections.

For chronic diffuse (central) pain such as fibromyalgia in patients with isolated musculoskeletal chest pain that is persistent and negatively affects the patient's quality of life, tricyclic antidepressants, selective serotonin and norepinephrine reuptake inhibitors, selective serotonin reuptake inhibitors, and/or selected anticonvulsants such as gabapentin/pregabalin can be used similarly to dosing in fibromyalgia or myofascial pain syndrome.

Opioid use is not recommended in patients with chest pain due to musculoskeletal etiology.

Persistent pain from posterior chest wall syndrome requiring intercostal nerve block or facet joint injection, persistent pain from other isolated musculoskeletal conditions requiring local glucocorticoid injection, uncertainty in diagnosis, and lack of improvement after one to three months of interventions require consultation or referral.

## REFERENCES

Almansa, C., Wang, Benjamin, Achem, Sami R. (2010). Noncardiac Chest Pain and Fibromyalgia. *Medical Clinics of North America, 94*(2). doi:10.1016/j.mcna. 2010.01.002.

Brunse, M. H., Stochkendahl, M. J., Vach, W., Kongsted, A., Poulsen, E., Hartvigsen, J., & Christensen, H. W. (2010). Examination of musculoskeletal chest pain - an inter-observer reliability study. *Man. Ther., 15*(2), 167-172. doi:10.1016/ j.math.2009.10.003.

Chopra, R., Chaudhary, N. and Kay, J. (2013). Relapsing Polychondritis. *Rheumatic Disease Clinics of North America*, 263-276. doi:http://dx. doi.org/10.1016 /j.rdc.2013.03.002.

David G. Borenstein, & Korn, S. (2003). Efficacy of a low-dose regimen of cyclobenzaprine hydrochloride in acute skeletal muscle spasm: Results of two placebo-controlled trials. *Clinical Therapeutics, 25*(4), 1056-1073.

Depasquale, R., Kumar, N., Lalam, R. K., Tins, B. J., Tyrrell, P. N. M., Singh, J., & Cassar-Pullicino, V. N. (2012). SAPHO: What radiologists should know. *Clinical Radiology, 67*(3), 195-206. Retrieved from <Go to ISI>://WOS:000300808100001.

Disla, E., Rhim, H. R., Reddy, A., Karten, I., & Taranta, A. (1994). Costochondritis - a Prospective Analysis in an Emergency Department Setting. *Archives of Internal Medicine, 154*(21), 2466-2469. Retrieved from <Go to ISI>://WOS: A1994PR04300011.

E Wolf, S. S. (1976). Costosternal syndrome: its frequency and importance in differential diagnosis of coronary heart disease. *Archives of Internal Medicine*. doi:10.1001/archinte.136.2.189.

Hayem, G., Bouchaud-Chabot, A., Benali, K., Roux, S., Palazzo, E., Silbermann-Hoffman, O., . . . Meyer, O. (1999). SAPHO syndrome: A long-term follow-up study of 120 cases. *Seminars in Arthritis and Rheumatism, 29*(3), 159-171. Retrieved from <Go to ISI>://WOS: 000084397000004.

Jurik, A. G. (1992). Seronegative anterior chest wall syndromes. A study of the findings and course at radiography. *Acta Radiol. Suppl., 381*, 1-42. Retrieved from https://www.ncbi.nlm.nih.gov/pubmed/1488919.

Murga, A., Copeland, H., Hargrove, R., Wallen, J. M., & Zaheer, S. (2017). Treatment for sternoclavicular joint infections: a multi-institutional study. *Journal of Thoracic Disease, 9*(6), 1503-1508. Retrieved from <Go to ISI>://WOS:000405815000038.

Nguyen, M. T., Borchers, A., Selmi, C., Naguwa, S. M., Cheema, G., & Gershwin, M. E. (2012). The SAPHO syndrome. *Semin. Arthritis Rheum., 42*(3), 254-265. doi:10.1016/j.semarthrit.2012.05.006.

Ramonda, R., Lorenzin, M., Lo Negro, A., Vio, S., Zucchetta, P., Frallonardo, P., . . . Punzi, L. (2012). Anterior Chest Wall Involvement in Early Stages of Spondyloarthritis: Advanced Diagnostic Tools. *Journal of Rheumatology, 39*(9), 1844-1849. Retrieved from <Go to ISI>://WOS:000308774000015.

Rodriguez-Henriquez, P., Solano, C., Pena, A., Leon-Hernandez, S., Hernandez-Diaz, C., Gutierrez, M., & Pineda, C. (2013). Sternoclavicular Joint Involvement in Rheumatoid Arthritis: Clinical and Ultrasound Findings of a Neglected Joint. *Arthritis Care & Research, 65*(7), 1177-1182. Retrieved from <Go to ISI>://WOS:000321184000019.

Wang, W., Sun, Y. H., Wang, Y. Y., Wang, Y. T., Wang, W., Li, Y. Q., & Wu, S. X. (2012). Treatment of functional chest pain with antidepressants: a meta-analysis. *Pain Physician, 15*(2), E131-142. Retrieved from https://www.ncbi.nlm.nih.gov/pubmed/22430659.

Yelland, M. J. (2001). Back, chest and abdominal pain: How good are spinal signs at identifying musculoskeletal causes of back, chest or abdominal pain? *Australian Family Physician, 30*(9), 908-912.

In: Musculoskeletal Pain (Common Clinical Presentations) ISBN: 978-1-68507-410-4
Editors: Mehmet Cenk Turgut and Serdar Toy 

*Chapter 5*

# FIBROMYALGIA

***Gonca Sağlam****
Department of Physical Medicine and Rehabilitation,
Karadeniz Technical University Faculty of Medicine, Trabzon, Turkey

## ABSTRACT

Fibromyalgia syndrome is the third most frequent painful musculoskeletal condition after lumbar pain and osteoarthritis, in terms of prevalence. It is a complicated disease that causes severe impairment in quality of life and function, as well as significant financial costs. Although its diagnosis has improved with the development of more precise diagnostic criteria, there may be missed diagnoses of fibromyalgia. Once a diagnosis has been determined, clinicians should enhance patient function and reduce the severity of pain by nonpharmacological and pharmacological treatments. A multi-modal therapy strategy is required due to the various components of the etiology and maintenance of the disease. The rate of disability is shown to be considerably decreased with effective treatment.

**Keywords:** Fibromyalgia, pathogenesis, diagnosis, exercise, treatment

## INTRODUCTION

Fibromyalgia is defined as a chronic syndrome, frequently observed across the world, which substantially impairs quality of life, and is characterized by widespread body pain, a decreased pain threshold, hyperalgesia, and allodynia. Its etiology has not yet been fully determined. Among its possible causes are genetic, neurological, psychological, sleep-

* Corresponding Author's E-mail: goncasaglam@ktu.edu.tr.

related, and immunological factors (Bair and Krebs 2020). The duration of diagnosis of fibromyalgia, which has been defined as a real syndrome according to the American College of Rheumatology (ACR) 1990 classification criteria, may be prolonged owing to the subjectivity of the symptoms and the fact that the evaluation is based on patients' statements, and there are no objective diagnostic tests to confirm the diagnosis (Bazzichi et al., 2020). The diagnosis and treatment of fibromyalgia syndrome are constantly changing and renewed. There is a wide variety of treatment options including medications, exercises, and lifestyle changes to manage symptoms and to improve quality of life (Kia and Joy, 2017).

## Epidemiology and Pathophysiology

First described in the 19th century, fibromyalgia is the most prevalent rheumatic disease after osteoarthritis. Its prevalence in society varies depending on the diagnostic criteria used. Its prevalence has been reported to be between 0.2% and 6.6% in the general population. This rate has been stated to be between 2.4% and 6.8% in women (Marques et al., 2017). Its prevalence in the population is generally accepted as 2%. The disease is encountered 6-9 times more often in women (Macfarlane et al., 2017). Although fibromyalgia is usually observed in middle-aged women, it can also affect children, adolescents, and the elderly (Vincent et al., 2013). A history of chronic pain has also been revealed in the family members of patients with fibromyalgia.

Certain infections can cause fibromyalgia or other comparable conditions like chronic fatigue syndrome (e.g., Epstein-Barr virus, Lyme disease, Q fever, viral hepatitis) (Buskila et al., 2008). Fibromyalgia can also be triggered by traumas and psychological stressors. Fibromyalgia may appear in other chronic pain conditions such as osteoarthritis, rheumatoid arthritis, and systemic lupus erythematosus. Approximately 10% to 30% of patients with certain rheumatic diseases fulfill the fibromyalgia criteria (Phillips and Clauw, D.J., 2013).

It is thought that abnormal central and/or peripheral pain mechanisms play a role, together with genetic factors, in the development of widespread and chronic pain reported by patients with fibromyalgia, and fibromyalgia develops as a consequence of exposure of these individuals to physiological and psychological stresses. It is asserted that the main mechanisms leading to pain in fibromyalgia patients are hyperalgesia and allodynia. With the observation of the frequency of fibromyalgia and small-fiber polyneuropathy in recent studies, the view that the peripheral nervous system also contributes to the condition has gained currency (Chinn et al., 2016). Among the possibly modifiable risk factors for the development of fibromyalgia are poor sleep quality, obesity, physical inactivity, and work or life dissatisfaction (Clauw, D., 2014).

## CLINICAL CHARACTERISTICS

Fibromyalgia should be suspected in patients with widespread pain and patients whose pain cannot be explained by injury or inflammation. Musculoskeletal pain is the most evident presentation of fibromyalgia in most cases.

The general pain threshold can be evaluated caudally by firmly pressing on the hands and arms, several interphalangeal joints of each hand or adjacent phalanges, followed by palpation of the forearm muscles. Should there be a low central pain threshold, the patient will have tenderness in most of these regions or only in the forearm muscles. A systemic autoimmune illness should be explored if pain is limited to the interphalangeal joints and not the other areas (particularly if there is swelling over these joints).

Patients who develop fibromyalgia usually have several clinical histories in their bodies, such as widespread chronic pain, headache, dysmenorrhea, temporomandibular joint disorder, chronic fatigue, irritable bowel syndrome and other gastrointestinal disorders, interstitial cystitis or painful bladder syndrome, endometriosis and other regional pain syndromes. Fibromyalgia is a type of central pain, and pain is felt more than normally expected with a peripheral nociceptive input in central pain. The response of this pain to analgesic approaches is also low (Williams and Clauw, 2009). Because the physical symptoms of fibromyalgia cannot be fully explained, it is also considered to be in the group of functional somatic syndromes (Duruk et al., 2015).

**Table 1. Features of fibromyalgia and other centralized pain syndromes (Clauw, D., 2014)**

| |
|---|
| *Pain Character*<br><br>• Diffuse, multifocal and migration<br>• Often accompanied by dysesthesia or paresthesias presenting with numbness, tingling, or burning<br>• Discomfort with touch or wearing tight clothing |
| *Pain history of other body areas earlier in life* |
| *Accompanying symptoms also of central nervous system origin*<br><br>• Fatigue, sleep disturbances, memory, and mood difficulties<br>• Following suitable pharmacological or nonpharmacological therapy, several of these symptoms, as well as pain, will improve |
| *Symptoms suggesting more global sensory hyperresponsiveness*<br><br>• Light sensitivity, strong noise sensitivity, odor sensitivity, and visceral discomfort<br>• Often results in a "pan-positive assessment of symptoms," which has led to these people being labeled "somatizers," despite the fact that the biology of somatization is increasingly being recognized as sensory hyperresponsiveness |

## Diagnosis

The diagnosis of fibromyalgia is established by clinical evaluation; no laboratory tests, radiographic examination, and biomarkers have been identified for the disease yet. Diseases such as hypothyroidism and rheumatic diseases, which can mimic the symptoms of fibromyalgia, and drug-related conditions, such as statin-induced myopathy, should be considered and discarded (Annemans et al., 2008).

The initial diagnostic criteria set for fibromyalgia were published by the ACR in 1990 as research classification criteria. These criteria include widespread body pain for at least 3 months (both sides of the body in the upper and lower parts of the waist) and tenderness in at least 11 out of 18 tender spots (Bennett et al., 2007). In 2010, these criteria were updated to incorporate the more subjective widespread body pain scale and the symptom severity scale, which involve cognitive symptoms, sleep, fatigue, and additional somatic symptoms. The 2010 criteria include 19 pain spots and 41 somatic symptoms (Wolfe et al., 2010). In 2011, these criteria were also modified; sensitive spot examination was removed, and symptom-based evaluation was added with the concern that tender spot examination was not enough at the initial stage (Wolfe et al., 2011). In 2013, alternative criteria were developed. A new group of criteria was defined, including 28 pain regions and a 10-item assessment of symptom involvement. In the 28 pain regions, unlike the 19 regions, the back and waist regions were divided into three as right, left, and middle. Hands and wrists, knees, feet and ankles were added, and the abdomen was removed (Bennett, 2014). The ACR lastly presented the following diagnostic criteria in 2016 (Wolfe et al., 2016).

### Widespread Pain Index (WPI)

- Widespread pain (WP) is defined as pain in at least 4 out of 5 regions. The concept of widespread pain excludes jaw, chest, and abdominal pain.
- The number of regions in which the patient has had pain over the last week is noted. The score will range from 0 to 19.

### Symptom Severity Scale (SSS)

The SSS is the total of the severity scores (0-9) for the three symptoms (fatigue, waking unrefreshed, and cognitive symptoms) plus the sum (0-3) of the number of the following symptoms experienced by the patient in the preceding six months. The final SSS is between 0 and 12.

The fibromyalgia severity scale is the sum of the WPI and the SSS. Fibromyalgia is diagnosed in adults when all of the following criteria are met:

- Generalized pain, defined as pain in at least 4 out of 5 regions, is present.
- Symptoms have been present at a similar level for at least 3 months.

**Table 2. Widespread pain index**

<table>
<tr><th>Left upper region (region 1)</th><th>Right upper region (region 2)</th><th>Left lower region (region 3)</th></tr>
<tr><td>Jaw, left</td><td>Jaw, right</td><td>Hip (buttock, trochanter), left</td></tr>
<tr><td>Shoulder girdle, left</td><td>Shoulder girdle, right</td><td>Upper leg, left</td></tr>
<tr><td>Upper arm, left</td><td>Upper arm, right</td><td>Lower leg, left</td></tr>
<tr><td>Lower arm, left</td><td>Lower arm, right</td><td></td></tr>
<tr><th colspan="2">Right lower region (region 4)</th><th>Axial region (region 5)</th></tr>
<tr><td colspan="2">Hip (buttock, trochanter), right</td><td>Neck</td></tr>
<tr><td colspan="2">Upper leg, right</td><td>Back</td></tr>
<tr><td colspan="2">Lower leg, left</td><td>Waist</td></tr>
<tr><td colspan="2"></td><td>Chest</td></tr>
<tr><td colspan="2"></td><td>Abdomen</td></tr>
</table>

**Table 3. Symptom severity scale**

<table>
<tr><td>Fatigue (0-3)</td><td rowspan="3">0: No problem<br>1: Slight or mild problems, generally mild or intermittent<br>2: Moderate, considerable problems, often present and/or at a moderate level<br>3: Severe: pervasive, continuous, life-disturbing problems</td></tr>
<tr><td>Waking unrefreshed (0-3)</td></tr>
<tr><td>Cognitive symptoms (0-3), such as forgetfulness, concentration difficulties</td></tr>
<tr><td>Headaches (0-1)</td><td>0: No problem, 1: occurred during the previous 6 months</td></tr>
<tr><td>Pain or cramps in the lower abdomen (0-1)</td><td>0: No problem, 1: occurred during the previous 6 months</td></tr>
<tr><td>Depression (0-1)</td><td>0: No problem, 1: occurred during the previous 6 months</td></tr>
</table>

- The WPI is $\geq 7$ and the SSS score is $\geq 5$ OR there is a WPI of 4-6 and an SSS score of $\geq 9$.
- A diagnosis of fibromyalgia does not exclude the presence of other clinically important illnesses.

The fibromyalgia impact questionnaire, the fibromyalgia survey diagnostic criteria and the severity scale, medical outcomes study 36-item short-form health survey, the Pittsburg sleep quality index, the fatigue severity scale, and the Beck depression index can also be used to evaluate the severity of the syndrome (Evcik et al., 2018).

## NONPHARMACOLOGICAL THERAPIES

Currently, there are no treatments ensuring recovery from fibromyalgia. The aim is to reduce symptoms and maintain and improve life quality and functions. Clinicians administer drug therapies together with non-drug therapy, and approaches such as physical therapy, exercise, and cognitive-behavioral therapy, and treatment protocols that consider fibromyalgia as a systemic disease rather than a regional or multifocal muscle disorder are preferred (Sarzi-Puttini et al., 2020, Nüesch et al., 2013). It has been reported that multidisciplinary pharmacological and rehabilitative approaches and cognitive-behavioral treatments are the most effective methods in the treatment of fibromyalgia. Non-drug therapies basically include education, exercise and physical therapy modalities, and cognitive-behavioral therapy (Arnold and Clauw, 2017).

Patient education is the first step of treatment in fibromyalgia. Informing patients about their condition, and cooperation, affect their compliance with and response to treatment. Recommendations to patients on their compliance with treatment may positively influence the results (Conversano et al., 2019). Patients are informed about the disease and treatment options during the education process. Wrong expectations and information about the disease are addressed, and the fact that this is not a life-threatening condition is clarified. Patients should be told that factors such as stress, anxiety, depression, sleep disturbance, seasonal changes, working conditions, bad posture, and trauma may increase their complaints. Self-management training allows patients to take charge of the activities that will help them control their symptoms and enhance their problem-solving abilities (Rooks et al., 2007, Hammond and Freeman, 2006).

### Exercises

It is known that fibromyalgia patients have decreased muscle strength and muscle condition. In this disease, the main purposes behind exercises are to reduce stress, maintain and increase muscle strength and endurance, and ensure appropriate posture. The low condition also increases the risk of being influenced by microtraumas for the muscle, causing pain and fatigue. Exercise can provide an analgesic effect by increasing serum beta-endorphin levels. An increase has been detected in post-exercise pain in fibromyalgia patients due to decreased muscle blood flow, muscle contractions and post-exercise changes in pain modulation. Therefore, it is reported that appropriately planned and personalized exercises can increase blood flow in the muscles and serum adrenocorticotropic hormone and cortisol levels and be beneficial for patients. Moreover, impairment of the growth hormone response to exercise has also been reported. As stated, there is dysfunction in the hypothalamus-pituitary and adrenal axis in fibromyalgia, and implementing an exercise program can affect the hormone levels and thus symptoms

(Genc et al., 2015). The fact that inadequacy is more apparent in activities requiring long-term static contractions has suggested that exercises requiring long-term static contractions may be more important (Gowans and Dehueck, 2004).

Low-intensity aerobic workouts and exercise regimens that may be coupled with other therapeutic modalities are now commonly recommended. Exercise programs should be planned individually and specifically for the patient by starting below the patient's exercise capacity and increasing gradually. Adjustments should be made according to the patient's tolerance status. When a general exercise program is to be prepared, activities can start with basic neck joint range of motion and posture correction exercises. Then, whole-body strengthening and aerobic exercises can be added and intensified gradually (Sosa-Reina et al., 2017).

The effectiveness of aerobic, strengthening, stretching, relaxation and aquatic exercises in fibromyalgia has been investigated and found to be useful. It has been concluded that physical activity and exercise are beneficial at mild to moderate levels in respect of reducing pain severity and improving physical functions in general, and enhancing the quality of life (Geneen et al., 2017). Aerobic exercises are usually recommended to patients. In the publications evaluated, aerobic and strengthening exercises were found to be effective in general, and aquatic and floor exercises also had similar efficiency (Bidonde et al., 2014).

## Aerobic Exercises

Aerobic exercises include land-based and water-based exercises. Activities such as walking, cycling, games, dancing, boxing, and running in water are among these exercises. Most of the studies on this subject have shown that aerobic exercises have a positive effect on fibromyalgia patients. In a review evaluating exercise in the treatment of fibromyalgia, aerobic exercises were found to achieve a 35% and 34% improvement in pain and physical functions, respectively (Busch 2007). In another review, in fibromyalgia, the efficiency of exercise therapy was proven to be low for pain severity, fatigue, stiffness and physical function and to be moderate for quality of life. As a result, aerobic exercises improve quality of life, physical functions and pain (Bidonde et al., 2017).

## Muscle Strengthening Exercises

In fibromyalgia, it is claimed that a combination exercise program (aerobic and/or strengthening and/or stretching activities) improves pain and physical functioning even more (Busch et al., 2017). In a review, it was reported that strengthening exercises applied for 12 weeks could provide significant improvement in pain, tender spots, depression and overall well-being. However, no change occurred in physical functions. In another review of five studies, low-quality evidence showed that moderate and moderate-to-intensive strengthening exercises brought about significant improvement in pain, tenderness, functions, and muscle strength. A low level of evidence has been put forward regarding the fact that fibromyalgia patients can perform moderate-to-intensive exercises safely. Aerobic activities have been proven to be more helpful than moderate strength exercises in reducing pain (Busch, 2013).

## Flexibility Exercises

Flexibility exercises include controlled static stretching. Stretching in a flexibility exercise program should be repeated 3-4 times, continued for 20-30 seconds and performed at least two days a week. Although there is not much evidence about stretching exercises in fibromyalgia, pain, pain-related quality of life, and functions have been observed to improve. There was an improvement in aerobic capacity, pain, and physical functioning in both stretching and aerobic exercise groups in a research study, although aerobic activities were shown to be more beneficial (Lorena et al., 2015).

## Hydrotherapy

It has been revealed that in-water exercises are tolerated well and have positive effects on mood and sleep as well as pain. As is concluded, the effectiveness is at a similar level with terrestrial exercises (Bidonde et al., 2014). Balneotherapy and non-exercise spa therapy are also effective, safe, and possible alternative treatments that can heal patients with fibromyalgia (Langhorst, 2009).

## Electrotherapeutic Interventions

Along with other treatment modalities, physical therapy modalities in fibromyalgia aim to improve disease symptoms, physical function, general health and emotional well-being. These methods are generally applied to facilitate stretching and reduce muscle tone. Through the modification of pain with hot, cold and electrotherapy methods, patients' compliance with exercise can be increased. All physical therapy modalities in use nowadays can be applied in the treatment of fibromyalgia (Ediz and Hiz, 2011).

Transcutaneous electrical nerve stimulation (TENS) is usually recommended for the treatment of localized pain in fibromyalgia. Although it was concluded that electrical stimulation significantly reduced pain, no difference was detected in quality of life and fatigue, and the level of evidence was low (Salazar et al., 2017). There are studies indicating that pulsed electromagnetic fields and rTMS reduce pain and/or improve quality of life in fibromyalgia patients (Short et al., 2014). Transcranial direct current stimulation, one of the non-invasive brain stimulation methods, is a safe and simple procedure that has been demonstrated to help with pain and functions in a small number of clinical trials and a review (Zhu et al., 2017). The significance of low-dose laser therapy in the treatment of fibromyalgia is controversial. It is claimed to reduce pain by causing photochemical reactions that alter the activity of neurons. In a study, 75 patients were compared with placebo and amitriptyline, and laser therapy was reported to be effective in reducing pain (Gür et al., 2002). In a study conducted to evaluate the efficiency of ultrasound therapy in fibromyalgia patients, ultrasound and laser therapy were compared, and a reduction was observed in pain, stiffness and the number of tender spots via both methods. In another study, improvement was achieved in pain, functions, and sleep. In fibromyalgia, pulsed ultrasound therapy can be applied at 1 MHz and 2.5 W/cm2 (Almeida et al., 2003).

## Acupuncture

Acupuncture uses heat, pressure, lasers, and tiny needles to stimulate particular areas of the body in order to have a therapeutic impact. An analysis evaluating the role of acupuncture in fibromyalgia revealed that adding acupuncture to standard treatments resulted in a 30% reduction in pain (Deare et al., 2013). With acupuncture, pain reduction is achieved in a short time, but data on its long-term effects are inadequate. A reduction has been determined in pain and fatigue with electroacupuncture, and the possible undesirable effects have been reported to be mild and temporary in general. In a multicenter, randomized, single-blind study, acupuncture and sham acupuncture were compared, and a 14% pain reduction was achieved with acupuncture. In the study, it was stated that the pain reduction lasted for one year, and the undesirable effects were at a mild level (Vas et al., 2016).

## Cognitive-Behavioral Therapy

Cognitive-behavioral therapy (CBT) is applied when the behavioral and physiological reactions arising for protection during acute pain persist in chronic pain and become harmful and ineffective, and aims to help the patient get rid of these negative reactions. It is known that particularly long-lasting pain can lead to widespread and important mental problems, and the ability of patients to cope with this situation can have positive effects on treatment. Patients who learn coping methods can live with pain more productively (Okifuji, 2016).

In CBT, cognitively, it is aimed to modify the maladaptive thoughts that affect the patient's mood and behavior, to correct the errors in thought, to try to instill a more realistic thinking system, to reduce patients' pain severity and to increase their functions, whereas, behaviorally, it is attempted to change maladaptive behaviors with behavioral modification techniques. Behavioral techniques are applied by teaching behavioral activation techniques such as encouraging patients to increase their activity level and to exercise, regulating the speed of activity, improving the ability to cope with pain, preventing behaviors that cause secondary gain, and providing sleep hygiene and relaxation techniques such as progressive muscle relaxation. It has been reported that CBT mildly reduces pain and disability and its benefits endure for a long period (Bernardy et al., 2013).

## Pharmacological Therapies

In fibromyalgia patients, drug therapy should be selected according to the patient's clinical characteristics, side effect profile and response to treatment. When initiating drug therapy, first, it is necessary to confirm the diagnosis and identify comorbidities such as depression, anxiety, and sleep disturbance. Patients who start drug therapy should be checked frequently. If the drug is used for the first time, patients should be checked after 7-10 days to evaluate the side effects and patient compliance. Then, they should be checked every 2 weeks until symptom control and dose adjustment are achieved, and every 2 months when patients' symptoms are reduced by at least 50% and the effective dose/combination is reached. The drug dose should be adjusted according to patients' responses. It is recommended to initiate the treatment at low doses and gradually titrate doses. A few studies on medication combinations suggest starting with monotherapy (Evcik et al., 2018). Tricyclic antidepressants (TSA), cyclobenzaprine, tramadol, serotonin-noradrenaline reuptake inhibitors (SNRI), and certain antiepileptics have all been proven to be helpful in the treatment of fibromyalgia. It is stated that NSAIDs are not effective enough in fibromyalgia (Macfarlane et al., 2017).

### Antiepileptics

In the reviews of pregabalin and gabapentin studies, it is reported that the data obtained with gabapentin are limited, and there are more data on the efficiency of pregabalin. In general, it is stated that pain is reduced with antiepileptics, other symptoms may decrease, and they are moderately effective. Pregabalin has been shown to reduce pain, fix sleep disturbance and improve functions, and have a positive effect on sleep disturbance. In a safety review of eight studies, it was concluded that, despite the observation of undesirable effects such as somnolence, drowsiness, weight gain and peripheral edema with pregabalin, these effects were mild to moderate, and the treatment was tolerated well.

In a review conducted to compare pregabalin, duloxetine, and milnacipran, it was concluded that these three drugs had similar discontinuation rates due to a 30% pain reduction and undesirable effects (Clair and Emir 2016). Duloxetine and pregabalin had a higher effect on pain and sleep disturbance than milnacipran. While the effect of duloxetine on depressive mood was higher than that of the other two drugs, milnacipran and pregabalin reduced fatigue more than duloxetine. The side-effect profiles of the drugs also differed. Consequently, it was suggested that attention should be paid to the patient's symptoms and possible side effects when selecting a drug. In a review on the use of gabapentin in fibromyalgia, the level of evidence was concluded to be insufficient (Cooper et al., 2017).

## Selective Serotonin Reuptake Inhibitors

Eight reviews focused on the effectiveness of selective serotonin reuptake inhibitors (SSRI) in fibromyalgia. The majority of these studies researched antidepressants in fibromyalgia in a broad sense. SSRIs were shown to have a lesser impact than TSAs in several studies examining the use of antidepressants in fibromyalgia. In a review of 7 placebo-controlled studies (2 citalopram, 3 fluoxetine, 2 paroxetine), it was concluded that SSRIs were more effective in the main symptoms of fibromyalgia, namely pain, fatigue and sleep problems, than the placebo, and they could be used in the treatment of depression in people with fibromyalgia (Walitt et al., 2015).

## Serotonin-Noradrenaline Reuptake Inhibitors

Serotonin-noradrenaline reuptake inhibitors are hypothesized to work by blocking serotonin and noradrenaline, both of which are important in fibromyalgia's descending pain inhibition pathways. In the Cochrane review, which included five studies on duloxetine and five studies on milnacipran, along with 6,038 patients, pain was found to improve with both drugs slightly more than the placebo. No significant difference was observed in symptoms compared to the placebo or between both drugs. While duloxetine was evaluated to be more effective than milnacipran in most symptoms in three reviews, duloxetine was revealed to be more effective in pain and sleep disturbance, and milnacipran to be more effective in reducing fatigue in another review (Hauser et al.,

2011). Regarding the effect of duloxetine on diabetic peripheral neuropathy doses, low-quality evidence has been obtained. It has been reported that the improvement in mental symptoms might be greater than that in physical symptoms. While minor undesirable effects are common with duloxetine, severe undesirable effects have rarely been encountered (Bair and Krebs, 2020).

## Cyclobenzaprine

Cyclobenzaprine is a muscle relaxant with a central effect, structurally similar to tricyclic antidepressants. A single systematic review of 312 patients revealed that 85% of patients experienced undesirable effects, and 71% could complete the study. Undesirable effects of cyclobenzaprine consist of confusion, skin lesions, and liver toxicity. In a review, it was stated that pain and sleep disturbance improved with cyclobenzaprine, but further studies were required (Tofferi, 2004).

## Tramadol

Tramadol, a weak opioid, also has a mild serotonin-noradrenaline reuptake inhibitory effect. In a review, two studies evaluating the efficiency of tramadol in fibromyalgia were reviewed. In these studies, which respectively evaluated monotherapy and combination with paracetamol, it was concluded that tramadol reduced pain in fibromyalgia patients. It is stated that tramadol can be administered at a dose of 150 mg/day (Schmidt-Wilcke and Diers, 2017).

## Tricyclic Antidepressants

Amitriptyline, a tricyclic antidepressant, is said to be beneficial in multiple ways by blocking adrenoceptor and 5-HT receptors and perhaps histaminic and muscarinic receptors, by stimulating peripheral adenosine A1 receptors, by binding to opioid and N-Methyl-D-Aspartate receptors and by interacting with sodium, potassium and calcium channels in fibromyalgia patients (Lawson, 2017). Amitriptyline, given at a dose of 25-50 mg/day, was shown to have a moderate effect on pain and sleep disruption, as well as an ability to reduce tiredness, according to the results of a review of five trials. Amitriptyline was reported to have positive effects on pain, sleep, and fatigue when administered at a dose of 25 mg for 6-8 weeks. Side effects such as dry mouth, somnolence, gastrointestinal complaints, and weight gain increase when the dose increases should not be forgotten (Kia and Choy, 2017).

## Conclusion

Fibromyalgia is a chronic disease that negatively affects physical and mental functioning, activities of daily living, personal relationships, work productivity, career development, and quality of life. Despite the ACR guidelines, it may take years to establish an accurate diagnosis. Establishing no diagnosis, and delays eventually result in patient dissatisfaction and disappointment, inadequate medical care, inadequate compliance and an increased healthcare burden.

Owing to the difficulty of fibromyalgia treatment and the inability to achieve enough efficiency with single administrations of drug and non-drug therapies, multidisciplinary and interdisciplinary treatment approaches, which combine psychosocial and behavioral treatment methods and educational practices, have started to be applied, and multidisciplinary and interdisciplinary treatment has been determined as the most effective method. Treatment plans integrating lifestyle changes, disease education involving patients and family members, aerobic exercises, sleep hygiene, strength training, dietary counseling aimed at weight loss, complementary and alternative medicines, cognitive behavioral therapy, and pharmacotherapy are recommended. In the co-use of drug and non-drug therapies, short-term relief is achieved in patients with drug therapies, whereas the co-application of both treatment approaches targets the long-term symptoms of fibromyalgia, such as physical dysfunction, psychological stress, and decrease in muscle condition and strength. It is known that the multidisciplinary pharmacological, rehabilitative approach and cognitive-behavioral treatments are the most effective methods in fibromyalgia.

## References

Annemans, L., Wessely, S., Spaepen, E., Caekelbergh, K., Caubère, J. P., Lay, K. L. & Taïeb, C. (2008). Health economic consequences related to the diagnosis of fibromyalgia syndrome. *Arthritis & Rheumatism: Official Journal of the American College of Rheumatology*, *58*(3), 895-902.

Arnold, L. M. & Clauw, D. J. (2017). Challenges of implementing fibromyalgia treatment guidelines in current clinical practice. *Postgraduate medicine*, *129*(7), 709–714.

Bair, M. J. & Krebs, E. E. (2020). Fibromyalgia. *Annals of internal medicine*, *172*(5), ITC33–ITC48.

Bazzichi, L., Giacomelli, C., Consensi, A., Giorgi, V., Batticciotto, A., Di Franco, M. & Sarzi-Puttini, P. (2020). *One year in review 2020: fibromyalgia. Clinical and experimental rheumatology*, *38*, Suppl 123(1), 3–8.

Bennett, R., Friend, R., Marcus, D., Bernstein, C., Han, B. K., Yachoui, R. & Jones, K. (2014). Criteria for the diagnosis of fibromyalgia: validation of the modified 2010 preliminary ACR criteria and the development of alternative criteria. *Arthritis Care Res*, *66*(9), 1364-1373.

Bernardy, K., Klose, P., Busch, A. J., Choy, E. H. & Häuser, W. (2013). Cognitive behavioural therapies for fibromyalgia. *Cochrane Database of Systematic Reviews*, (9).

Bidonde, J., Busch, A. J., Schachter, C. L., Overend, T. J., Kim, S. Y., Góes, S. M. & Foulds, H. J. (2017). Aerobic exercise training for adults with fibromyalgia. *Cochrane Database of Systematic Reviews*, (6).

Bidonde, J., Busch, A. J., Webber, S. C., Schachter, C. L., Danyliw, A., Overend, T. J. & Rader, T. (2014). Aquatic exercise training for fibromyalgia. *Cochrane Database of Systematic Reviews*, (10).

Busch, A. J., Barber, K. A., Overend, T. J., Peloso, P. M. J. & Schachter, C. L. (2007). Exercise for treating fibromyalgia syndrome. *Cochrane database of systematic reviews*, (4).

Busch, A. J., Webber, S. C., Richards, R. S., Bidonde, J., Schachter, C. L., Schafer, L. A. & Overend, T. J. (2013). Resistance exercise training for fibromyalgia. *Cochrane database of systematic reviews*, (12).

Buskila, D., Atzeni, F. & Sarzi-Puttini, P. (2008). Etiology of fibromyalgia: the possible role of infection and vaccination. *Autoimmunity reviews*, *8*(1), 41-43.

Chinn, S., Caldwell, W. & Gritsenko, K. (2016). Fibromyalgia pathogenesis and treatment options update. *Current pain and headache reports*, *20*(4), 25.

Clair, A. & Emir, B. (2016). The safety and efficacy of pregabalin for treating subjects with fibromyalgia and moderate or severe baseline widespread pain. *Current medical research and opinion*, *32*(3), 601-610.

Clauw D. J. (2014). Fibromyalgia: a clinical review. *JAMA*, *311*(15), 1547–1555.

Conversano, C., Poli, A., Ciacchini, R., Hitchcott, P., Bazzichi, L. & Gemignani, A. (2019). A psychoeducational intervention is a treatment for fibromyalgia syndrome. *Clinical and experimental rheumatology*, *37*, Suppl 116(1), 98–104.

Cooper, T. E., Derry, S., Wiffen, P. J. & Moore, R. A. (2017). Gabapentin for fibromyalgia pain in adults. *Cochrane Database of Systematic Reviews*, (1).

Deare, J. C., Zheng, Z., Xue, C. C., Liu, J. P., Shang, J., Scott, S. W. & Littlejohn, G. (2013). Acupuncture for treating fibromyalgia. *Cochrane Database of Systematic Reviews*, (5).

Duruk, B., Sertel Berk, H. Ö. & Ketenci, A. (2015). Are fibromyalgia and failed back surgery syndromes actually "functional somatic syndromes" in terms of their symptomatological, familial and psychological characteristics? *A comparative study with chronic medical illness and healthy controls. Agri*, *27*(3), 123-131.

Ediz, L. & Hiz, Ö. (2011). Physical Therapy in Treating Fibromyalgia Syndrome: A Brief Review. *Journal of Physical Medicine & Rehabilitation Sciences/Fiziksel Tup ve Rehabilitasyon Bilimleri Dergisi*, *14*(1).

Evcik, D., Ketenci, A. & Sindel, D. (2019). The Turkish Society of Physical Medicine and Rehabilitation (TSPMR) guideline recommendations for the management of fibromyalgia syndrome. *Turkish journal of physical medicine and rehabilitation*, *65*(2), 111.

Genc, A., Tur, B. S., Aytur, Y. K., Oztuna, D. & Erdogan, M. F. (2015). Does aerobic exercise affect the hypothalamic-pituitary-adrenal hormonal response in patients with fibromyalgia syndrome?. *Journal of physical therapy science*, *27*(7), 2225-2231.

Geneen, L. J., Moore, R. A., Clarke, C., Martin, D., Colvin, L. A. & Smith, B. H. (2017). Physical activity and exercise for chronic pain in adults: an overview of Cochrane Reviews. *Cochrane Database of Systematic Reviews*, (4).

Gowans, S. E. & dehueck, A. (2004). Effectiveness of exercise in management of fibromyalgia. *Current opinion in rheumatology*, *16*(2), 138-142.

Gür, A., Karakoc, M., Nas, K., Cevik, R., Sarac, A. & Ataoglu, S. (2002). Effects of low power laser and low dose amitriptyline therapy on clinical symptoms and quality of life in fibromyalgia: a single-blind, placebo-controlled trial. *Rheumatology international*, *22*(5), 188-193.

Hammond, A. & Freeman, K. (2006). Community patient education and exercise for people with fibromyalgia: a parallel group randomized controlled trial. *Clinical rehabilitation*, *20*(10), 835-846.

Kia, S. & Choy, E. (2017). Update on treatment guideline in fibromyalgia syndrome with focus on pharmacology. *Biomedicines*, *5*(2), 20.

Langhorst, J., Musial, F., Klose, P. & Häuser, W. (2009). Efficacy of hydrotherapy in fibromyalgia syndrome—a meta-analysis of randomized controlled clinical trials. *Rheumatology*, *48*(9), 1155-1159.

Lawson, K. (2017). A brief review of the pharmacology of amitriptyline and clinical outcomes in treating fibromyalgia. *Biomedicines*, *5*(2), 24.

Lorena, S. B. D., Lima, M. D. C. C. D., Ranzolin, A. & Duarte, Â. L. B. P. (2015). Effects of muscle stretching exercises in the treatment of fibromyalgia: a systematic review. *Revista brasileira de reumatologia*, *55*(2), 167-173.

Macfarlane, G. J., Kronisch, C., Dean, L. E., Atzeni, F., Häuser, W., Fluß, E., et al. (2017). EULAR revised recommendations for the management of fibromyalgia. *Ann Rheum Dis.*, *76*(2), 318-328.

Macfarlane, G. J., Kronisch, C., Dean, L. E., Atzeni, F., Häuser, W., Fluß, E. & Jones, G. T. (2017). EULAR revised recommendations for the management of fibromyalgia. *Annals of the rheumatic diseases*, *76*(2), 318-328.

Marques, A. P., Santo, A. D. S. D. E., Berssaneti, A. A., Matsutani, L. A. & Yuan, S. L. K. (2017). Prevalence of fibromyalgia: literature review update. *Revista brasileira de reumatologia*, *57*(4), 356-363.

Nüesch, E., Häuser, W., Bernardy, K., Barth, J. & Jüni, P. (2013). Comparative efficacy of pharmacological and non-pharmacological interventions in fibromyalgia syndrome: network meta-analysis. *Annals of the rheumatic diseases*, *72*(6), 955-962.

Okifuji, A., Gao, J., Bokat, C. & Hare, B. D. (2016). Management of fibromyalgia syndrome in 2016. *Pain management*, *6*(4), 383-400.

Phillips, K. & Clauw, D. J. (2013). Central pain mechanisms in rheumatic diseases: future directions. *Arthritis and rheumatism*, *65*(2), 291.

Rooks, D. S., Gautam, S., Romeling, M., Cross, M. L., Stratigakis, D., Evans, B. & Katz, J. N. (2007). Group exercise, education, and combination self-management in women with fibromyalgia: a randomized trial. *Archives of internal medicine*, *167*(20), 2192-2200.

Salazar, A. P., Stein, C., Marchese, R. R., Plentz, R. D. & Pagnussat, A. S. (2017). Electric Stimulation for Pain Relief in Patients with Fibromyalgia: A Systematic Review and Meta-analysis of Randomized Controlled Trials. *Pain Physician*, *20*(2), 15-25.

Saral, I., Sindel, D., Esmaeilzadeh, S., Sertel-Berk, H. O. & Oral, A. (2016). The effects of long-and short-term interdisciplinary treatment approaches in women with fibromyalgia: a randomized controlled trial. *Rheumatology international*, *36*(10), 1379-1389.

Sarzi-Puttini, P., Giorgi, V., Marotto, D. & Atzeni, F. (2020). Fibromyalgia: an update on clinical characteristics, aetiopathogenesis and treatment. Nature reviews. *Rheumatology*, *16*(11), 645–660.

Schmidt-Wilcke, T. & Diers, M. (2017). New insights into the pathophysiology and treatment of fibromyalgia. *Biomedicines*, *5*(2), 22.

Sosa-Reina, M. D., Nunez-Nagy, S., Gallego-Izquierdo, T., Pecos-Martín, D., Monserrat, J. & Álvarez-Mon, M. (2017). Effectiveness of Therapeutic Exercise in Fibromyalgia Syndrome: A Systematic Review and Meta-Analysis of Randomized Clinical Trials. *BioMed research international*, 2017, 2356346.

Tofferi, J. K., Jackson, J. L. & O'Malley, P. G. (2004). Treatment of fibromyalgia with cyclobenzaprine: A meta-analysis. *Arthritis Care & Research*, *51*(1), 9-13.

Vas, J., Santos-Rey, K., Navarro-Pablo, R., Modesto, M., Aguilar, I., Campos, M. Á. & Behrens, N. (2017). *Acupuncture for fibromyalgia in primary care: a randomised controlled trial.*

Walitt, B., Urrútia, G., Nishishinya, M. B., Cantrell, S. E. & Häuser, W. (2015). Selective serotonin reuptake inhibitors for fibromyalgia syndrome. *Cochrane Database of Systematic Reviews*, (6).

Williams, D. A. & Clauw, D. J. (2009). Understanding fibromyalgia: lessons from the broader pain research community. *The Journal of Pain*, *10(*8), 777-791.

Wolfe, F., Clauw, D. J., Fitzcharles, M. A., Goldenberg, D. L., Häuser, W., Katz, R. S. & Winfield, J. B. (2011). Fibromyalgia criteria and severity scales for clinical and epidemiological studies: a modification of the ACR Preliminary Diagnostic Criteria for Fibromyalgia. *The Journal of rheumatology*, *38*(6), 1113-1122.

Wolfe, F., Clauw, D. J., Fitzcharles, M. A., Goldenberg, D. L., Katz, R. S., Mease, P. & Yunus, M. B. (2010). The American College of Rheumatology preliminary diagnostic criteria for fibromyalgia and measurement of symptom severity. *Arthritis care & research*, *62*(5), 600-610.

Zhu, C. E., Yu, B., Zhang, W., Chen, W. H., Qi, Q. & Miao, Y. (2017). Effectiveness and safety of transcranial direct current stimulation in fibromyalgia: a systematic review and meta-analysis. *Journal of rehabilitation medicine*, *49*(1), 2-9.

In: Musculoskeletal Pain (Common Clinical Presentations) ISBN: 978-1-68507-410-4
Editors: Mehmet Cenk Turgut and Serdar Toy 

*Chapter 6*

# OSTEOARTHRITIS OF THE HIP

***Özkan Öztürk**, MD***
Department of Orthopedics and Traumatology,
Erzurum City Hospital, Erzurum, Turkey

## ABSTRACT

Osteoarthritis of the hip is a common degenerative arthritis and a common reason for disability. Common etiological factors are femoroacetabular impingement, dysplastic hip, trauma and osteonecrosis. The diagnosis is clinical and radiological. The most common symptoms are decreased range of motion and pain around the hip. Narrowing of joint spaces and osteophytes are the common radiological findings. The first line of treatment is conservative. Lifestyle modifications, weight loss, and physiotherapy are the choices. If these measures fail, then surgical treatment must be done.

## INTRODUCTION

Osteoarthritis (OA) of the hip is the degenerative arthritis of the hip. It affects 9.2% of adults older than 45 years in the US (Jordan et al., 2009), and the global prevalence of hip arthritis is 0.85% (Cross et al., 2014). OA of the hip and knee is the 11th highest contributor to global disability (Cross et al., 2014).

The treatment modalities for hip OA are lifestyle modifications, physiotherapy, pharmacological agents, intra-articular injections, and surgery (Aresti et al., 2016).

This section will summarize the epidemiology, etiology and pathogenesis, diagnosis, and treatment options of hip OA.

* Corresponding Author's E-mail: ortopedikcerrahi@gmail.com.

## EPIDEMIOLOGY

The hip is the second most common joint affected by degenerative arthritis, just after the knee (Aresti et al., 2016). Symptomatic hip arthritis prevalence is reported as between 1% (Nevitt et al., 2002) and 10% (Jordan et al., 2009). These prominent differences may occur because of the diversity of samples. 25% of adults will suffer from hip OA until the 85th year of age (L. B. Murphy et al., 2010). Radiological hip OA is more common than symptomatic hip OA (Kim et al., 2014).

## ETIOLOGY AND PATHOGENESIS

Hip OA can be grouped as primary or secondary according to the etiology. Primary OA is an exclusion diagnosis, meaning that no etiological factor is found.

Risk factors are suggested to be categorized into joint-level and person-level (N. J. Murphy et al., 2016) (Table 1).

**Table 1. Risk factors for hip OA**

| Joint-level | Person-level |
|---|---|
| Abnormal joint morphology<br>Joint injury<br>Poor hip muscular function | Age<br>Weight<br>Genetics<br>Ethnicity<br>Occupation<br>Inflammatory arthritis |

Abnormal joint morphology can result from developmental dysplasia of the hip (DDH), acetabular fractures, femoroacetabular impingement (FAI), slipped capital femoral epiphysis (SCFE), osteonecrosis (ON) of the femoral head, and Legg-Calvé-Perthes disease (LCPD).

DDH is a well-known precursor of hip OA (Figure 1). In a study conducted on patients treated with unilateral total hip arthroplasty (THA) under 55 years of age, patients with DDH had a two-third risk of undergoing THA (Wyles et al., 2017).

Acetabular fractures can also distort the hip joint's morphology and induce OA (Figure 2). One-quarter of the surgically treated and anatomically reduced acetabular fracture patients develop posttraumatic OA (Gänsslen et al., 2012, 2013). Posttraumatic OA accounts for 1.6% of all symptomatic hip OA patients (Brown et al., 2006). 10% of the femoral neck fractures treated with closed reduction and percutaneous fixation will be converted to THA in five years (Kahlenberg et al., 2018).

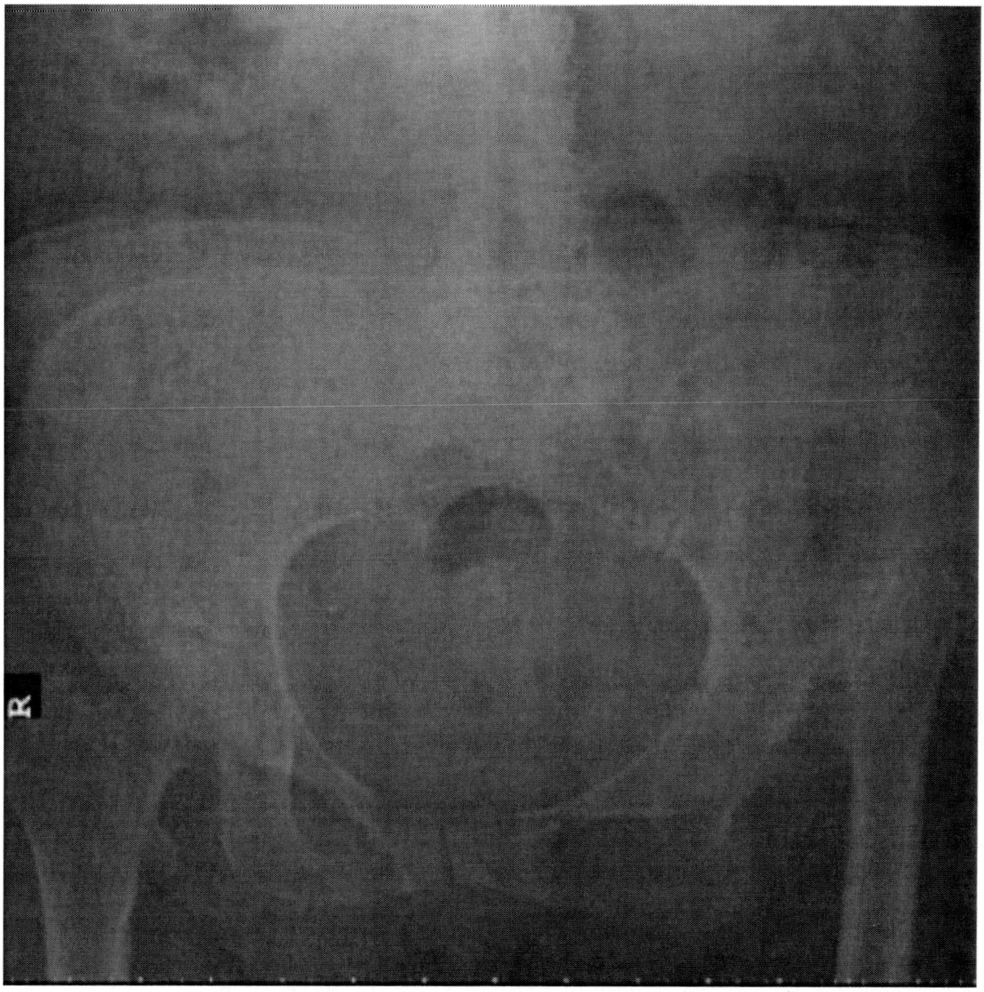


Figure 1. Degenerative OA of the left hip secondary to DDH. Author's own archive.

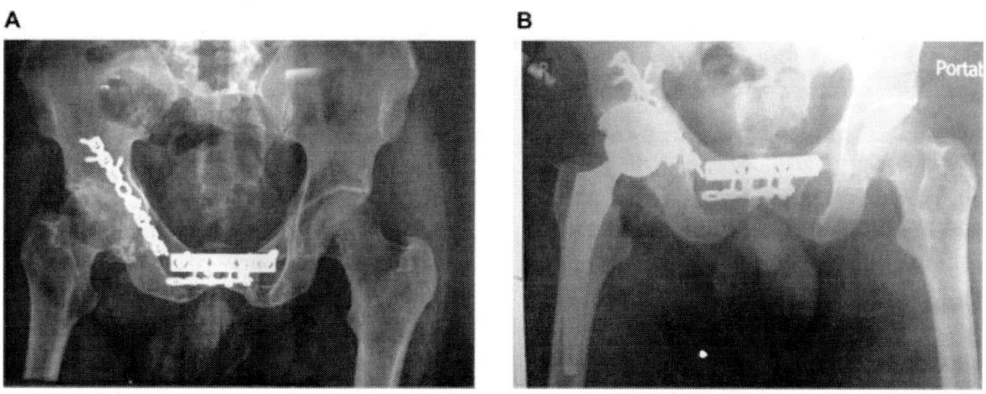


Figure 2. A. A 62-year-old male operated for acetabular fracture and symphysis pubis separation. He developed posttraumatic OA in the right hip. B. The OA was treated with cementless THA. The picture is taken from (Taheriazam & Saeidinia, 2019) under the Creative Commons 3.0 license.

The relationship between FAI and hip OA is well-known (Ganz et al., 2003).

The annual incidence of SCFE is 10 in 100,000 children, and 2% to 28% of them progress to end-stage OA after surgical treatment (Mathew & Larson, 2019).

ON of the femoral head is the reason for THA in 10% of the female and 24.4% of the male patients (Uluçay et al., 2013).

LCPD is another risk factor for hip OA. 7% of conservatively treated LCPDs had undergone THA within 40 years (Perpich et al., 1983), and 21% of them had surgery between the ages of 30 and 50 (McAndrew & Weinstein, 1984).

Weakness of hip flexors and adductors is associated with hip OA (Loureiro et al., 2013).

The other risk factors for hip OA are age (Jordan et al., 2009), obesity (Jiang et al., 2011), genetics (Pelt et al., 2015), Caucasian race (Dudda et al., 2011), inflammatory arthritis (Hoaglund & Steinbach, 2001), heavy manual work (Harris & Coggon, 2015) and elite athleticism (Gouttebarge et al., 2015) (Table 1).

Sex (Srikanth et al., 2005) and diet (N. J. Murphy et al., 2016) are not associated with hip OA.

While physiological loading is crucial for the homeostasis of the joints (Guilak et al., 2004), altered load distribution disturbs the balance between joint tissue synthesis and degradation (Eyre, 2004) in favor of degradation and leads to hip OA. The etiological risk factors mentioned above all participate in this process (Table 1).

Altered load distribution leads to subchondral bone remodeling. Cartilage damage leads the proinflammatory cytokines to pass from the subchondral bone to the cartilage (N. J. Murphy et al., 2016). The inflammatory process secondary to osteochondral microdamage leads to apoptosis of the subchondral bone (Charlier et al., 2016), which is responsible for subchondral cysts.

Lymphocyte-dominant synovitis can explain the generalized nature of the OA, while microtrauma is local (Benito et al., 2005).

# DIAGNOSIS

## Symptoms and Medical History

The most common symptom of hip OA is pain around the groin and inguinal region. Movement can increase the pain. Stiffness of the hip may harden the daily activities and mobilization. Loose cartilage in the joint may cause a "click" sound while walking. Decreased range of motion (ROM) may cause limping.

A thorough medical history is essential for differential diagnosis. The nature and onset of the pain must be reviewed. Risk factors, including family history, trauma, and others mentioned above, should be investigated.

Hip bursitis, labral tears, occult femoral neck fractures, malignancies, ON, Paget disease, piriformis syndrome, septic arthritis, and rheumatological diseases are all differential diagnoses (Cibulka et al., 2009). Radiating pain from the L2-L3 roots must also be evaluated.

## Physical Examination

Edema, swelling, localized tumors, muscle wasting, and previous surgical scars should be investigated in the inspection. Leg length discrepancies must also be measured.

Gait evaluation may show limping, and Trendelenburg gait may be observed.

Active and passive ROM and muscle strength must be examined.

Patrick's test, or the FABERE test, may show labral tears (Mitchell et al., 2003). While the patient is supine, the hip is passively flexed to 90°, abducted, and externally rotated. Pain provoked with this test is accepted as positive. This test may be positive with intra-articular pathologies, and sacroiliac joint problems (Wilson & Furukawa, 2014).

The onset of pain after the 90° flexion, adduction and external rotation (FADIR test) suggests FAI (Leibold et al., 2008).

Provocative sacroiliac tests (van der Wurff et al., 2006) show possible sacroiliac problems. A straight leg raise test and femoral nerve stretch test must also be performed for thoracolumbar spinal problems (Tokuhashi et al., 2001).

## Radiological Evaluation

Conventional X-rays are still the first choice of diagnostic tools. It is crucial for both the differential diagnosis and choosing the suitable treatment option.

Classical findings in hip OA are joint space narrowing, subchondral sclerosis, osteophytes around the joint and subchondral cysts (Weber et al., 2016) (Figure 3). In advanced stages, deformities and enlargement of the femoral head may be visible (Figure 3). Underlying deformities such as DDH (Figure.1), trauma (Figure 2) and ON can be visible with standing anteroposterior X-rays.

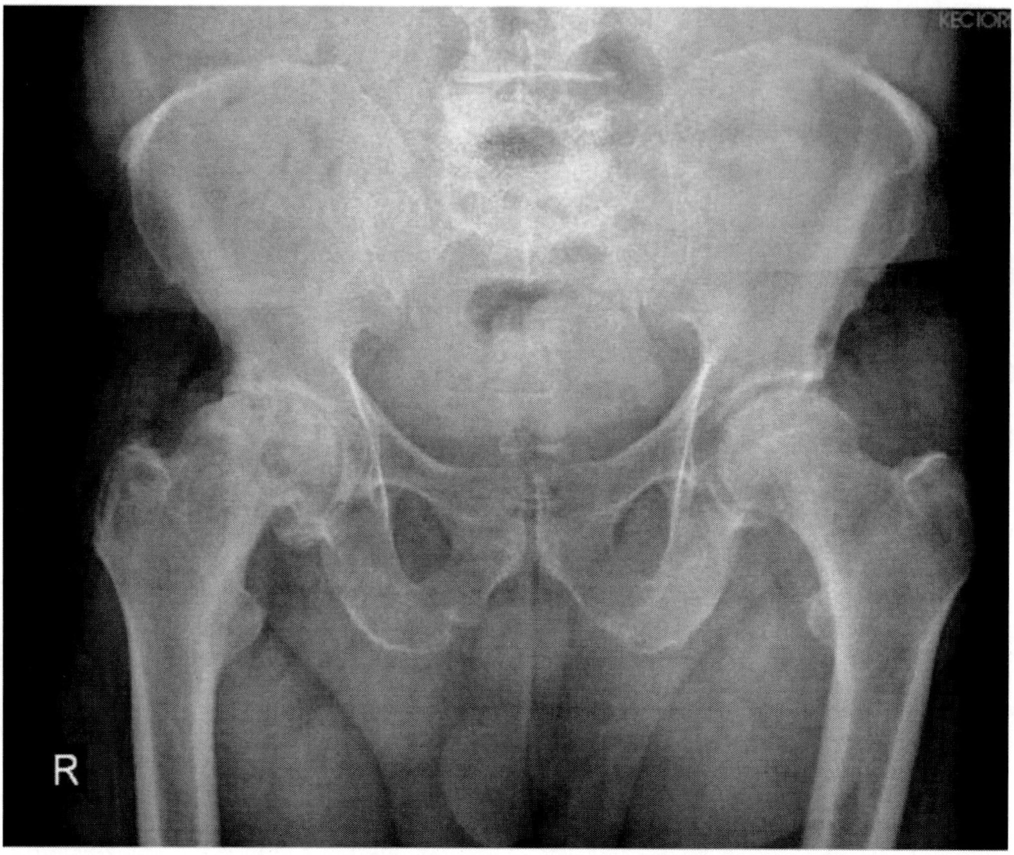


Figure 3. Standing anteroposterior X-ray of a hip OA patient. Note the joint space narrowing, subchondral sclerosis, subchondral cysts, and osteophytes in the right hip. The femoral head is also enlarged. Author's own archive.

**Table 2. Kellgren-Lawrence Classification System**

| | |
|---|---|
| Grade 0 (none) | No X-ray change |
| Grade 1 (doubtful) | Possible osteophytes and doubtful joint space narrowing |
| Grade 2 (minimal) | Definite osteophytes and possible joint space narrowing |
| Grade 3 (moderate) | Multiple osteophytes, narrowing of joint space and some sclerosis |
| Grade 4 (severe) | Large osteophytes, marked narrowing of joint space |

The Kellgren-Lawrence Classification system is widely used for radiological classification (Kellgren & Lawrence, 1957). This classification is based on joint space narrowing and osteophytes (Table 2). Another widely-used classification system is defined by Tönnis (Tönnis, 1976). The main handicap of these systems is that the radiological level is not correlated with the clinical situation (Cubukcu et al., 2012).

Computerized tomography is not routinely used for the diagnosis. However, it is a powerful tool for the surgeon for the preoperative planning of hip OA with significant bony defects, protrusio acetabuli, DDH, and ankylosis.

Magnetic resonance imaging (MRI) may show labral tears, early-stage osteochondral defects and synovial problems (Weber et al., 2016). Several MRI techniques monitor cartilage, such as T2 mapping and delayed gadolinium-enhanced MRI of cartilage (dGEMRIC) (Huang et al., 2019). The findings of these novel methods may help the surgeon to decide on joint preserving surgical techniques (Huang et al., 2019).

## TREATMENT

There is no standard treatment option for hip OA, but the symptoms can be treated, and progression can be decelerated. The treatment options may be grouped as nonpharmacological, pharmacological, and surgical.

### Nonpharmacological Modalities

Strengthening exercises for the muscles around the hip may decrease the symptoms (Bartels et al., 2016). Aquatic exercises are also moderately efficient in decreasing pain (Bartels et al., 2016).

Physiotherapy is the mainstream treatment for mild to moderate hip OA (Lespasio et al., 2018), and transcutaneous electrical nerve stimulation is an adjunct for that (Hochberg et al., 2012).

While obesity is a risk factor for hip OA, weight loss may be efficient for relief (Curtis et al., 2017).

Assistive devices like sticks, walkers, and canes decrease the load on the joint and relieve pain (Lespasio et al., 2018).

### Pharmacological Modalities

Acetaminophen is the first-line medical treatment for mild OA (Lespasio et al., 2018). It diminishes the pain in the short term. Combination with local nonsteroidal anti-inflammatory drugs (NSAID) may be helpful (Lespasio et al., 2018).

Oral NSAIDs are efficient when acetaminophen cannot dissolve pain (da Costa et al., 2017). Diclofenac and etoricoxib are the most potent NSAIDs for pain relief (Hochberg et al., 2012). These drugs must be used cautiously because of side effects like gastrointestinal bleeding and cardiac events.

Opioids may diminish the pain when NSAIDs are inefficient but must be used cautiously because of the abuse risk.

Intra-articular corticosteroid, platelet-rich plasma, or hyaluronic acid injections are not advised (Kolasinski et al., 2020) because of the lack of evidence. Some further research is needed.

## Surgical Management

Hip arthroscopy may reduce symptoms in the early stages of OA (Andronic et al., 2021). While primarily performed for FAI and labral tears (Kyin et al., 2021), conversion to THA will be mandatory for 2.4 to 40% of the patients (Kyin et al., 2021).

Hip resurfacing arthroplasty was designed for young OA patients. Very few high-quality studies about the outcomes exist, and revision rates are high (van Gerwen et al., 2010). Recall of some implants from the market because of metallosis raises concern (Girard, 2017). We can conclude that its usage is limited to a selected group of patients.

THA is the mainstream of surgical management. It is indicated for severe hip pain not relieved by conservative modalities and radiological end-stage OA. It is cost-effective (Daigle et al., 2012), and diminishes the pain while improving the functions, and implants survive for a long time (Lespasio et al., 2018). Survival of the implants may be 25 to 30 years (Shon et al., 2019). Patients can return to daily life after this procedure (Shon et al., 2019). Delays in THA for end-stage hip OA may worsen the clinical outcome (Daigle et al., 2012).

# Conclusion

Hip OA is a common reason for disability. Altered joint anatomy and increased load on the joint end up with end-stage OA. A positive family history, obesity, heavy manual labor, DDH, FAI, fractures, and ON are the main risk factors. A thorough evaluation, including a detailed patient history, physical examination, and standing AP radiograms, is mandatory for the diagnosis. Lifestyle modifications and physiotherapy are the first-line treatment options. Analgesic drugs must be used carefully, and if these fail the most efficient treatment option is THA.

# References

Andronic, O., Claydon, L., Cubberley, R., Sunil-Kumar, K. H., & Khanduja, V. (2021). Outcomes of Hip Arthroscopy in Patients with Femoroacetabular Impingement and Concomitant Tönnis Grade II Osteoarthritis or Greater: Protocol for a Systematic

Review. *International Journal of Surgery Protocols*, *25*(1), 1–6. https://doi.org/10.29337/ijsp.26.

Aresti, N., Kassam, J., Nicholas, N., & Achan, P. (2016). Hip osteoarthritis. *BMJ*, *354*. https://doi.org/10.1136/bmj.i3405.

Bartels, E. M., Juhl, C. B., Christensen, R., Hagen, K. B., Danneskiold-Samsøe, B., Dagfinrud, H., & Lund, H. (2016). Aquatic exercise for the treatment of knee and hip osteoarthritis. *The Cochrane Database of Systematic Reviews*, *3*, CD005523. https://doi.org/10.1002/ 14651858.CD005523.pub3.

Benito, M. J., Veale, D. J., FitzGerald, O., van den Berg, W. B., & Bresnihan, B. (2005). Synovial tissue inflammation in early and late osteoarthritis. *Annals of the Rheumatic Diseases*, *64*(9), 1263–1267. https://doi.org/10.1136/ard.2004.025270.

Brown, T. D., Johnston, R. C., Saltzman, C. L., Marsh, J. L., & Buckwalter, J. A. (2006). Posttraumatic osteoarthritis: a first estimate of incidence, prevalence, and burden of disease. *Journal of Orthopaedic Trauma*, *20*(10), 739–744. https://doi.org/10.1097/01. bot.0000246468.80635.ef.

Charlier, E., Relic, B., Deroyer, C., Malaise, O., Neuville, S., Collée, J., Malaise, M. G., & De Seny, D. (2016). Insights on Molecular Mechanisms of Chondrocytes Death in Osteoarthritis. *International Journal of Molecular Sciences*, *17*(12). https://doi.org/10.3390/ ijms17122146.

Cibulka, M. T., White, D. M., Woehrle, J., Harris-Hayes, M., Enseki, K., Fagerson, T. L., Slover, J., & Godges, J. J. (2009). Hip pain and mobility deficits--hip osteoarthritis: clinical practice guidelines linked to the international classification of functioning, disability, and health from the orthopaedic section of the American Physical Therapy Association. *The Journal of Orthopaedic and Sports Physical Therapy*, *39*(4), A1-25. https://doi.org/10.2519/jospt.2009. 0301.

Cross, M., Smith, E., Hoy, D., Nolte, S., Ackerman, I., Fransen, M., Bridgett, L., Williams, S., Guillemin, F., Hill, C. L., Laslett, L. L., Jones, G., Cicuttini, F., Osborne, R., Vos, T., Buchbinder, R., Woolf, A., & March, L. (2014). The global burden of hip and knee osteoarthritis: estimates from the global burden of disease 2010 study. *Annals of the Rheumatic Diseases*, *73*(7), 1323–1330. https://doi.org/10.1136/annrheumdis-2013-204763.

Cubukcu, D., Sarsan, A., & Alkan, H. (2012). Relationships between Pain, Function and Radiographic Findings in Osteoarthritis of the Knee: A Cross-Sectional Study. *Arthritis*, *2012*, 984060. https:// doi.org/10.1155/2012/984060.

Curtis, G. L., Chughtai, M., Khlopas, A., Newman, J. M., Khan, R., Shaffiy, S., Nadhim, A., Bhave, A., & Mont, M. A. (2017). Impact of Physical Activity in Cardiovascular and Musculoskeletal Health: Can Motion Be Medicine? *Journal of Clinical Medicine Research*, *9*(5), 375–381. https://doi.org/10.14740/jocmr3001w.

da Costa, B. R., Reichenbach, S., Keller, N., Nartey, L., Wandel, S., Jüni, P., & Trelle, S. (2017). Effectiveness of non-steroidal anti-inflammatory drugs for the treatment of pain in knee and hip osteoarthritis: a network meta-analysis. *Lancet (London, England)*, *390*(10090), e21–e33. https://doi.org/10.1016/S0140-6736(17)31744-0.

Daigle, M. E., Weinstein, A. M., Katz, J. N., & Losina, E. (2012). The cost-effectiveness of total joint arthroplasty: a systematic review of published literature. *Best Practice & Research. Clinical Rheumatology*, *26*(5), 649–658. https://doi.org/10.1016/j.berh. 2012. 07.013.

Dudda, M., Kim, Y.-J., Zhang, Y., Nevitt, M. C., Xu, L., Niu, J., Goggins, J., Doherty, M., & Felson, D. T. (2011). Morphologic differences between the hips of Chinese women and white women: could they account for the ethnic difference in the prevalence of hip osteoarthritis? *Arthritis and Rheumatism*, *63*(10), 2992–2999. https://doi.org/10.1002/art.30472.

Eyre, D. R. (2004). Collagens and cartilage matrix homeostasis. *Clinical Orthopaedics and Related Research*, *427 Suppl*, S118-22. https://doi. org/10.1097/01.blo.0000144855.48640.b9.

Gänsslen, A., Frink, M., Hildebrand, F., & Krettek, C. (2012). Both column fractures of the acetabulum: epidemiology, operative management and long-term-results. *Acta Chirurgiae Orthopaedicae et Traumatologiae Cechoslovaca*, *79*(2), 107–113.

Gänsslen, A., Hildebrand, F., & Kretek, C. (2013). Transverse + posterior wall fractures of the acetabulum: epidemiology, operative management and long-term results. *Acta Chirurgiae Orthopaedicae et Traumatologiae Cechoslovaca*, *80*(1), 27–33.

Ganz, R., Parvizi, J., Beck, M., Leunig, M., Nötzli, H., & Siebenrock, K. A. (2003). Femoroacetabular impingement: a cause for osteoarthritis of the hip. *Clinical Orthopaedics and Related Research*, *417*, 112–120. https://doi.org/10.1097/01.blo.0000096804.78689.c2.

Girard, J. (2017). Hip Resurfacing: International Perspectives: Review Article. *HSS Journal : The Musculoskeletal Journal of Hospital for Special Surgery*, *13*(1), 7–11. https://doi.org/10.1007/s11420-016-9511-y.

Gouttebarge, V., Inklaar, H., Backx, F., & Kerkhoffs, G. (2015). Prevalence of osteoarthritis in former elite athletes: a systematic overview of the recent literature. *Rheumatology International*, *35*(3), 405–418. https://doi.org/10.1007/s00296-014-3093-0.

Guilak, F., Fermor, B., Keefe, F. J., Kraus, V. B., Olson, S. A., Pisetsky, D. S., Setton, L. A., & Weinberg, J. B. (2004). The role of biomechanics and inflammation in cartilage injury and repair. *Clinical Orthopaedics and Related Research*, *423*, 17–26. https://doi. org/10.1097/01.blo.0000131233.83640.91.

Harris, E. C., & Coggon, D. (2015). HIP osteoarthritis and work. *Best Practice & Research. Clinical Rheumatology*, *29*(3), 462–482. https://doi.org/10.1016/j.berh.2015.04.015.

Hoaglund, F. T., & Steinbach, L. S. (2001). Primary osteoarthritis of the hip: etiology and epidemiology. *The Journal of the American Academy of Orthopaedic Surgeons*, *9*(5), 320–327. https://doi.org/10. 5435/00124635-200109000-00005.

Hochberg, M. C., Altman, R. D., April, K. T., Benkhalti, M., Guyatt, G., McGowan, J., Towheed, T., Welch, V., Wells, G., & Tugwell, P. (2012). American College of Rheumatology 2012 recommendations for the use of nonpharmacologic and pharmacologic therapies in osteoarthritis of the hand, hip, and knee. *Arthritis Care & Research*, *64*(4), 465–474. https://doi.org/10.1002/acr.21596.

Huang, B. K., Tan, W., Scherer, K. F., Rennie, W., Chung, C. B., & Bancroft, L. W. (2019). Standard and Advanced Imaging of Hip Osteoarthritis. What the Radiologist Should Know. *Seminars in Musculoskeletal Radiology*, *23*(3), 289–303. https://doi.org/10. 1055/ s-0039-1681050.

Jiang, L., Rong, J., Wang, Y., Hu, F., Bao, C., Li, X., & Zhao, Y. (2011). The relationship between body mass index and hip osteoarthritis: a systematic review and meta-analysis. *Joint Bone Spine*, *78*(2), 150–155. https://doi.org/10.1016/ j.jbspin.2010.04.011.

Jordan, J. M., Helmick, C. G., Renner, J. B., Luta, G., Dragomir, A. D., Woodard, J., Fang, F., Schwartz, T. A., Nelson, A. E., Abbate, L. M., Callahan, L. F., Kalsbeek, W. D., & Hochberg, M. C. (2009). Prevalence of hip symptoms and radiographic and symptomatic hip osteoarthritis in African Americans and Caucasians: the Johnston County Osteoarthritis Project. *The Journal of Rheumatology*, *36*(4), 809–815. https://doi.org/10.3899/jrheum.080677.

Kahlenberg, C. A., Richardson, S. S., Schairer, W. W., & Cross, M. B. (2018). Rates and Risk Factors of Conversion Hip Arthroplasty After Closed Reduction Percutaneous Hip Pinning for Femoral Neck Fractures—A Population Analysis. *The Journal of Arthroplasty*, *33*(3), 771–776. https://doi.org/https://doi.org/10.1016/j.arth.2017. 10.004.

Kellgren, J. H., & Lawrence, J. S. (1957). Radiological assessment of osteo-arthrosis. *Annals of the Rheumatic Diseases*, *16*(4), 494–502. https://doi.org/10.1136/ ard.16.4.494.

Kim, C., Linsenmeyer, K. D., Vlad, S. C., Guermazi, A., Clancy, M. M., Niu, J., & Felson, D. T. (2014). Prevalence of radiographic and symptomatic hip osteoarthritis in an urban United States community: the Framingham osteoarthritis study. *Arthritis & Rheumatology (Hoboken, N.J.)*, *66*(11), 3013–3017. https://doi.org/10.1002/art. 38795.

Kolasinski, S. L., Neogi, T., Hochberg, M. C., Oatis, C., Guyatt, G., Block, J., Callahan, L., Copenhaver, C., Dodge, C., Felson, D., Gellar, K., Harvey, W. F., Hawker, G., Herzig, E., Kwoh, C. K., Nelson, A. E., Samuels, J., Scanzello, C., White, D., ... Reston, J. (2020). 2019 American College of Rheumatology/Arthritis Foundation

Guideline for the Management of Osteoarthritis of the Hand, Hip, and Knee. *Arthritis Care & Research*, *72*(2), 149–162. https://doi.org/10.1002/acr.24131.

Kyin, C., Maldonado, D. R., Go, C. C., Shapira, J., Lall, A. C., & Domb, B. G. (2021). Mid- to Long-Term Outcomes of Hip Arthroscopy: A Systematic Review. *Arthroscopy : The Journal of Arthroscopic & Related Surgery : Official Publication of the Arthroscopy Association of North America and the International Arthroscopy Association*, *37*(3), 1011–1025. https://doi.org/10.1016/j.arthro.2020.10.001.

Lau, E. M., Lin, F., Lam, D., Silman, A., & Croft, P. (1995). Hip osteoarthritis and dysplasia in Chinese men. *Annals of the Rheumatic Diseases*, *54*(12), 965–969. https://doi.org/10.1136/ard.54.12.965.

Leibold, M. R., Huijbregts, P. A., & Jensen, R. (2008). Concurrent criterion-related validity of physical examination tests for hip labral lesions: a systematic review. *The Journal of Manual & Manipulative Therapy*, *16*(2), E24-41. https://doi.org/10.1179/jmt. 2008.16.2.24E.

Lespasio, M. J., Sultan, A. A., Piuzzi, N. S., Khlopas, A., Husni, M. E., Muschler, G. F., & Mont, M. A. (2018). Hip Osteoarthritis: A Primer. *The Permanente Journal*, *22*, 17–84. https://doi.org/10.7812/TPP/17-084.

Loureiro, A., Mills, P. M., & Barrett, R. S. (2013). Muscle weakness in hip osteoarthritis: A systematic review. *Arthritis Care \& Research*, *65*(3), 340–352. https://doi.org/https://doi.org/10.1002/acr.21806.

Mathew, S. E., & Larson, A. N. (2019). Natural History of Slipped Capital Femoral Epiphysis. *Journal of Pediatric Orthopedics*, *39*(Issue 6, Supplement 1 Suppl 1), S23–S27. https://doi.org/10.1097/ BPO.0000000000001369.

McAndrew, M. P., & Weinstein, S. L. (1984). A long-term follow-up of Legg-Calvé-Perthes disease. *JBJS*, *66*(6). https://journals.lww.com/ jbjsjournal/Fulltext/ 1984/66060/A_long_term_follow_up_of_Legg_Calv__Perthes.6.aspx.

Mitchell, B., McCrory, P., Brukner, P., O'Donnell, J., Colson, E., & Howells, R. (2003). Hip joint pathology: clinical presentation and correlation between magnetic resonance arthrography, ultrasound, and arthroscopic findings in 25 consecutive cases. *Clinical Journal of Sport Medicine : Official Journal of the Canadian Academy of Sport Medicine*, *13*(3), 152–156. https://doi.org/10.1097/00042752-200305000-00005.

Murphy, L. B., Helmick, C. G., Schwartz, T. A., Renner, J. B., Tudor, G., Koch, G. G., Dragomir, A. D., Kalsbeek, W. D., Luta, G., & Jordan, J. M. (2010). One in four people may develop symptomatic hip osteoarthritis in his or her lifetime. *Osteoarthritis and Cartilage*, *18*(11), 1372–1379. https://doi.org/10.1016/j.joca. 2010.08.005.

Murphy, N. J., Eyles, J. P., & Hunter, D. J. (2016). Hip Osteoarthritis: Etiopathogenesis and Implications for Management. *Advances in Therapy*, *33*(11), 1921–1946. https://doi.org/10.1007/s12325-016-0409-3.

Nevitt, M. C., Xu, L., Zhang, Y., Lui, L.-Y., Yu, W., Lane, N. E., Qin, M., Hochberg, M. C., Cummings, S. R., & Felson, D. T. (2002). Very low prevalence of hip osteoarthritis among Chinese elderly in Beijing, China, compared with whites in the United States: The Beijing osteoarthritis study. *Arthritis \& Rheumatism*, *46*(7), 1773–1779. https://doi.org/https://doi.org/10.1002/art.10332.

Pelt, C. E., Erickson, J. A., Peters, C. L., Anderson, M. B., & Cannon-Albright, L. (2015). A Heritable Predisposition to Osteoarthritis of the Hip. *The Journal of Arthroplasty*, *30*(9 Suppl), 125–129. https://doi.org/10.1016/j.arth.2015.01.062.

Perpich, M., McBeath, A., & Kruse, D. (1983). Long-Term Follow-up of Perthes Disease Treated with Spica Casts. *Journal of Pediatric Orthopaedics*, *3*(2). https://journals.lww.com/pedorthopaedics/Fulltext/1983/05000/Long_Term_Follow_up_of_Perthes_Disease_Treated.3.aspx.

Shon, W. Y., Park, B.-Y., R, R. N., Park, P. S., Im, J. T., & Yun, H. H. (2019). Total Hip Arthroplasty: Past, Present, and Future. What Has Been Achieved? *Hip & Pelvis*, *31*(4), 179–189. https://doi.org/10. 5371/hp.2019.31.4.179.

Srikanth, V. K., Fryer, J. L., Zhai, G., Winzenberg, T. M., Hosmer, D., & Jones, G. (2005). A meta-analysis of sex differences prevalence, incidence and severity of osteoarthritis. *Osteoarthritis and Cartilage*, *13*(9), 769–781. https://doi.org/10.1016/j .joca.2005.04.014.

Taheriazam, A., & Saeidinia, A. (2019). Conversion to total hip arthroplasty in posttraumatic arthritis: short-term clinical outcomes. *Orthopedic Research and Reviews*, *11*, 41–46. https://doi.org/10. 2147/ORR.S184590.

Tokuhashi, Y., Matsuzaki, H., Uematsu, Y., & Oda, H. (2001). Symptoms of thoracolumbar junction disc herniation. *Spine*, *26*(22), E512-8. https://doi.org/10. 1097/00007632-200111150-00021.

Tönnis, D. (1976). Normal values of the hip joint for the evaluation of X-rays in children and adults. *Clinical Orthopaedics and Related Research*, *119*, 39–47.

Uluçay, C., Ozler, T., Güven, M., Akman, B., Kocadal, A. O., & Altıntaş, F. (2013). Etiology of coxarthrosis in patients with total hip replacement. *Acta Orthopaedica et Traumatologica Turcica*, *47*(5), 330–333. https://doi.org/10.3944/aott.2013.3103.

van der Wurff, P., Buijs, E. J., & Groen, G. J. (2006). A multitest regimen of pain provocation tests as an aid to reduce unnecessary minimally invasive sacroiliac joint procedures. *Archives of Physical Medicine and Rehabilitation*, *87*(1), 10–14. https://doi.org/10.1016/j. apmr.2005.09.023.

van Gerwen, M., Shaerf, D. A., & Veen, R. M. (2010). Hip resurfacing arthroplasty. *Acta Orthopaedica*, *81*(6), 680–683. https://doi.org/10. 3109/17453674.2010.501742.

Weber, M.-A., Merle, C., Rehnitz, C., & Gotterbarm, T. (2016). Modern Radiological Imaging of Osteoarthritis of The Hip Joint With Consideration of Predisposing Conditions. *RoFo : Fortschritte Auf Dem Gebiete Der Rontgenstrahlen Und Der Nuklearmedizin*, *188*(7), 635–651. https://doi.org/10.1055/s-0042-104511.

Wilson, J. J., & Furukawa, M. (2014). Evaluation of the patient with hip pain. *American Family Physician*, *89*(1), 27–34.

Wyles, C. C., Heidenreich, M. J., Jeng, J., Larson, D. R., Trousdale, R. T., & Sierra, R. J. (2017). The John Charnley Award: Redefining the Natural History of Osteoarthritis in Patients With Hip Dysplasia and Impingement. *Clinical Orthopaedics and Related Research*, *475*(2), 336–350. https://doi.org/10.1007/s11999-016-4815-2.

Yoshimura, N., Campbell, L., Hashimoto, T., Kinoshita, H., Okayasu, T., Wilman, C., Coggon, D., Croft, P., & Cooper, C. (1998). Acetabular dysplasia and hip osteoarthritis in Britain and Japan. *British Journal of Rheumatology*, *37*(11), 1193–1197. https://doi.org/10.1093/ rheumatology/37.11.1193.

In: Musculoskeletal Pain (Common Clinical Presentations) ISBN: 978-1-68507-410-4
Editors: Mehmet Cenk Turgut and Serdar Toy 

*Chapter 7*

# FEMOROACETABULAR IMPINGEMENT

***Feyzi Kılıç**, MD***
Department of Orthopedics and Traumatology,
Gaziosmanpaşa Training and Research Hospital, Istanbul, Turkey

## ABSTRACT

Femoroacetabular impingement (FAI) is a hip pathology that has been known to orthopedic surgeons for nearly 90 years, but for which gold standards have not yet been established in terms of its mechanism, clinical symptoms, diagnosis, and treatment. Diagnosis is attempted with different examination methods and radiological parameters, and in clinical practice, it is mostly seen in the athlete patient group. Conservative and surgical methods are used in its treatment. There is not yet a consensus on the optimal surgical procedure.

## INTRODUCTION

The concept of hip impingement was first suggested by Smith-Petersen in 1936. However, FAI (femoroacetabular impingement) was first described by Myers et al. in 1999 (Zhou et al., 2020). Ganz et al. defined FAI as a condition resulting from the proximal femur and/or acetabulum in patients or from the movement of the hip beyond its physiological limits (Ganz et al., 2001).

FAI is a clinical picture that occurs due to contact surfaces having deteriorated as a result of abnormal morphology in the acetabulum and femoral head-neck junction (Hale

* Corresponding Author's E-mail: drkilicfeyzi@gmail.com.

et al., 2019). This condition is one of the most common causes of hip pain and a predisposing factor for hip osteoarthritis (Nakashima et al. 2019).

In clinical practice, FAI presents with groin pain, pain with hip movement, limitation of activity, and decreased range of motion of the joint (Mallets et al., 2019).

It may occur in 3 different clinical forms: the cam type, pincer type, and mixed type. While pathology is in the femoral head and neck junction in the cam type, it is in the acetabulum in the pincer type and in both anatomical regions in the mixed type (Zhou et al., 2020).

Diagnosis can be made using clinical evaluation and radiological examinations such as direct radiography, computed tomography, and magnetic resonance imaging (Rhee et al., 2017).

Its treatment is divided into conservative and surgical methods. In the literature, there is no clear conclusion about the superiority of methods over each other. Surgical methods are divided into open and closed (arthroscopic) methods (Mallets et al., 2019, Hoit et al., 2020).

**Table 1. Typical features of Cam and Pincer-Type FAI (Pfirrmann et al. 2006)**

| | **Cam FAI** | **Pincer FAI** |
|---|---|---|
| Sex | Male | Female |
| Age | Young | Middle age |
| Mechanism | Separation forces affecting the interior of the joint damage the acetabular cartilage | Linear effect on the acetabulum and femur head-neck junction causes impaction injury |
| Activity | High-level athletes | Individuals who do not play sports professionally |
| Deformity | Cam-type deformity: Lateral enlargement on the femoral neck | Increased coverage of the femoral head: Coxa profunda, protrusion acetabuli, acetabular retroversion |
| Early intra-articular damage | Delamination of the acetabular cartilage, cartilage lesions from outside to inside | It may range from mild labral injury to extensive labral injury |
| Late intra-articular damage | Large full-thickness anterosuperior cartilage defect; labral injury accompanied by sub-surface tears, cartilage lesions of the femoral head | Ossified labrum with the ossified bone acetabular lip; cartilage injury in the acetabular lip; acetabulum injury in theposteroinferior quadrant of the contrecoup |

## Prevalence and Clinical Findings

Although FAI is mostly observed between the ages of 20 and 45, its prevalence is 10-15% in the general population (Hoit et al., 2020). In a cross-sectional study conducted by Diesel et al., the prevalence of FAI was found to be 53% (Diesel et al., 2015).

It was found to be 79% in a study in which symptomatic patients with hip or groin pain were examined (Bowler et al., 2012). In another study, the prevalence of cam and pincer type deformities was found to be between 37% and 67% in the asymptomatic patient group. In patients with the clinical picture of hip pain, radiological findings were found to be positive in 60.5% of patients (Hoit et al., 2020).

The prevalence of FAI was found to be higher in athletes, especially football players, compared to other individuals in the same age group who did not do sports (Marom et al., 2020).

FAI manifests itself with pain as a clinical symptom, which negatively affects the quality of life of the individual. The onset of symptoms in patients is mostly insidious, and symptoms are usually observed with physical activity (Clohisy et al., 2009). Groin pain (83%) is mostly observed in patients. The mean time between the patient's diagnosis of FAI and clinical symptoms was reported to be 3 years (Clohisy et al., 2009). The features of cam and pincer-type FAI are presented in Table 1.

The FABER (flexion, abduction, external rotation) test is performed on the supine position of the patient. The examined hip is brought to position 4, the unexamined pelvis is manually fixed on the table, and the examined leg is pressed against the table. This procedure is performed bilaterally. While pressing the leg, the distance between the knee and the examined table is measured. The test is considered to be positive if the distance on the affected side is greater than that of the hip without pathology. The sensitivity of this test for FAI was reported to be high (Philippon et al., 2007).

A decrease in the hip joint range of motion can be observed in FAI. It is recommended to use the FADIR (flexion, adduction, internal rotation) test as a sensitive test in the examination of the patient. The patient's complaints are aggravated with the FADIR test. The negative aspect of the FADIR test is that its specificity is low, and the test may be positive in other clinical situations (Brunner et al. 2016) (Figure 1). When we ask about the patient's complaint, the "grip or C sign" made to show the aching region is valuable in terms of showing the pathology inside the hip (Byrd et al., 2014) (Figure 2).

The Drehmann sign is the passive movement of the patient's hip to an irresistible external rotation position while the hip joint is placed in the flexion position in a patient with FAI (Tannast et al., 2007).

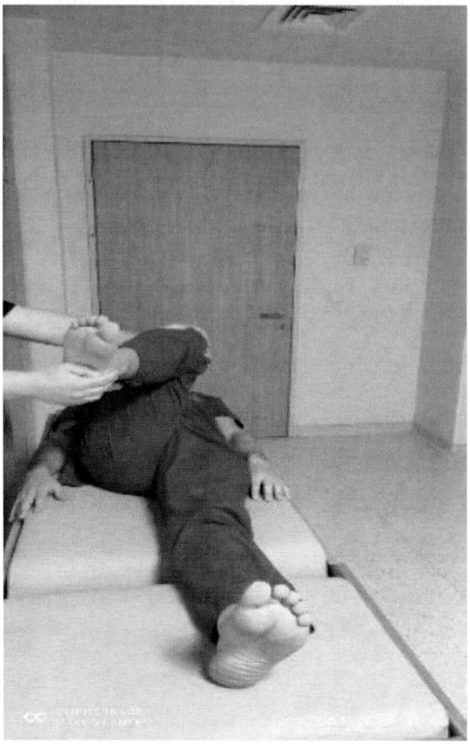

Figure 1. FADIR test.

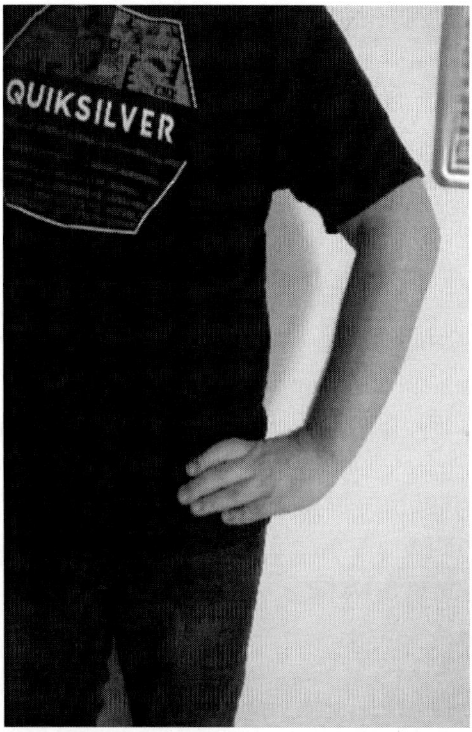


Figure 2. C sign.

The rolling test refers to the patient's discomfort in the hip while lying on the examination table in the supine position during inward and outward turning or rolling of the thigh on the hip side, which is considered as a pathology. This maneuver moves the femoral head and joint capsule, and pathologies in other anatomical structures are not aggravated (Byrd et al., 2014).

## PREDISPOSING FACTORS

Torsional abnormalities of the femur, along with the cam- and pincer-type pathologies, are one of the three factors that are considered to affect the development of FAI (Rienmüller et al., 2017). There are different combinations of torsional changes with cam- and/or pincer-type FAI (Tibor et al., 2013). Advanced torsional abnormalities were detected in only 17% of patients admitted to the outpatient clinic with hip pain (Sutter et al., 2017). Since abnormalities can also be observed in femoral torsion measurements in different hip pathologies, measurements should be performed in all patients with hip complaints (Sutter et al., 2017).

Malunions observed after fracture are among the most common causes of FAI-related hip pain, which results in a cam-type deformity and is observed in the adult age group (Morris et al., 2018).

Some hip pathologies that can be observed in childhood may also be effective in the development of FAI. LCPD (Legg-Calve-Perthes-Disease) may coexist with a cam-type deformity and result in osteoarthritis manifested by hip pain (Morris et al., 2018, Accadbled et al., 2014). SCFE (slipped capital femoral epiphysis) is defined as the posterior and inferior displacement of the femoral head after the separation between the epiphysis of the femoral head and the neck. Acam-type deformity is frequently observed after SCFE (Morris et al., 2018).

The relationship between the development of FAI and professional sports is quite high. Athletes between the ages of 12 and 21 were included in a study of 300 athletes and 290 non-athlete control groups with athletes being highly engaged in sports branches such as basketball, football, ice hockey, and football. The prevalence of cam-type lesions was found to be 2 to 8 times higher in athletes. While the prevalence of a cam-type deformity was 41% in male athletes, this ratio was 17% when the control group was examined (Nepple et al., 2015).

A high activity level during growth plate closure is an important factor in the development of a cam-type deformity. In a prospective study in which 63 football players were followed for at least 2 years, the development of a cam-type deformity gradually increased until the growth plate was closed. The development of a cam-type deformity was observed in individuals with normal hips during the period between the age of 12 and the end of growth. On the other hand, there was no significant increase in the prevalence of a cam-type deformity after the growth plate was closed (Agricola et al., 2014).

In the development of FAI, performing an activity above the physiologically accepted limits in terms of the range of motion of the joint can be considered as a factor. Classical osseous conditions of FAI due to high performance do not occur in athletes involved in ballet dancing, ice skating, or martial arts. Atypical hip impingement may occur due to a high range of motion of the joint (Duthon et al., 2013, Kang et al., 2009). Although osseous changes are not observed in most people involved in this type of sport, professional ballet dancers have a higher incidence of pincer-type impingement, superolateral defect of the acetabular cartilage, and labral tear compared to asymptomatic ballet dancers (Kolo et al., 2013).

## Radiological Diagnosis

The diagnosis of FAI is not only made radiologically as it is a condition in which dynamic factors play a role. We attempt to make a diagnosis with instant data by obtaining only static imaging in the radiological examination. The clinical picture of FAI can be observed if a person with an anatomically normal hip increases the range of motion of the joint above the physiological limits (Sutter et al., 2017). When we consider the opposite of this situation, the person may have pathology radiologically. However, the clinical picture of FAI may not be observed if he/she does not perform movements that require an excessive range of motion of the joint (Sutter et al., 2017).

**Table 2. Radiological findings according to the types of FAI (Hale et al. 2021)**

| Type | Radiological findings |
|---|---|
| Cam | Typical pistol grip deformity and/or an alpha angle >55° |
| Pincer | Crossover sign and/or a lateral center-edge angle (LCEA) ≥40° and/or a Tönnis angle <0° |
| Mixed | Cam-and pincer-type features |

Diagnosis can be made using direct radiography, CT (computerized tomography), and MRI (magnetic resonance imaging) examinations (Rhee et al., 2017). The findings in Table 2 with these methods are significant in the classification of FAI. While MRI is used to identify pathologies such as chondral lesions and labral lesions, the use of CT comes to the forefront in the detection of osseous pathologies.

# Treatment

## Conservative Treatment

Conservative treatment of FAI includes non-steroidal anti-inflammatory drugs, activity modification, prevention of excessive movement of the hip joint and/or rest, osteopathy and coreopraxy, intra-articular steroid injections, and physical treatment modalities (Wall et al., 2013).

While there are studies with a moderate level of evidence reporting that surgical treatment is not superior to conservative treatment in short-term follow-ups, it is observed that studies have a low level of evidence when this effect is examined in the medium term (Bastos et al., 2021). When the literature is reviewed, there is limited literature indicating that conservative treatment is beneficial for patients. Although there are publications advocating conservative treatment, there is a need for high-quality randomized and controlled studies (Wall et al., 2013).

## Surgical Treatment

Open and arthroscopic surgeries are used in the surgery of FAI. Open methods can also be divided into open and mini-explicit surgery (Matsuda et al., 2011). In terms of its effect on pain and its contribution to short-to-medium-term functions in FAI, all methods of surgery provide benefits in appropriate indications. Performing the open method with trochanteric osteotomy is the cause of major complications compared to the others (Matsuda et al., 2011). In the mini-open method, iatrogenic damage to the lateral femoral cutaneous nerve can be observed (Matsuda et al., 2011).

When arthroscopic surgery was performed by experienced surgeons, it was observed that the complication rates were low and that it had equal or better results compared to other methods (Matsuda et al., 2011). As in all surgical procedures, it is very important to decide on the timing, and the patients who will benefit from arthroscopic surgery. For example, while obesity, female gender, and hip joint degeneration can be considered as factors that negatively affect the surgical outcomes and clinical scores, the age of the patient is not a contraindication for the application of hip arthroscopy (Naal et al., 2017, Lin et al., 2021, Javed et al., 2011, Dick et al., 2020, Gupta et al., 2015).

Preoperative, intraoperative, and postoperative radiological evaluations are important for clinical outcomes. It was demonstrated that intra-articular treatments might be insufficient in mildly and moderately dysplastic hips (Larson et al., 2016). Inadequate surgical correction may be associated with poor clinical outcomes and the need for revision surgery (Domb et al., 2020). In the literature, it was observed that acetabular retroversion might adversely affect the results of FAS surgery, and there was an indication that it would be useful to perform periacetabular osteotomy in this patient group (Vahedi et al., 2019). The clinical outcomes were observed to be worse in patients with Tönnis grade 1 and patients with a range of motion of the joint narrower than 2 mm (Domb et al., 2015).

Although complication rates are reported to be lower compared to open surgeries, severe complications may also be encountered in arthroscopic surgery. Neurological complications such as pudendal nerve injury and lateral femoral cutaneous nerve injury due to traction use, and complications such as chondral and labral injuries, perineal skin injuries, deep vein thrombosis, heterotopic ossification, hip dislocation, hypothermia, and extra-articular fluid extravasation may be encountered in arthroscopic surgery (Weber et al., 2015).

The cost of a doctor's examination, medical treatment, diagnosis of the disease, and conservative treatment in FAI was indicated to be 2,456.97 dollars per patient (Kahlenberg et al., 2014). The cost increases to 21,700 dollars in patients who undergo surgical treatment with hip arthroscopy (Shearer et al., 2012). When these data are considered, we can see the economic importance of the early diagnosis and treatment of FAI.

## CONCLUSION

FAI is a hip pathology that is mostly observed in the young to middle-aged group and athletes and one of the predisposing factors for osteoarthritis. Primary and secondary causes are effective in the etiology of FAI. Hip pain and groin pain are common clinical findings. It is diagnosed by using clinical and radiological methods together. Conservative and surgical methods are used in its treatment. Surgical methods are divided into open and arthroscopic methods.

## REFERENCES

Accadbled, F., Pailhé, R., Launay, F., Nectoux, E., Bonin, N., & Gicquel, P. (2014). "Femoroacetabular impingement." Legg-Calve-Perthes disease: From childhood to adulthood. *Orthopaedics & Traumatology: Surgery & Research*, 100(6), 647-649.

Agricola, R., Heijboer, M. P., Ginai, A. Z., Roels, P., Zadpoor, A. A., Verhaar, J. A., & Waarsing, J. H. (2014). A cam deformity is gradually acquired during skeletal maturation in adolescent and young male soccer players: a prospective study with minimum 2-year follow-up. *The American Journal of Sports Medicine*, 42(4), 798-806.

Bastos, R. M., de Carvalho Júnior, J. G., da Silva, S. A. M., Campos, S. F., Rosa, M. V., & de Moraes Prianti, B. (2021). Surgery is no more effective than conservative treatment for Femoroacetabular impingement syndrome: Systematic review and meta-analysis of randomized controlled trials. *Clinical Rehabilitation*, 35(3), 332-341.

Bowler, D. J., & Flandry, F. (2012). Prevalence of femoroacetabular impingement in younger patients undergoing total hip arthroplasty. *Journal of Surgical Orthopaedic Advances*, 21(3), 122-125.

Brunner, R., Maffiuletti, N. A., Casartelli, N. C., Bizzini, M., Sutter, R., Pfirrmann, C. W., & Leunig, M. (2016). Prevalence and functional consequences of femoroacetabular impingement in young male ice hockey players. *The American Journal of Sports Medicine*, 44(1), 46-53.

Byrd, J. T. (2014). Femoroacetabular impingement in athletes: current concepts. *The American Journal of Sports Medicine*, 42(3), 737-751.

Clohisy, J. C., Knaus, E. R., Hunt, D. M., Lesher, J. M., Harris-Hayes, M., & Prather, H. (2009). Clinical presentation of patients with symptomatic anterior hip impingement. *Clinical Orthopaedics and Related Research*, 467(3), 638-644.

Dick, A. G., Smith, C., Bankes, M. J., & George, M. (2020). The impact of mental health disorders on outcomes following hip arthroscopy for femoroacetabular impingement syndrome: a systematic review. *Journal of Hip Preservation Surgery*, 7(2), 195-204.

Diesel, C. V., Ribeiro, T. A., Scheidt, R. B., de Souza Macedo, C. A., & Galia, C. R. (2015). The prevalence of femoroacetabular impingement in radiographs of asymptomatic subjects: a cross-sectional study. *Hip International*, 25(3), 258-263.

Domb, B. G., Annin, S., Chen, J. W., Kyin, C., Rosinsky, P. J., Maldonado, D. R., & Shapira, J. (2020). Optimal treatment of cam morphology may change the natural history of femoroacetabular impingement. *The American Journal of Sports Medicine*, 48(12), 2887-2896.

Domb, B. G., Gui, C., & Lodhia, P. (2015). How much arthritis is too much for hip arthroscopy: a systematic review. *Arthroscopy: The Journal of Arthroscopic & Related Surgery*, 31(3), 520-529.

Duthon, V. B., Charbonnier, C., Kolo, F. C., Magnenat-Thalmann, N., Becker, C. D., Bouvet, C., & Menetrey, J. (2013). Correlation of clinical and magnetic resonance imaging findings in hips of elite female ballet dancers. *Arthroscopy: The Journal of Arthroscopic & Related Surgery*, 29(3), 411-419.

Ganz, R., Gill, T. J., Gautier, E., Ganz, K., Krügel, N., & Berlemann, U. (2001). Surgical dislocation of the adult hip: a technique with full access to the femoral head and acetabulum without the risk of avascular necrosis. *The Journal of Bone and Joint Surgery. British volume*, 83(8), 1119-1124.

Gupta, A., Redmond, J. M., Hammarstedt, J. E., Lindner, D., Stake, C. E., & Domb, B. G. (2015). Does Obesity Affect Outcomes After Hip Arthroscopy?: A Cohort Analysis. *JBJS*, 97(1), 16-23.

Hale, R. F., Melugin, H. P., Zhou, J., La Prade, M. D., Bernard, C., Leland, D., & Krych, A. J. (2021). Incidence of Femoroacetabular Impingement and Surgical Management Trends over Time. *The American Journal of Sports Medicine*, 49(1), 35-41.

Hoit, G., Whelan, D. B., Dwyer, T., Ajrawat, P., & Chahal, J. (2020). Physiotherapy as an initial treatment option for femoroacetabular impingement: a systematic review of the literature and meta-analysis of 5 randomized controlled trials. *The American Journal of Sports Medicine*, 48(8), 2042-2050.

Javed, A., & O'Donnell, J. M. (2011). Arthroscopic femoral osteochondroplasty for cam femoroacetabular impingement in patients over 60 years of age. *The Journal of Bone and Joint Surgery. British volume*, 93(3), 326-331.

Kahlenberg, C. A., Han, B., Patel, R. M., Deshmane, P. P., & Terry, M. A. (2014). Time and cost of diagnosis for symptomatic femoroacetabular impingement. *Orthopaedic Journal of Sports Medicine*, 2(3), 2325967114523916.

Kang, C., Hwang, D. S., & Cha, S. M. (2009). Acetabular labral tears in patients with sports injury. *Clinics in Orthopedic Surgery*, 1(4), 230-235.

Kolo, F. C., Charbonnier, C., Pfirrmann, C. W., Duc, S. R., Lubbeke, A., Duthon, V. B., & Becker, C. D. (2013). Extreme hip motion in professional ballet dancers: dynamic and morphological evaluation based on magnetic resonance imaging. *Skeletal Radiology*, 42(5), 689-698.

Larson, C. M., Ross, J. R., Stone, R. M., Samuelson, K. M., Schelling, E. F., Giveans, M. R., & Bedi, A. (2016). Arthroscopic management of dysplastic hip deformities: predictors of success and failures with comparison to an arthroscopic FAI cohort. *The American Journal of Sports Medicine*, 44(2), 447-453.

Lin, L. J., Akpinar, B., Bloom, D. A., & Youm, T. (2021). Age and outcomes in hip arthroscopy for femoroacetabular impingement: a comparison across 3 age groups. *The American Journal of Sports Medicine*, 49(1), 82-89.

Mallets, E., Turner, A., Durbin, J., Bader, A., & Murray, L. (2019). Short-term outcomes of conservative treatment for femoroacetabular impingement: a systematic review and meta-analysis. *International Journal of Sports Physical Therapy*, 14(4), 514.

Marom, N., Dooley, M. S., Burger, J. A., Chang, B., Coleman, S. H., Ranawat, A. S., & Nawabi, D. H. (2020). Characteristics of Soccer Players Undergoing Primary Hip Arthroscopy for Femoroacetabular Impingement: A Sex-and Competitive Level-Specific Analysis. *The American Journal of Sports Medicine*, 48(13), 3255-3264.

Matsuda, D. K., Carlisle, J. C., Arthurs, S. C., Wierks, C. H., & Philippon, M. J. (2011). Comparative systematic review of the open dislocation, mini-open, and arthroscopic surgeries for femoroacetabular impingement. *Arthroscopy: The Journal of Arthroscopic & Related Surgery*, 27(2), 252-269.

Morris, W. Z., Li, R. T., Liu, R. W., Salata, M. J., & Voos, J. E. (2018). Origin of cam morphology in femoroacetabular impingement. *The American Journal of Sports Medicine*, 46(2), 478-486.

Naal, F. D., Müller, A., Varghese, V. D., Wellauer, V., Impellizzeri, F. M., & Leunig, M. (2017). Outcome of hip impingement surgery: does generalized joint hypermobility matter?. *The American Journal of Sports Medicine*, 45(6), 1309-1314.

Nakashima, H., Tsukamoto, M., Ohnishi, Y., Utsunomiya, H., Kanezaki, S., Sakai, A., & Uchida, S. (2019). Clinical and radiographic predictors for unsalvageable labral tear at the time of initial hip arthroscopic management for femoroacetabular impingement. *The American Journal of Sports Medicine*, 47(9), 2029-2037.

Nepple, J. J., Vigdorchik, J. M., & Clohisy, J. C. (2015). What is the association between sports participation and the development of proximal femoral cam deformity? A systematic review and meta-analysis. *The American Journal of Sports Medicine*, 43(11), 2833-2840.

Pfirrmann, C. W., Mengiardi, B., Dora, C., Kalberer, F., Zanetti, M., Hodler, J. Cam and pincer femoroacetabular impingement: characteristic MR arthrographic findings in 50 patients. *Radiology* 2006;240 (03):778-785.

Philippon, M. J., Maxwell, R. B., Johnston, T. L., Schenker, M., & Briggs, K. K. (2007). Clinical presentation of femoroacetabular impingement. *Knee Surgery, Sports Traumatology, Arthroscopy*, 15(8), 1041-1047.

Rhee, C., Le Francois, T., Byrd, J. T., Glazebrook, M., & Wong, I. (2017). Radiographic diagnosis of pincer-type femoroacetabular impingement: a systematic review. *Orthopaedic Journal of Sports Medicine*, 5(5), 2325967117708307.

Rienmüller, T. M., Makarenko, V. N., Bockeria, O. L., Rychina, I. E., Bereznitsky, V., Baumgartner, C., & Rienmüller, R. (2017, February). A multiple regression analysis of determinants of myocardial perfusion as measured by CT. In: *ECR 2017*.

Ross, J. R., Larson, C. M., Adeoyo, O., Kelly, B. T., & Bedi, A. (2015). Residual deformity is the most common reason for revision hip arthroscopy: a three-dimensional CT study. *Clinical Orthopaedics and Related Research®*, 473(4), 1388-1395.

Shearer, D. W., Kramer, J., Bozic, K. J., & Feeley, B. T. (2012). Is hip arthroscopy cost-effective for femoroacetabular impingement?. *Clinical Orthopaedics and Related Research®*, 470(4), 1079-1089.

Sutter, R., & Pfirrmann, C. W. (2017, November). Update on femoroacetabular impingement: what is new, and how should we assess it?. In: *Seminars in Musculoskeletal Radiology* (Vol. 21, No. 05, pp. 518-528). Thieme Medical Publishers.

Tannast, M., Siebenrock, K. A., & Anderson, S. E. (2007). Femoroacetabular impingement: radiographic diagnosis - what the radiologist should know. *American Journal of Roentgenology*, 188(6), 1540-1552.

Tibor, L. M., Liebert, G., Sutter, R., Impellizzeri, F. M., & Leunig, M. (2013). Two or more impingement and/or instability deformities are often present in patients with hip pain. *Clinical Orthopaedics and Related Research®*, 471(12), 3762-3773.

Vahedi, H., Aalirezaie, A., Schlitt, P. K., & Parvizi, J. (2019). Acetabular retroversion is a risk factor for less optimal outcome after femoroacetabular impingement surgery. *The Journal of Arthroplasty*, 34(7), 1342-1346.

Wall, P. D., Fernandez, M., Griffin, D. R., & Foster, N. E. (2013). Nonoperative treatment for femoroacetabular impingement: a systematic review of the literature. *PM&R*, 5(5), 418-426.

Weber, A. E., Harris, J. D., & Nho, S. J. (2015). Complications in hip arthroscopy: a systematic review and strategies for prevention. *Sports Medicine and Arthroscopy Review*, 23(4), 187-193.

Zhou, J., Melugin, H. P., Hale, R. F., Leland, D. P., Bernard, C. D., Levy, B. A., & Krych, A. J. (2020). The prevalence of radiographic findings of structural hip deformities for femoroacetabular impingement in patients with hip pain. *The American Journal of Sports Medicine*, 48(3), 647-653.

In: Musculoskeletal Pain (Common Clinical Presentations) ISBN: 978-1-68507-410-4
Editors: Mehmet Cenk Turgut and Serdar Toy 

*Chapter 8*

# PIRIFORMIS SYNDROME

***Cengiz Kazdal**, *MD***
Department of Orthopedics and Traumatology,
Ağrı Training and Research Hospital, Ağrı, Turkey

## ABSTRACT

Although there is no consensus on the diagnosis of piriformis syndrome, it can generally be defined as sciatic nerve compression by the piriformis muscle. Even though there is no specific maneuver for the diagnosis of piriformis syndrome, physical examination might be helpful in diagnostics. Apart from that, electrodiagnostic tests and alternative radiological imaging techniques can be utilized to diagnose piriformis syndrome. In terms of treatment, while conservative approaches are primary choices, alternative surgical methods can be utilized for patients who are unresponsive to conservative treatment and patients with persistent complaints.

## INTRODUCTION

Piriformis syndrome (PS) is described as sciatic nerve compression by the piriformis muscle. 6%-8% of all sciatic pains are caused by piriformis syndrome (Hallin, R.P., 1983). It was first defined in 1928, and the term piriformis syndrome was first used in 1947 (Probst et al., 2019). The general population's lifetime prevalence of sciatic pain is 12-27%, with an annual prevalence of 2.2%-19.5% (Konstantinou et al., 2008). While defining piriformis syndrome, confusion continues during the diagnosis in the literature and daily practice. Incomplete or misdiagnosis can often be made for more common

* Corresponding Author's E-mail: zzengizz@gmail.com.

conditions like facet joint arthropathy, lumbar disc pathologies, sacroiliitis, and radiculopathy (Kirkaldy-Willis, W.H. and Hill, R.J., 1979).

On the other hand, in the isolated pathology of the region, disagreements continue among clinicians about whether piriformis syndrome is caused by muscle hypertrophy or myofascial pain, or sciatic nerve compression by the piriformis muscle (Kirschner et al., 2009). The definition of deep gluteal syndrome is also used as an alternative for piriformis syndrome because of the etiologically different anatomical variations seen in the pathology of piriformis syndrome and the potential anatomical regions where the sciatic nerve is under pressure (Probst et al., 2019). Ultrasonography (US), electromyography (EMG), computed tomography (CT), and magnetic resonance imaging (MRI) can be used in the piriformis syndrome diagnosis (Kirschner et al., 2009). Medical treatment, stretching exercises, local anesthetic and corticosteroid injections, ESWT (extracorporeal shock wave therapy), and botulinum injection can be used in conservative treatment. In surgical treatment, the release of the piriformis muscle and sciatic neurolysis can be applied (Han et al., 2017).

## Anatomy

The piriformis muscle is a flat, pear-shaped muscle (Kirschner et al., 2009). It originates from the sacrum and sacrotuberous ligament, proceeds laterally into the greater sciatic foramen, and terminates on the superior-internal part of the greater trochanter (Jenkins, D.B., 2009). The muscle performs external rotation when the hip joint is in extension and abduction when the hip is in flexion. Its innervation is from the posterior ventral rami of S1-S2 (Probst et al., 2019).

Beaton and Anson's study on 240 cadavers described six different anatomical variations of the sciatic nerve and piriformis muscle. 90% of the cadavers had a piriformis-sciatic relationship defined as normal. Other variations were defined as the sciatic nerve, passing over, under, and through the piriformis muscle in orientation, and being single or bipartite in integrity. In the systematic review, including 6602 cadavers, the variation rate was stated as 16.9% (Beaton, L.A. & Anson, B.J., 1938). In an MR study, an aberrant relationship was defined between the piriformis muscle and the sciatic nerve in 19.2% of 783 hips, supporting these studies (Martin et al., 2014). The opinion that "the observed variations do not affect the frequency of piriformis syndrome" was shared (Probst et al., 2019).

Studies on the piriformis muscle itself are also available in the literature. In a study of 112 cadavers, the width of the piriformis tendon was measured between 3 mm and 9 mm. The insertion point was in the traditional region in 53.6% of the cases; in 29.5% of cases, the piriformis tendon joined the gemellus superior and merged with the internal obturator tendon to insert into the trochanter major. In 13.4% cases, the piriformis tendon merged with the gluteus medius and the obturator internus and inserted into the medial of the trochanter major. In the remaining 3.6% of cases, the piriformis tendon fused with the gluteus medius fibers and terminated in the trochanter major. In joining with the obturator internus muscle, the piriformis muscle may cause impingement in the sciatic nerve when the hip is in internal rotation, or its contraction may result in hip pain in the case of the obturator internus thickening or stiffening (Windisch et al., 2007). In 6 patients examined intraoperatively, the Laseque test was performed with the suspicion of piriformis syndrome, and the structure causing impingement was not the piriformis muscle but the obturator internus muscle (Meknas et al., 2003). In a patient with piriformis syndrome, injected into the piriformis muscle, complaints were partially healed after the injection. However, the complaints of the same patient were completely regressed after injection into the obturator internus muscle. This situation indicates that the obturator internus muscle also contributes to the pathology (Dalmau-Carola, J., 2005).

## Clinical Findings

Although there is no specific maneuver for the diagnosis of piriformis syndrome, physical examination helps us diagnose and exclude different diagnoses. In suspected piriformis syndrome, the lumbar region, pelvis, hip, and lower extremities should be carefully evaluated.

Robinson listed six criteria for the diagnosis of piriformis syndrome in his study in 1947. These include a trauma history to the sacroiliac-gluteal region, difficulty in walking due to changes in gait and the piriformis muscle length, pain in the sacroiliac joint and the greater sciatic notch, acute worsening when lifting something from the ground, and relief by pulling on the affected leg, the palpable piriformis muscle, a positive Laseque sign and finally, gluteal muscle atrophy depending on the complaint duration (Robinson, D.R., 1947).

Freiberg suggested three criteria in his study for the definition of piriformis muscle-based sciatic pain. These include tenderness on palpation of the sciatic notch, a positive Laseque sign, and improvement with conservative treatment. However, it is seen that Frieberg's criteria are quite superficial, while Robinson's criteria are quite specific and do not cover all types of piriformis syndrome (Freiberg, A.H., 1937).

Piriformis syndrome patients often present with hip pain, pain in the buttocks, dyspareunia in women, and sciatic pain (Halpin, R.J. & Ganju, A., 2009). The pain increases with sitting for a long time, driving a car, and standing up from a sitting position (Windisch et al., 2007).

In the case of weakness and loss of sensation, a diagnosis of piriformis syndrome should be avoided, except in long-term chronic cases. On physical examination, tenderness in the greater sciatic notch corresponding to the body of the piriformis muscle gives us a clue (Kirschner et al., 2009). In Durrani's study, 92% positivity was reported with tenderness at this point (Durrani, Z. & Winnie, A.P., 1991). Tenderness with palpation on the outer surface of the greater sciatic notch is one of the most common examination findings of piriformis syndrome (Probst et al., 2019). Another method of palpation is the pelvic or rectal evaluation of the deep lateral extension of the muscle. There may be a trigger point in the sciatic axis above the piriformis muscle, or a mass may be palpated, and gluteal atrophy and a positive Laseque sign may be seen (Robinson, D.R., 1997). However, the relatively small and deep structure of the piriformis muscle raises questions in terms of palpability (Windisch et al., 2007).

Several maneuvers have been described to aid the diagnosis of piriformis syndrome. The general purpose of the tests is to assess the pressure on the sciatic nerve by passive stretching of the piriformis muscle.

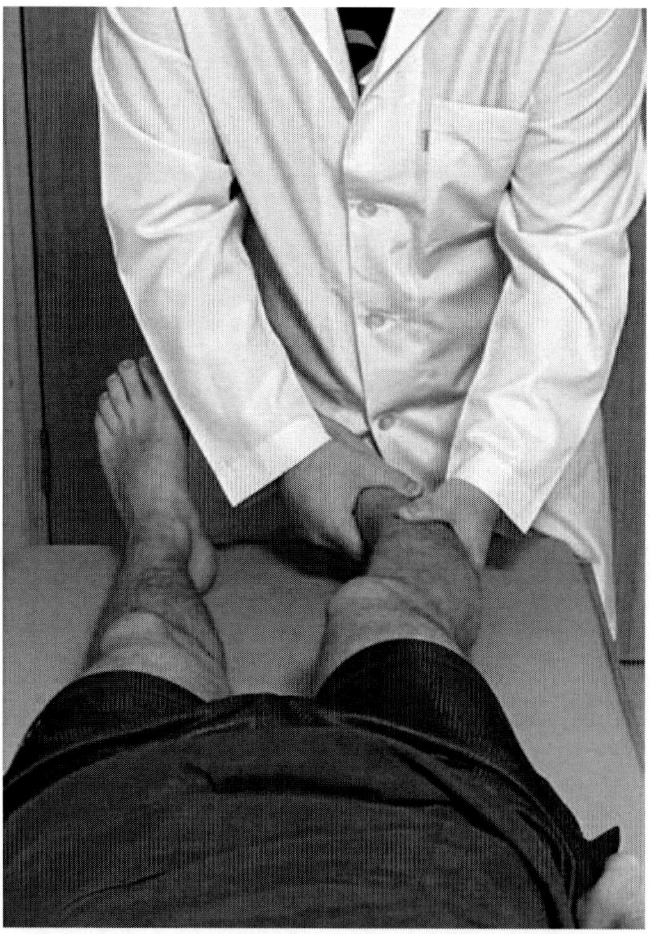

Figure 1. Sciatic nerve compression by irritating the piriformis muscle with the Freiberg maneuver (author's own archive).

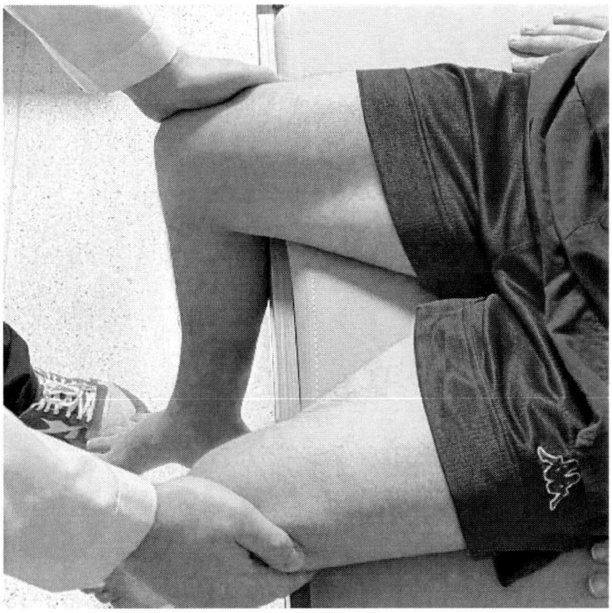

Figure 2. Inducing pain by resisting hip abduction with the Pace maneuver (author's own archive).

The Freiberg maneuver aims to aggravate sciatic nerve compression by irritating the patient's piriformis muscle with the performance of forced internal rotation of the affected leg while the patient is in the supine or lateral decubitus position (Figure 1) (Beatty, R.A., 1994). A study of 130 cadavers revealed that passive hip internal rotation compresses the piriformis while external rotation relaxes it. In addition, electrophysiological studies have shown that the adduction, flexion, and internal rotation position of the hip creates maximal compression in the sciatic nerve (Pec'ina, M., 1979).

The pace maneuver aims to aggravate pain by resisting hip abduction while the patient is in a sitting position. This movement stretches the piriformis muscle (Figure 2) (Pace, J.B. & Nagle, D., 1976).

The Beatty test is performed with the patient lying on the unaffected side in the lateral decubitus position (Figure 3). An increase in hip pain is seen with thigh abduction. In the case of lumbar disc pathology, low back and leg pain are observed during this maneuver (Beatty, R.A., 1994).

The active piriformis test is performed while the patient is lying in the lateral decubitus position. The examiner resists the patient's hip abduction and external rotation movements. The sensitivity and specificity of the test are 0.78 and 0.80, respectively (Figure 4) (Martin et al., 2014).

In the FAIR test, the patient is laid in the supine position with the affected hip on top. The hip is fixed by passively placing the lower extremity in a 90-degree flexion, adduction, and internal rotation. A positive test occurs with the pain and paresthesia in the sciatic region when internal rotation and adduction are forced by pressing the knee (Figure 5).

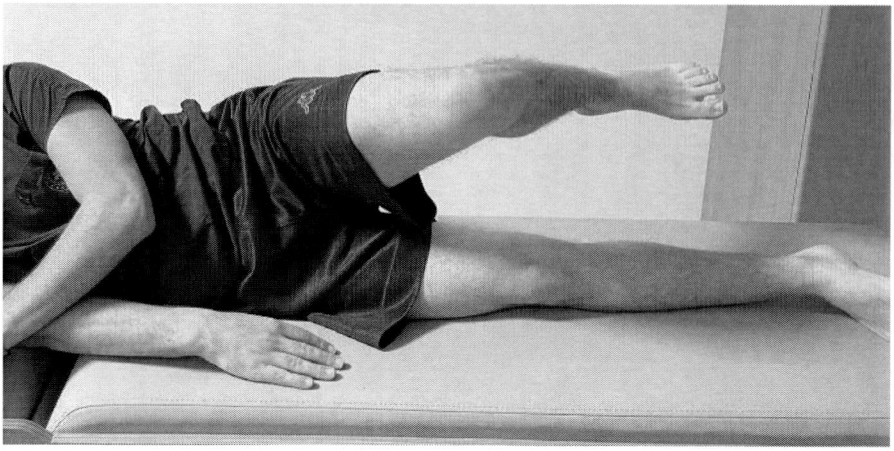

Figure 3. Beatty Test (author's own archive).

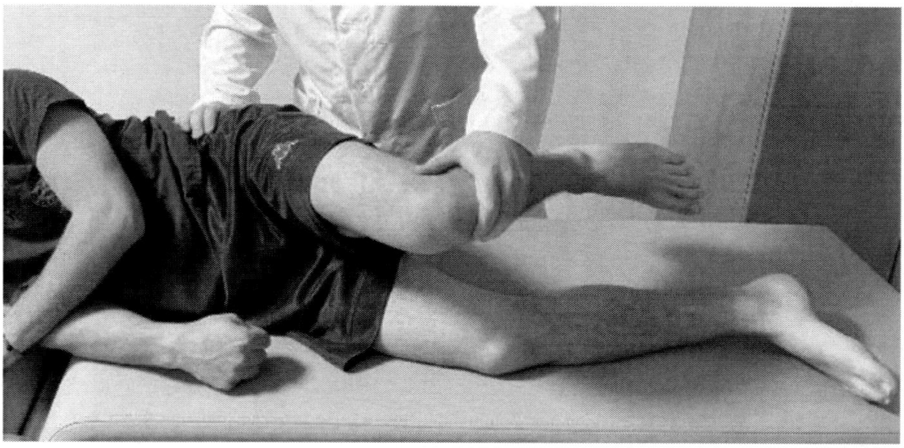

Figure 4. Active piriformis test (author's own archive).

In the seated piriformis stretch test, the patient sits on the examination table, with the hip flexed to 90 degrees and the knee in the extended position. The examiner internally rotates and adducts the hip while palpating the greater sciatic notch. The sensitivity and specificity of the test are 0.53 and 0.90, respectively (Martin et al., 2014).

In the Laseque test, the knee and hip are flexed to 90 degrees while the patient is lying on his back. Then, a positive test occurs with the pain due to sciatic nerve compression by the piriformis during the slow extension of the knee joint (Martin et al., 2014). The sensitivity and specificity of the Laseque test are 0.15 and 0.95, respectively. With the combined application of the seated piriformis stretch test and the active piriformis test, sensitivity and specificity increase to 0.91 and 0.80, respectively (an endoscopic sign of sciatic nerve compression) (Martin et al., 2015).

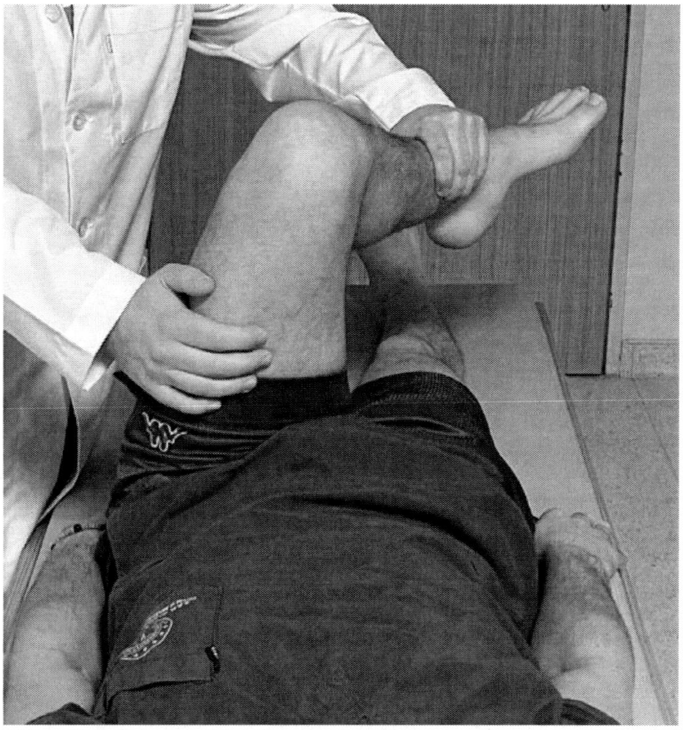

Figure 5. FAIR test (author's own archive).

## Electrodiagnostic Studies

Electrodiagnostic test results are usually normal in piriformis syndrome but may be helpful to exclude lumbosacral pathologies (Probst et al., 2019). Nerve conduction studies in piriformis syndrome are usually regular. Occasionally, slowing conduction velocity and a decrease in sensory nerve action potentials and combined motor action potentials can be observed. The amount of slowing in the conduction rate is directly proportional to the duration of the symptoms (Chang et al., 2006).

In a study of 1,014 legs of 918 patients, a delay in the H reflex was observed in the FAIR position. The method's sensitivity is 0.88 and the specificity is 0.83, considering the piriformis syndrome diagnostic criteria (Fishman et al., 2002).

Needle EMG results are usually normal in piriformis syndrome. Depending on long-term nerve compression, denervations can be observed in the muscles innervated by the nerve. EMG can distinguish lumbosacral radiculopathies from peripheral nerve lesions (Probst et al., 2019).

## RADIOLOGICAL IMAGING

Computed tomography can be used to exclude causes such as tumor, hematoma, and abscess causing sciatic nerve compression. However, despite the benefits of tomography, MRI is the recommended imaging modality for diagnosing piriformis syndrome (Miller et al., 2012).

MRI provides us with important advantages in determining the cause of spinal stenosis and radiculopathy-based gluteal region pain, with good imaging of the spinal canal and good detection of the vertebra and spinal canal pathologies. It is also advantageous in imaging anatomical abnormalities, effective in the piriformis syndrome etiology (Lee et al., 2004).

By evaluating the piriformis muscle comparatively, changes in the piriformis muscle dimension can be observed. Although 19% of the patients were asymptomatic in a study, piriformis muscle hypertrophy was observed. Therefore, the piriformis muscle hypertrophy is not pathognomonic (Probst et al., 2019).

MR neurography allows imaging of the tissues around the nerve. MR neurography was performed in 14 patients with unexplained sciatic pain, and an increased signal was observed in the STIR sequence of 12 patients (Lewis et al., 2006). Conversely, an abnormal signal was detected at the level of the piriformis muscle and sciatic notch in 8 out of 12 patients. In a study of 239 individuals, MR neurography was performed on patients having pain in the sciatic nerve distribution region and failed back surgery. In 94% of patients, edema or hyperintensity of the sciatic nerve on the painful side was seen, and symptoms increased at the FAIR position in 88% (Filler et al., 2005).

In evaluating the diagnostic efficiency of MR neurography, piriformis muscle asymmetry at the level of the sciatic notch and sciatic nerve hyperintensity were assessed. It has 93% sensitivity and 64% specificity in differentiating piriformis syndrome patients from patients without similar symptoms. Furthermore, the literature has stated that the evaluation of the treatment's effectiveness can also be observed with MR (Filler et al., 2005).

Ultrasound is effective in observing myofascial trigger points in the resting piriformis muscle. Thus, ultrasound is helpful in the evaluation of sciatic nerve sections, but additional tests are needed for diagnosis in a suspected piriformis syndrome with ultrasound evaluation (Probst et al., 2019).

# TREATMENT

## Conservative Treatment

In the piriformis syndrome diagnosis, a conservative-multidisciplinary approach is primarily preferred as a treatment modality. Muscle relaxants, non-steroidal anti-inflammatory drugs, and neuropathic molecules such as pregabalin and gabapentin can be used in medical treatment. In addition, physical therapy has an important place in piriformis syndrome treatment (Miller et al., 2012).

The length and tension of the piriformis muscle determined by the physical therapy physician are valuable in guiding the treatment. The most common finding is the shortening of the piriformis muscle. A shortening in muscle length may be accompanied by taut bands or myofascial trigger points. These conditions create tension in the muscle, cause the hip to go into external rotation, and shorten the hip external rotator muscles. In some patients, the hip is in the internal rotation due to excessive tension in the piriformis muscle, regardless of the pathologies causing tension in the muscle. Bands creating tension in the piriformis muscle can be detected by palpation, and different treatment methods can be applied, including the injection of anesthetic to the trigger point, dry needling, acupuncture, and manual massage. In addition, heat and muscle stimulation may also be used in treatment. Physical therapy aims to restore healthy muscle length and tries to release the muscle (Probst et al., 2019).

The treatment should also focus on biomechanical stabilization by strengthening the spine, pelvis, and hip joint. In the patient group with shortened external rotators, the treatment should not be focused on the shortening of the piriformis muscle alone. The femoral head and the acetabulum relationship should also be carefully evaluated. Relative repetitive anterior displacement of the femoral head beside the acetabulum and a persistence of this condition result in stiffness in the posterior capsule. This situation may cause pain in the distal legs of patients (Butler, D., 1991).

In a study conducted with 250 patients with piriformis syndrome, the symptoms were observed to be regressed by 51.2% with medical treatment and physical therapy (Michel et al., 2013). In a study of 665 patients, simultaneous injection of triamcinolone acetonide into the piriformis muscle with physical therapy ensured at least 50% relief of complaints in 79% of patients. This study should be carefully evaluated regarding the lack of a control group and supporting intramuscular steroid injections (Fishman et al., 2002).

## Injections

Injections can be used for both the diagnosis and treatment of piriformis syndrome. The injections can be applied without imaging methods or performed with EMG, fluoroscopy, ultrasound, MRI, or CT guidance (Halpin, R.J. & Ganju, A., 2009).

The methods used by the practitioner may have advantages over each other. For example, a 30% success rate was achieved in the anatomical markers and fluoroscopy-guided injections, while this increased to 95% in the ultrasound-guided injections (Finnoff et al., 2008).

In a study of 162 piriformis syndrome patients, injections into the piriformis muscle were performed under MRI guidance. Complete recovery was achieved in 15% of the patients without recurrence and 8%, with an additional injection after a recovery period of 2-4 months. However, in 37% of the patients, recurrence was observed after 2-4 months, and in less than two weeks in 24%; no improvement was observed despite the injection in 16% of the patients (Filler et al., 2005).

A reduction in pain scores has been observed in piriformis syndrome with the intramuscular injection of steroids and a combination of steroids and local anesthetics. In a randomized, double-blind study of 57 patients, patients had a positive FAIR test, unilateral hip pain, and piriformis muscle tenderness. Lidocaine or a betamethasone-lidocaine combination was applied to the piriformis muscle under USG guidance. A significant reduction in pain was observed in both injection-administered groups. There was no statistical difference between the two groups in pain scores. Due to the similar level of improvement in pain scores and considering the side effects of steroids, the authors only recommended local anesthetic application and, in limited cases, steroid application (Misirlioglu et al., 2015).

There are also studies in the literature on pain relief after Botox application in piriformis syndrome. With MRI, a decrease in muscle thickness and volume was observed following Botox injection into the piriformis muscle. In the light of this information, it can be said that Botox application is effective in piriformis syndrome treatment (Al-Al-Shaikh et al., 2015).

In a double-blind, randomized, controlled study, Botox injection effectively reduced pain more than the steroid-lidocaine combination. In addition, the combination of Botox injection and physical therapy resulted in more than a 50% improvement in pain scores in 24 out of 27 patients, and their VAS scores declined from 6.7 to 2.3 (Fishman et al., 2004).

In a study of 122 patients with piriformis syndrome whose complaints did not regress at the desired level with physical therapy and medical treatment, good to very good improvement in pain scores was observed in 77% of the patients with Botox injection (Michel et al., 2013).

## Surgical Interventions

Conservative treatment is the primary choice in the treatment of piriformis syndrome. However, in patients whose complaints do not regress with conservative treatment, surgical treatment should be applied. The main aim of surgical treatment is to relieve compression of the sciatic nerve by relaxing the piriformis muscle (Cass, S.P., 2015). There are two main surgical methods, open and endoscopic.

Among the previous studies, Frieberg's study of 12 patients resulted in failed surgery in 3 patients (Freiberg, A.H., 1937), while satisfactory surgical results were reported in Mizuguchi's study of 14 patients in 1976 (Mizuguchi, 1976).

Filler et al. performed surgery on 64 patients with piriformis syndrome, and 82% of patients benefited from surgery in the short-term follow-up. This rate was reported as 76% in the long-term follow-ups (Filer et al., 2005). Han et al. performed surgery on 12 patients with a mean age of 61 (45-71), and the VAS scores of 83% of the patients showed a significant improvement to the preoperative period (Han et al., 2017). In a case series of 19 patients, tenotomy was performed on all patients, and recovery was observed in 8 patients during an average follow-up of 8 (1-16) years. In addition, complaints improved in two-thirds of the patients compared to the baseline (Indrekvam, 2002).

The endoscopic method has significant advantages over open surgery. In endoscopic surgery, there is less postoperative pain, it has aesthetic advantages due to the smaller incisions used, the postoperative recovery time is short, and the surgical field can be seen as wider with appropriate maneuvers (Dezawa et al., 2003). On the other hand, the requirement of surgical experience, difficulty in bleeding control in a large area, and the risk of pressure on the sciatic nerve from possible post-surgical bleeding are among its disadvantages (Knudsen et al., 2016).

In the study of 15 patients who underwent piriformis release by endoscopic surgery, the patients were followed up for at least two years after surgery. The Harris hip score (HHS) of the patients with a mean age of 40.2 increased from 46.8 to 84.9, and the visual analog scale (VAS) score decreased from 7.4 to 1.86. Benson's score was excellent in 11 patients, good in 3 patients and reasonable in 1 patient (Illizaliturri et al., 2018). In the study of 60 patients who underwent endoscopic surgery, a significant improvement was observed in the VAS scores and HHS of the patients. The authors stated that endoscopic sciatic nerve decompression is a safe and effective procedure (Park et al., 2016). In a study of 35 patients with a mean age of 47 years, the endoscopic release was applied to the patients, and the patients' VAS and HHS scores were improved after surgery (Martin et al., 2011).

Due to the lack of large case series in the literature on the surgical treatment of piriformis syndrome, it is currently difficult to reach a clear conclusion about the procedure to be followed. However, the publications on endoscopic surgery in the literature are promising about this method.

## CONCLUSION

Piriformis syndrome is a clinical picture mainly occurring due to compression in an area along the sciatic nerve tracing. Confusion still exists in the clinical diagnosis, and there is no definitive examination method for diagnosis. Imaging methods can be used to diagnose and treat piriformis syndrome. Conservative treatment is the primary option. Open or endoscopic surgical methods may be preferred in the group of patients who do not benefit from conservative treatment and whose complaints persist for a long time.

## REFERENCES

Al-Al-Shaikh, M., Michel, F., Parratte, B., Kastler, B., Vidal, C., & Aubry, S. (2015). An MRI evaluation of changes in piriformis muscle morphology induced by botulinum toxin injections in the treatment of piriformis syndrome. *Diagnostic and interventional imaging*, *96*(1), 37-43.

Bartret, A. L., Beaulieu, C. F., & Lutz, A. M. (2018). Is it painful to be different? Sciatic nerve anatomical variants on MRI and their relationship to piriformis syndrome. *European radiology*, *28*(11), 4681-4686.

Beaton L. A., Anson B. J. The sciatic nerve and the piriformis muscle: their interrelation a possible cause of coccygodynia. *J Bone Joint Surg*. 1938;20(3):686-688.

Beatty R. A. The piriformis muscle syndrome: a simple diagnostic maneuver. *Neurosurgery* 1994;34:512–514.

Butler, D. (1991). Mobilisation of the Nervous System. Edinburgh: Churchill Livingstone. Council J, Ahem D, Follick M and Kline C (1988): Expectancies and functional impairment in chronic low back pain. *Pain*, *33*, 323-333.

Cass, S. P. (2015). Piriformis syndrome: a cause of nondiscogenic sciatica. *Current sports medicine reports*, *14*(1), 41-44.

Chang, C. W., Shieh, S. F., Li, C. M., Wu, W. T., & Chang, K. F. (2006). Measurement of motor nerve conduction velocity of the sciatic nerve in patients with piriformis syndrome: a magnetic stimulation study. *Archives of physical medicine and rehabilitation*, *87*(10), 1371-1375.

Dalmau-Carola J. Myofascial pain syndrome affecting the piriformis and the obturator internus muscle. *Pain Pract*. 2005;5 (4):361-363.

Durrani Z., Winnie A. P. Piriformis muscle syndrome: an underdiagnosed cause of sciatica. *J Pain Symptom Manage*. 1991;6(6): 374-379.

Filler, A. G., Haynes, J., Jordan, S. E., Prager, J., Villablanca, J. P., Farahani, K., ... & Johnson, J. P. (2005). Sciatica of nondisc origin and piriformis syndrome: diagnosis by magnetic resonance neurography and interventional magnetic resonance imaging with outcome study of resulting treatment. *Journal of Neurosurgery: Spine*, *2*(2), 99-115.

Finnoff J. T., Hurdle M. F., Smith J. Accuracy of ultrasound-guided versus fluoroscopically guided contrast-controlled piriformis injections: a cadaveric study. *J Ultrasound Med.* 2008;27(8):1157-1163.

Fishman L. M., Dombi G. W., Michaelsen C., et al. Piriformis syndrome: diagnosis, treatment, and outcome--a 10-year study. *Arch Phys Med Rehabil.* 2002;83(3):295-301.

Fishman L. M., Zybert P. A. Electrophysiologic evidence of piriformis syndrome. *Arch Phys Med Rehabil* 1992;73:359 –364.

Fishman, L. M., Konnoth, C., & Rozner, B. (2004). Botulinum neurotoxin type B and physical therapy in the treatment of piriformis syndrome: a dose-finding study. *American journal of physical medicine & rehabilitation*, *83*(1), 42-50.

Freiberg A. H. Sciatic pain and its relief by operations on muscle and fascia. *Arch Surg.* 1937;34(2):337-350.

Hallin R. P. Sciatic pain and the piriformis muscle. *Postgrad Med.* 1983;74(2):69-72.

Halpin R. J., Ganju A. Piriformis syndrome a real pain in the buttock? *Neurosurgery.* 2009;65(suppl 4):A197-A202.

Han, S. K., Kim, Y. S., Kim, T. H., & Kang, S. H. (2017). Surgical treatment of piriformis syndrome. *Clinics in orthopedic surgery*, *9*(2), 136.

Ilizaliturri Jr, V. M., Arriaga, R., Villalobos, F. E., & Suarez-Ahedo, C. (2018). Endoscopic release of the piriformis tendon and sciatic nerve exploration. *Journal of hip preservation surgery*, *5*(3), 301-306.

Indrekvam, K., & Sudmann, E. (2002). Piriformis muscle syndrome in 19 patients treated by tenotomy–a 1-to 16-year follow-up study. *International orthopaedics*, *26*(2), 101-103.

Jenkins D. B. *Functional Anatomy of the Limbs and Back.* 9th ed. St. Louis, MO: Saunders Elsevier; 2009.

Kirkaldy-Willis W. H., Hill R. J. A more precise diagnosis for low-back pain. *Spine* 1979;4:102–109.

Kirschner, J. S., Foye, P. M., & Cole, J. L. (2009). Piriformis syndrome, diagnosis and treatment. *Muscle & nerve*, *40*(1), 10-18.

Knudsen, J. S., Mei-Dan, O., & Brick, M. J. (2016). Piriformis syndrome and endoscopic sciatic neurolysis. *Sports medicine and arthroscopy review*, *24*(1), e1-e7.

Konstantinou K., Dunn K. M. Sciatica: review of epidemiological studies and prevalence estimates. *Spine.* 2008;33(22):2464-2472.

Lee, E. Y., Margherita, A. J., Gierada, D. S., & Narra, V. R. (2004). MRI of piriformis syndrome. *American Journal of Roentgenology*, *183*(1), 63-64.

Lewis, A. M., Layzer, R., Engstrom, J. W., Barbaro, N. M., & Chin, C. T. (2006). Magnetic resonance neurography in extraspinal sciatica. *Archives of Neurology, 63*(10), 1469-1472.

Martin H. D., Kivlan B. R., Palmer I. J., Martin R. L. Diagnostic accuracy of clinical tests for sciatic nerve entrapment in the gluteal region. *Knee Surg Sports Traumatol Arthrosc.* 2014;22(4):882-888.

Martin H. D., Reddy M., Gómez-Hoyos J. Deep gluteal syndrome. *J Hip Preserv Surg.* 2015;2(2):99-107.

Martin, H. D., Shears, S. A., Johnson, J. C., Smathers, A. M., & Palmer, I. J. (2011). The endoscopic treatment of sciatic nerve entrapment/deep gluteal syndrome. *Arthroscopy: The Journal of Arthroscopic & Related Surgery, 27*(2), 172-181.

Meknas K., Christensen A., Johansen O. The internal obturator muscle may cause sciatic pain. *Pain.* 2003;104(1–2):375-380.

Michel F., Decavel P., Toussirot E., et al. Piriformis muscle syndrome: diagnostic criteria and treatment of a monocentric series of 250 patients. *Ann Phys Rehabil Med.* 2013;56(5):371-383.

Miller, T. A., White, K. P., & Ross, D. C. (2012). The diagnosis and management of Piriformis Syndrome: myths and facts. *Canadian journal of neurological sciences, 39*(5), 577-583.

Misirlioglu T. O., Akgun K., Palamar D., Erden M. G., Erbilir T. Piriformis syndrome: comparison of the effectiveness of local anesthetic and corticosteroid injections: a double-blinded, randomized controlled study. *Pain Physician.* 2015;18(2):163-171.

Mizuguchi, T. (1976). Division of the pyriformis muscle for the treatment of sciatica: postlaminectomy syndrome and osteoarthritis of the spine. *Archives of Surgery, 111*(6), 719-722.

Pace J. B., Nagle D. Piriformis syndrome. *West J Med* 1976;124: 435– 439.

Papadapoulos E. C., Khan S. N. Piriformis syndrome and low back pain: a new classification and review of the literature. *Orthop Clin N Am* 2004;35:65–71.

Park, M. S., Yoon, S. J., Jung, S. Y., & Kim, S. H. (2016). Clinical results of endoscopic sciatic nerve decompression for deep gluteal syndrome: mean 2-year follow-up. *BMC musculoskeletal disorders, 17*(1), 1-7.

Pec'ina M. Contribution to the etiological explanation of the piriformis syndrome. *Acta Anat* 1979;105:181–187.

Probst, D., Stout, A., & Hunt, D. (2019). Piriformis syndrome: a narrative review of the anatomy, diagnosis, and treatment. *PM&R, 11*, S54-S63.

Robinson D. R. Pyriformis syndrome in relation to sciatic pain. *Am J Surg.* 1947;73(3):355-358.

Smoll N. R. Variations of the piriformis and sciatic nerve with clinical consequence: a review. *Clin Anat.* 2010;23(1):8-17.

Windisch G., Braun E. M., Anderhuber F. Piriformis muscle: clinical anatomy and consideration of the piriformis syndrome. *Surg Radiol Anat.* 2007;29(1):37-45.

In: Musculoskeletal Pain (Common Clinical Presentations) ISBN: 978-1-68507-410-4
Editors: Mehmet Cenk Turgut and Serdar Toy 

*Chapter 9*

# Coccydynia

***Halil Sezgin Semis**, MD***
Department of Orthopedics and Traumatology, Private Buhara Hospital, Erzurum, Turkey

## Abstract

Coccydynia is seen in all age groups and both sexes, it is more common in the 40s and five times more common in women than men. Coccydynia describes pain in the coccyx or tailbone. The coccyx is a bone formed by the fusion of 3-5 vertebrae in the distal segment of the vertebral column. The coccyx bone, forming the terminal segment of the vertebral column, has great functional importance as it is the attachment site of many muscles, tendons, and ligaments. Besides, the coccyx bone also serves as positional support to the anus.

A direct fall on the coccyx and repetitive microtraumas are the most common causes of coccydynia, but the etiology could not be determined in 30% of coccydynia patients. The Postacchini-Massobrio classification based on sacrococcygeal angulation is the most commonly used classification system in the coccyx fracture classification. Coccydynia patients have pain in the lumbar region and around the coccyx. The pain becomes evident after sitting for a long time or during getting up from sitting. Besides, pain may also increase during defecation or sexual intercourse.

Conservative treatment is primarily applied, and 90% of the patients respond well to conservative treatment. Surgical treatment can be applied in resistant coccydynia patients who are unresponsive to conservative treatment. Coccygectomy is applied as surgical treatment.

* Corresponding Author's E-mail: sezginsemis@gmail.com.

## INTRODUCTION

The term coccydynia was first suggested by Simpson in the mid-1800s and described pain in the coccyx region. Although coccydynia is seen in all age groups and both sexes, it is more common in the 40s and five times more common in women than men. (Fogel et al., 2004). Coccydynia describes pain in the coccyx or tailbone. The tail bone got its name from the Greek word coccyx, and the term dynia meaning chronic pain. The pain felt around the coccyx, usually due to hypermobility of this bone, increasing typically with pressure on this area, is called coccydynia. (Emerseon S S, and Hodges S D., 2012).

The coccyx is a cone-shaped segment located at the most distal part of the vertebral column, mainly consisting of 4 segments. These segments are usually mobile in the infantile period and fuse from distal to proximal during adolescence. The sacrococcygeal joint usually remains mobile for life without fusion. (Sugar, 1995). According to the literature, 1% of all spinal pain disorders are due to coccydynia. (Dampc B, and Slowinski, 2017).

## ANATOMY

The coccyx is a bone formed by the fusion of 3-5 vertebrae in the distal segment of the vertebral column (Maigne et al., 1994). The coccyx has a concave structure on the anterior surface and a convex structure on the posterior surface. There are tubercular structures called articular processes on the posterior surface, and at the top of these tubercles is the coccygeal cornua. The coccygeal cornua articulates with the sacral cornua structure at the S5 level below the sacral apex. (Ravi et al., 2008).

The S5 nerve roots branch just above the first coccygeal vertebra, and the coccygeal nerve and anterior branches of the S4-S5 spinal nerves form the coccygeal plexus. While the coccygeal plexus is located anteriorly, a vast nerve network, including somatic and autonomic nerve endings, is found behind the intrapelvic organs. This neural network includes the ganglion impar (Walther ganglion) used in nerve block treatment in patients with coccydynia. (Moore KL, and Jason T K W., 2012) S4-S5 and coccygeal nerves are sensory. While, pain is felt in the vaginal and anal area with S4 root stimulation, S5 and coccygeal nerve root stimulation centers around the coccyx. Rarely, coccydynia pain may also originate from the S3 nerve root (Çifçi et al., 2016).

The borders of the anterior part of the coccyx are formed by the levator ani muscle and the sacrococcygeal ligament structures. The lateral part's borders are formed by the coccygeal muscles, sacrospinous ligament, sacrotuberous ligament, and gluteus maximus muscle fibers. The coccyx bone, forming the terminal segment of the vertebral column, has great functional importance as it is the attachment site of many muscles, tendons, and ligaments. Besides, the coccyx bone also serves as positional support to the anus (Lesley et al., 2014).

## Etiology

A direct fall on the coccyx and repetitive microtraumas are the most common causes of coccydynia, but the etiology could not be determined in 30% of coccydynia patients (Deniz et al., 2014). The most common injury mechanism is axial loading on the most distal segment of the vertebral column (Pennekamp et al., 2005).

The incidence of coccydynia in women is five times higher than in men. Difficult delivery is one of the common causes of coccydynia in women. In the last trimester of pregnancy, the coccyx becomes more mobile and allows excessive flexion-extension, and causes coccydynia by creating inflammation in the surrounding tissues due to microtrauma. (Veli et al., 2014) Pressure during labor can also cause coccydynia. The most common reason for this is the use of forceps in difficult deliveries. The most common etiological cause of coccydynia in such patients is luxation and fracture of the coccyx (Maigne at al., 2012).

Sitting on hard ground for a long time and sports such as horse riding, cycling, and motorcycle riding can also cause coccydynia by creating microtrauma. (Pennekamp et al., 2005) Non-traumatic causes of coccydynia include degenerative disc or joint diseases, infectious pathologies such as tuberculosis or osteomyelitis, various anatomical variations of the coccyx, tumoral formations involving the coccyx, and some somatization disorders. (Nathan et al., 2010).

## Classification

Acute coccydynia develops due to trauma and is a coccyx pain usually occurring due to coccygeal disc or joint damage. Acute coccydynia responds very well to conservative treatment. Coccyx pain for more than two months is called chronic coccydynia, and it is more complicated to treat. Different classifications have been defined for coccydynia as follows (Table 1) (Jose De A, and Santiago C., 2004).

The Postacchini-Massobrio classification based on sacrococcygeal angulation is the most commonly used classification system in the coccyx fracture classification, one of the common causes of coccydynia. In the Postacchini-Massobrio classification, the angle between the line drawn from the midpoint of the upper endplate of the sacrum to the midpoint of the first coccygeal segment and the line drawn from the middle of the coccyx was taken as a reference (Figure 1).

**Table 1. The causes of coccydynia**

| | |
|---|---|
| **Etiological** | Idiopathic |
| | Traumatic |
| **Pathological** | Degenerative changes in the intercoccygeal and sacrococcygeal discs or joints |
| | Various morphological variations of the coccyx |
| | Anatomical malformation of the coccyx (hypermobility or subluxation) |
| | Referred pain; lumbar discopathy, infectious pathologies of sacral nerve endings, spasm of muscular structures around the coccyx, soft tissue inflammation around the coccyx |
| | Other: Tumors, crystallized deposits, infections |

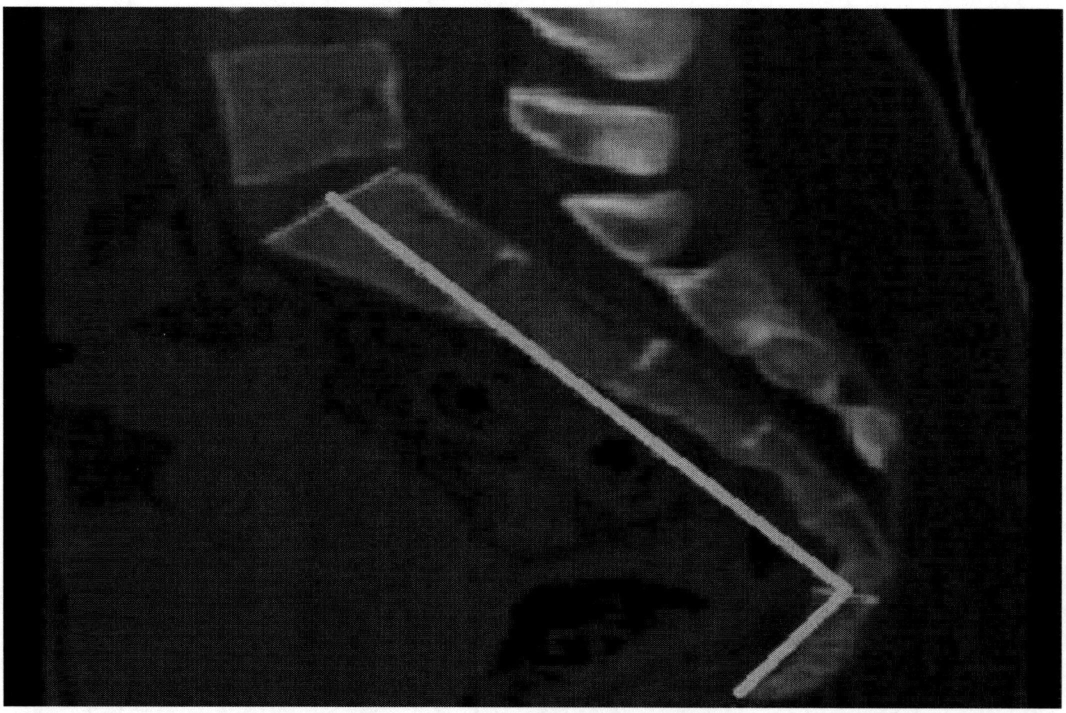

Figure 1. The angle between the line drawn from the midpoint of the upper endplate of the sacrum to the midpoint of the first coccygeal segment and the line drawn from the middle of the coccyx.

There are four types according to the Postacchini-Massobrio classification; (Postacchini F, and Massobrio M., 1983) (Figure 2).

Type 1: The injury is unexplained, and the coccyx is bent forward.

Type 2: Angled less than 90 degrees and bent markedly forward.

Type 3: 90-degree angulation is available.

Type 4: More than 90 degrees of angulation or subluxation of the sacrococcygeal joint is present.

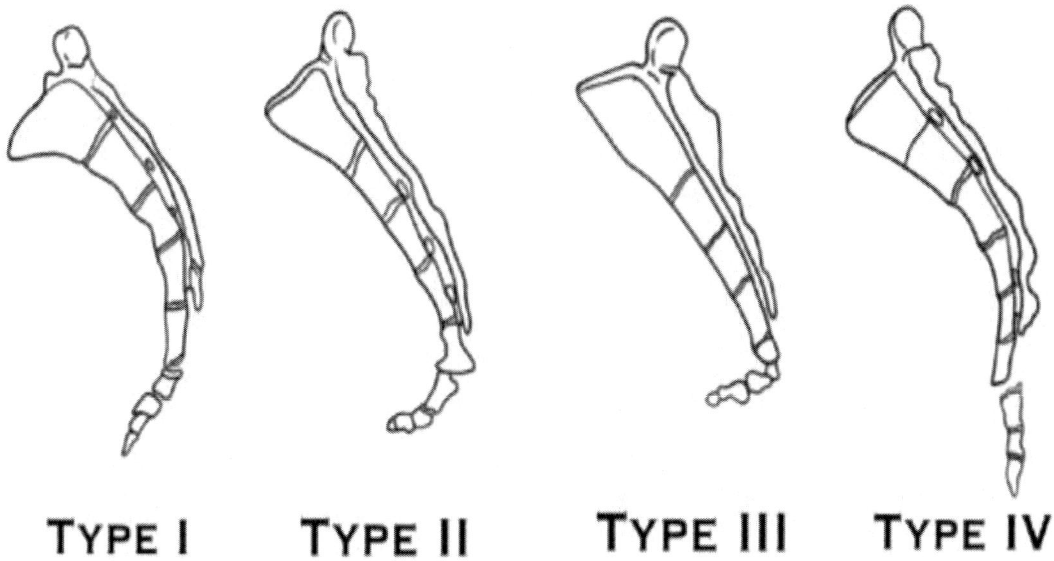


Figure 2. The Postacchini-Massobrio classification.

## Clinic and Diagnosis

Coccydynia patients have pain in the lumbar region and around the coccyx. The pain becomes evident after sitting for a long time or during getting up from sitting. Besides, pain may also increase during defecation or sexual intercourse. (Fogel et al., 2004) Ecchymosis or hematoma can be seen around the coccyx in coccydynia developing due to trauma. (Veli et al., 2014).

The first step in the diagnosis of coccydynia is a detailed anamnesis. Then, physical examination and radiographic imaging examinations are performed. In patients with coccydynia, trauma, sitting on hard ground, sports activities, and daily routines should be questioned in the anamnesis. (Maroy, 1988).

Diseases that accompany coccydynia or are considered in the differential diagnosis should be evaluated. Since low back pain in patients with coccydynia is higher than in the normal population, physical examination including sacroiliac pathologies, lumbar discopathy, and pelvic pathologies should be performed. (Postacchini F, and Massobrio M., 1983) Besides, soft tissue lesions like pilonidal sinus, anal abscesses, and hemorrhoids should be checked by palpation in physical examination. (Çifçi et al., 2016).

Risk factors must be determined in patients with coccydynia. Risk factors for coccydynia include: (Tekeoğlu İ., and Aydın Y., 2007).

- Past trauma
- Female gender

- Sports activities putting the coccyx under pressure for a long time
- History of low back pain
- High body mass index
- Spinal cord injuries
- Infectious diseases such as tuberculosis, brucellosis, or osteomyelitis involving the vertebral column
- Calcium storage diseases
- Rheumatological diseases such as ankylosing spondylitis
- Some psychiatric disorders.

Bidirectional lumbar, anterior-posterior pelvic, and lateral coccyx radiography should be taken in plain radiographs for diagnosis. In plain radiographs, fractures, degenerative diseases, sacrococcygeal luxation, tumoral formations, and infectious pathologies causing lytic lesions in the bone can be evaluated. (Jose De A, and Santiago C., 2004) Besides, dynamic radiographic evaluation is performed with radiographs taken while standing and sitting to measure coccygeal mobility. More than 25 degrees of angulation in the lateral plane is defined as coccygeal hypermobility in the dynamic radiographic examination. (Maigne et al., 2000).

Computed tomography and magnetic resonance imaging can also be used for diagnosis. Computed tomography is generally used for coccyx fractures, while magnetic resonance imaging is used for detecting cysts, tumoral lesions, and soft tissue pathologies. (Trouyin et al., 2013).

## TREATMENT

Conservative treatment is primarily applied, and 90% of the patients respond well to conservative treatment. (Wood K B, and Mehbod A A., 2004).

Using various types of seat cushions in the treatment of coccydynia can relieve pain by reducing the pressure on the coccyx during sitting. U- or wedge-shaped seat cushions with the open side falling on the coccyx to reduce the pressure on the coccyx are often beneficial. Although ring-shaped cushions are recommended more frequently, they have fewer clinical benefits because the back part of these cushions puts more pressure on the coccyx (Foye, 2015).

Ice therapy and topical drugs (topical non-steroidal anti-inflammatory drugs) may provide partial relief in coccydynia. However, local applications may cause hygiene problems due to the proximity of the coccyx to the anus. Although oral drugs provide clinical relief in patients, their effect on coccydynia pain is limited as they are systemically effective (Foye, 2015).

Local injection therapy techniques can minimize the side effects of systemically administered drugs and increase the effectiveness of local treatment. Injection treatments are done under fluoroscopy guidance. Fluoroscopy-guided injection therapy reduces the possibility of injection-induced damage to other tissues around the coccyx, such as the rectum, caudal epidural space, and vascular structures. Typical injection treatments for coccydynia include local corticosteroid injections, impar ganglion sympathetic nerve block, and nerve ablation therapy (Finsen, 2001).

In the manual manipulation technique used in the treatment of coccydynia, the clinician tries to manipulate the coccygeal bones and ligaments by inserting their first or second finger through the rectum. However, this treatment is not used much today due to its risk of causing joint diastases and coccyx fractures (Foye, 2015).

Surgical treatment can be applied in resistant coccydynia patients who are unresponsive to conservative treatment (Figure 3). Coccygectomy is applied as surgical treatment. The coccyx excision is performed according to the technique described by Key. The patients are placed in the prone position; then, the coccyx is palpated and entered with a longitudinal incision along the midline. All mobile coccyx and sacrococcygeal segments are resected after the coccyx is dissected adequately from the surrounding soft tissues and ligaments. (Capar et al., 2007).

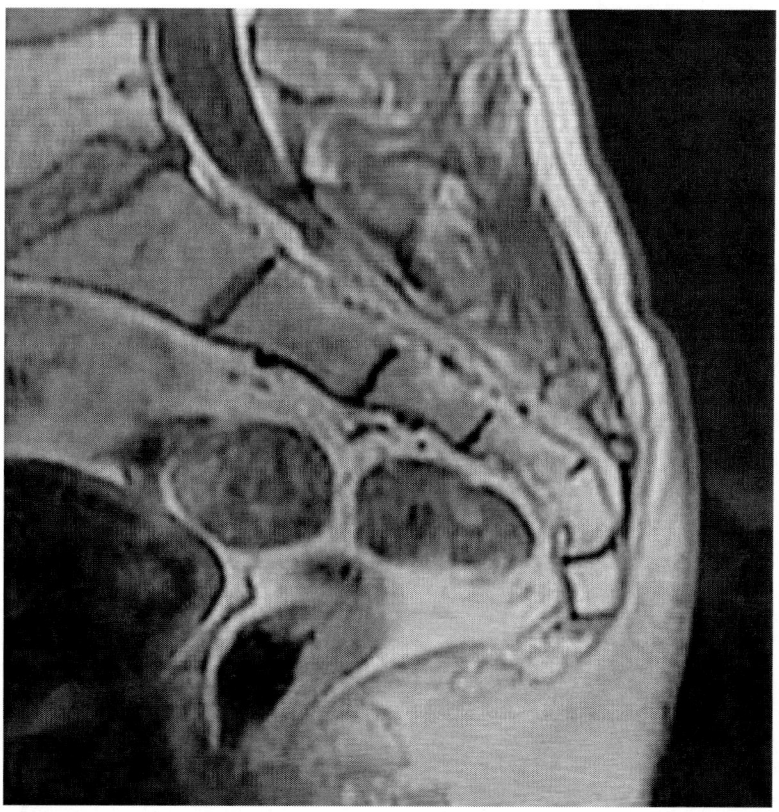

Figure 3. (Continued)

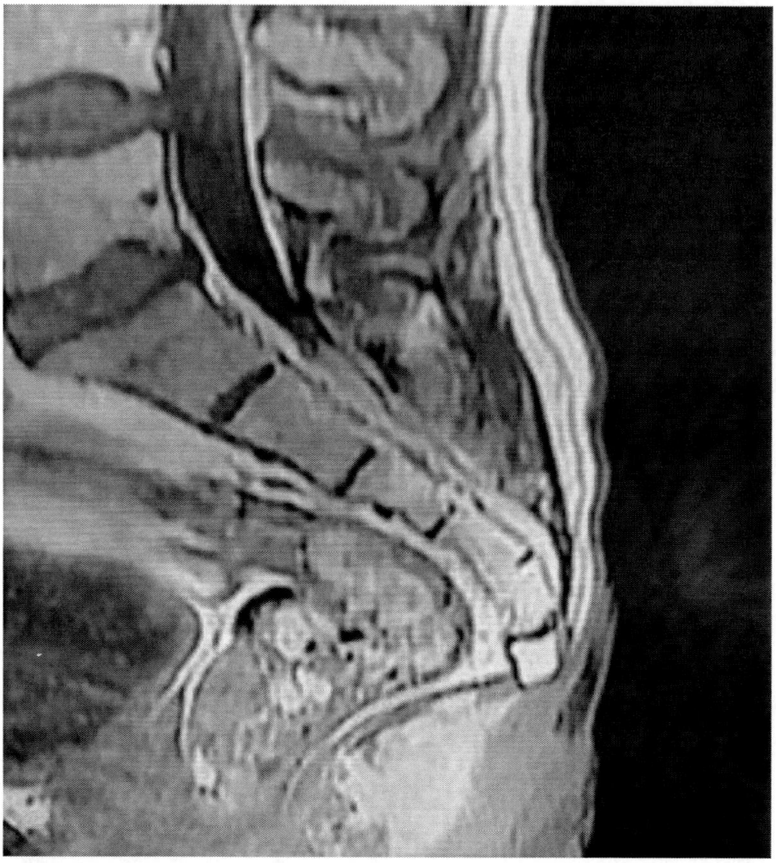

Figure 3. Pre and postoperative MRI images of a patient with coccydynia.

## Conclusion

In patients presenting with pain in the lumbar or sacrococcygeal region, coccydynia must be kept in mind in the differential diagnosis. In patients with coccydynia, imaging tests are performed after detailed anamnesis and physical examination. Conservative treatment is started after diagnosing coccydynia, and 90% of the patients respond well. In rare cases that do not respond to conservative treatment, surgical treatment is applied.

## References

Capar B, Akpinar N, Kutluay E, Müjde S, Turan A. (2007) "Coccygectomy in patients with coccydynia." *Acta Orthop. Traumatol. Turc.* Aug-Oct;41(4):277-80.

ÇIFTÇI, Betül; İKBALI AFŞAR, Sevgi; UZUNKULAOĞLU, Aslıhan. (2016) *"Koksidinia. Journal of Physical Medicine & Rehabilitation Sciences/Fiziksel Tup ve Rehabilitasyon Bilimleri Dergisi,"* 2016, 19.1.

Dampc B, Słowiński K. (2017) "Coccygodynia - pathogenesis, diagnostics and therapy. Review of the writing." *Pol. Przegl. Chir.*;89(4):33- 40. doi: 10.5604/01.3001.0010.3909.

Deniz R, Ozen G, Yilmaz-Oner S, (2014). "Ankylosing spondylitis and a diagnostic dilemma: coccydynia." *Clin. Exp. Rheumatol.;* 32(2):194-8.

Emerson S S, (2012) "Speece A J 3rd. Manipulation of the coccyx with anesthesia for the management of coccydynia." *J. Am. Osteopath. Assoc.*;112(12):805-7.

Finsen V. (2001) *"Corticosteroid injection for coccygodynia."* Tidsskr Nor Laegeforen;121(24):2832–3.

Fogel G, Cunningham P, Esses S. (2004) "Coccygodynia: evaluation and management." *J. Am. Acad. Orthop. Surg.*;12:49–54.

Foye P M. (2015) *"Cushions for tailbone pain. Tailbone pain relief now*!" Newark (NJ): Top Quality Publishing; p. 151–8.

Foye P M. (2015) *"Manipulation of the coccyx. Tailbone pain relief now!"* Newark (NJ): Top Quality Publishing; p. 169–74.

Foye P M. (2015) *"Medications for tailbone pain. Tailbone pain relief now!*" Newark (NJ): Top Quality Publishing; p. 159–68.

Hodges S D, Eck J C, Humphreys S C. (2004) "A treatment and outcomes analysis of patients with coccydynia." *Spine J.* 4(2):138-40.

Jason T K W, Mark D S. (2012) "Clinical anatomy of the coccyx: a systematic review." *Clinical anatomy;* 25:158-167.

Jose De A, Santiago C. (2004) "Coccygodynia: A Proposal for an algorithm for treatment." *The Journal of Pain* (5):257-266.

Lesley S L, Gassan C, Reda T, Hazem E. (2014) "Coccydynia: An Overview of the Anatomy, Etiology, and Treatment of Coccyx Pain." *The Ochsner Journal;*14:84-87.

Maigne JY, Guedj S, Straus C. (1994) "Lateral roentgenograms in the sitting position and coccygeal discography." *Spine* (Phila Pa 1976);19:930-934.

Maigne J Y, Lagauche D, Doursounian L. (2000) "Instability of the coccyx in coccydynia." *J. Bone Joint Surg. Br.* 82:1038- 1041.

Maigne J Y, Rusakiewicz F, Diouf M. (2012) "Postpartum coccydynia: a case series study of 57 women." *Eur. J. Phys. Rehabil. Med.*;48(3):387-92.

Maroy B. (1988) "Spontaneous and evoked cocygeal pain in depression." *Dis. Colon. Rectum.;*31:210-215.

Moore K L, Delley A F. (1999) *"Clinically Oriented Anatomy, 4th edition."* Philadelphia, PA, Lippincott Williams&Wilkins.

Nathan S T, Fisher B E, Roberts C S. (2010) "Coccydynia: a review of pathoanatomy, aetiology, treatment and outcome." *J. Bone Joint Surg. Br*; 92(12):1622-1627.

Pennekamp P H, Kraft C N, Stütz A. (2005) "Coccygectomy for coccygodynia: does pathogenesis matter?" *J. Trauma*; 59(6):1414.

Postacchini F, Massobrio M. Idiopathiccoccygodynia. (1983). "Analysis of fifty-oneoperative cases and a radiographicstudy of the normal coccyx." *J. Bone Joint Surg.* [Am] 65:112-123.

Ravi P, Anoop A, Peter G W. (2008) "Coccydynia." *Curr. Rev. Musculoskelet. Med.*;1:223-226.

Sugar O. (1995) "Coccyx. The bone namedfor a bird." *Spine*; 20:379- 83.

Tekeoğlu, İ., & AYDIN, Y. (2012) "Koksidini; Bel Ağrısının Az Bilinen Bir Nedeni." *Journal of Biotechnology and Strategic Health Research*, 1(3), 68-74. ["Coccydynia; A Little-Known Cause of Low Back Pain."]

Trouvin A P, Goeb V, Vandhuick T, Michelin P, Lequerré T, Vittecoq O.(2013) "Role for magnetic resonance imaging in coccydynia with sacrococygeal dislocation." *Joint Bone Spine*; 80(2):214-6.

Veli Ç, Şule O, Muhammet F S. (2014) "Literatür eşliğinde koksidinia." *Abant Medical Journal;* (3)3:306-312. ["Coccidinia in the accompaniment of literature."]

In: Musculoskeletal Pain (Common Clinical Presentations) ISBN: 978-1-68507-410-4
Editors: Mehmet Cenk Turgut and Serdar Toy 

*Chapter 10*

# RESTLESS LEGS SYNDROME

***Yunus Emre Aktaş*, MD***
Department of Neurology, Medical School of Atatürk University,
Erzurum, Turkey

## ABSTRACT

Restless legs syndrome (RLS) is a neurological disease that negatively affects daily activities and especially causes sleeping problems with a wide variety of symptoms such as pain, numbness, and tingling, a desire to move, and abnormal sensations, especially at night in the distal of both feet. Although there are certain symptoms of the disease, nonspecific symptoms often delay consulting the right outpatient clinic and diagnosis, therefore most of the patients reach the appropriate treatment later. Especially in some age groups, there are major difficulties in both diagnosis and treatment. Although iron deficiency is known to have a major role in pathophysiology, many genetic and environmental factors also have an effect. Even though dopamine agonists are still the first choice in treatment, it is clear that there will be new developments in both diagnosis and treatment in the upcoming period.

**Keywords**: restless leg syndrome; sleep; genetic; iron; dopamine

## INTRODUCTION

Restless legs syndrome, which was first defined in 1685 and described in detail with all its clinical features in 1944, is also known as Willis-Ekbom Disease, dedicated to these two names. Patients present with abnormal impulsive complaints such as pain,

* Corresponding Author's E-mail: cekicbey@gmail.com.

numbness, and tingling, and a desire to move, especially in the distal extremities. RLS can present itself both as primary or secondary. In particular, comorbid conditions such as peripheral artery disease, diabetes mellitus, peripheral neuropathy, cardiovascular diseases, and kidney failure can be seen. Although iron metabolism disorder and hypoxic pathway activation are emphasized in pathophysiology, studies on many genetic and environmental factors are ongoing. Today, despite the fact that dopamine agonists are still used as the first choice in the treatment, different options such as pregabalin, gabapentin, oxycodone-naloxone and iron supplements are used alternatively or in combination. Although RLS can be seen in any age group throughout life, it can also exacerbate at different stages of a person's life. The severity of the disease and the response to treatment vary according to the accompanying comorbid conditions. For instance, in the case of pregnancy, the severity of the disease increases and complaints that have been stable may increase in this period. Fluctuations and additional problems seen during the course of the disease cause difficulties in the treatment, especially the tolerance developed against dopamine agonists, adding alternative options to the treatment and causing new difficulties.

## Epidemiology

RLS is seen as between 5% and 10% in Europe, Caucasian countries and the American continent. This rate is lower in Asian countries. The disease is generally more common in the female gender, and older people are more affected than young people and children.

As it is more common in women than in men, the rate of RLS increases especially during pregnancy. As the number of births increases, the incidence of RLS increases.

There are two clinical presentations according to the age of onset of the first symptoms. The first is seen before the age of 45, also called early onset RLS, which is generally inherited in families and symptoms progress slowly. In the second, symptoms begin after the age of 45 and this is considered as late onset RLS. It has a rapid onset and there is an underlying comorbid condition, especially iron deficiency.

## Symptoms

RLS is a sensorimotor neurological problem that occurs with the desire to move the foot, especially in the late evening and all night long. Patients express their complaints with expressions such as restlessness, tension, twitching and itching when their feet remain still. This urge to move becomes irresistible, especially at night when it is bedtime. This causes sleep disorders to be added to the clinic of RLS. Patients frequently mention that they feel pain while describing these complaints.

RLS is usually seen in the distal of the lower extremities. It is mostly bilateral; but on one side, complaints may be more dominant. It is rarely seen in the arms and calf area.

The RLS clinic is divided into two: chronic and intermittent. Patients with fewer than two symptoms per week are called intermittent RLS, while patients with two or more symptoms per week are considered to be chronic RLS.

## Diagnosis

Although RLS has a classic clinical presentation, patients are often delayed in diagnosis. The reason for this is that the patients do not apply to the correct polyclinic and they lack the correct anamnesis. In order to avoid confusion in diagnosis, new diagnostic criteria were published by the International RLS Study Group (IRLSSG) in 2014. According to the diagnostic criteria described by the IRLSSG, the patient is diagnosed with the presence of 5 main clinical features, and no additional diagnostic procedure is required for diagnosis.

The International Study Group (IRLSSG) consensus of diagnostic criteria for restless leg syndrome/Willis-Ekbom disease (RLS/WED)[1] is as follows.

Essential diagnostic criteria (all must be met):

1) Not all the time, but usually, having the urge the move the legs, as a result or caused by the unpleasant feeling in the legs.
2) The unpleasant moving and feeling get started or get worse with resting such as sitting or napping.
3) The unpleasant moving and feeling start to fade away totally or partially as the mobilization starts to take over. Mobilization could be walking or exercising.
4) The unpleasant moving and feeling might occur especially at night, or get worse during the night time.
5) The listed features should not be related with other medical or behavioral situations such as muscle cramps or myalgia.

Specifiers for a clinical course of RLS/WED:

[1] Allen, R. P., Picchietti, D. L., Garcia-Borreguero, D., Ondo, W. G., Walters, A. S., Winkelman, J. W., ... & International Restless Legs Syndrome Study Group. (2014). Restless legs syndrome/Willis-Ekbom disease diagnostic criteria: updated International Restless Legs Syndrome Study Group (IRLSSG) consensus criteria–history, rationale, description, and significance. Sleepmedicine, 15(8), 860-873.)

A. Chronic-persistent RLS/WED: In the past year symptoms would appear at least twice a week (when no treatment is given).
B. Intermittent RLS/WED: In the past year symptoms would appear less than twice a week and 5 times in a lifetime (when no treatment is given).

Specifier for the clinical significance of RLS/WED:

RLS/WED symptoms result in major distress and deficiency in school and social life. This is the result of the disease on sleeping habits, vitality, mood and behavior.

a. Sometimes the urge to move the legs occurs without unpleasant feelings and not only the legs but other body parts move as well.
b. In the case of children, symptoms should be described in their own words.
c. In the case of severe disease, activity might not relieve the symptoms but it could have caused prevention before the severeness.
d. In the case of severe disease, the worsening in the evening and night time could not be noticed. But it must have been noticed before the symptoms got worse.
e. The conditions known as "RLS/WED mimics" are usually confused with RLS/WED in surveys. This is because the symptoms are close to meeting, or meet the criteria 1-4. The examples here in the list are from epidemiological studies and clinical experience. The list here gives some examples that have been noted as particularly significant in studies and clinical practice. RLS/WED may also occur with any of these conditions, but the RLS/WED symptoms will then be greater in degree, conditions of expression or character than those usually occurring as part of the other condition.
f. The clinical course criteria are not valid for pediatric cases. For the cases that increase the frequency of the disease such as pregnancy and drug-induced RLS/WED, the criteria do not apply and are limited to the duration of these conditions.

Since the patients' periodic limb movements of sleep (PLMS) occur especially at night, hospitalization in the sleep laboratory to observe these movements may help with diagnosis. Movements generally tend to be bilateral and can sometimes be seen in the arms. These movements do not always have to be synchronized. It can sometimes be seen while awake, and this condition is called periodic limb movements of wakefulness (PLMW).

In RLS patients with difficulty in diagnosis, the response to dopaminergic treatment is a good guide and PLMS can also be used as an aid in diagnosis. PLMS is thought to occur as a result of cardiovascular stimulation. Meanwhile, it has been determined that there are situations in which the patient may experience an increase in blood pressure and heart rate. This suggests that there may be a relationship between RLS and cardiovascular diseases, although no definite link is currently established.

In the differential diagnosis of RLS, localized vascular and neural pathologies, especially affecting peripheral limbs, should be taken into consideration. It should not be ignored that sometimes several clinical pictures can coexist. It should be kept in mind that the motor, sensory and circadian components of RLS in particular are indispensable in the anamnesis.

Other diseases that should be kept in mind in the differential diagnosis are; peripheral neuropathy, venous stasis, myopathy, radiculopathy, attention deficit, hyperactivity disorder and various akathisia.

Essential or primary RLS is defined as a condition seen without any other underlying disease, and secondary RLS is a condition that occurs in the presence of another condition proven to cause RLS. Although there is a definitional difference between the two conditions, it has been observed that the clinical presentation and treatment of both are exactly the same.

Since RLS occurs mainly at night, one of the most important problems in these patients is sleep problems. Patients who cannot maintain quality sleep at night have many problems such as daytime fatigue, sleepiness, irritability, and depressive mood.

It has been shown that RLS is associated with neurological diseases such as Parkinson's, migraine, and sleep disorders and systemic problems such as hypertension, diabetes, and metabolic syndrome.

Iatrogenic RLS is an important group that should not be forgotten among the causes of secondary RLS. In particular, RLS that develops due to drugs has a high rate that cannot be underestimated. Drugs may cause a new diagnosis of RLS as well as exacerbate existing RLS. The drugs that need particular attention are; antihistamines, dopamine receptor blockers, serotoninergic and noradrenergic receptor blockers, antidepressants and antiemetics. In detail, the diphenhydramine of antihistamines, olanzapine, and risperidone; the quetiapine of antipsychotics, amitriptyline, mirtazapine, and venlafaxine; the sertraline of antidepressants; and the metoclopramide of antiemetics are the drugs that should be questioned and given attention. If antidepressants are used in the treatment of these patients, antidepressants with dopaminergic activity such as bupropion and trazodone should be preferred.

## PATHOPHYSIOLOGY

The family history of RLS in more than half of the RLS patients reveals that the genetic inherited pattern of this disease is high. In this context, various genes are emphasized.

Two strong theses are still emphasized today in pathophysiology. The first one is iron deficiency and the second is disorders in dopamine metabolism. The suggestion of iron deficiency causing central hypoxia in certain regions of the brain has been accepted. Although dopamine levels were found to be high, it is believed that the disruption of the regional activity of the dopamine mechanism and a decrease in circadian rhythm trigger the symptoms. At the same time, it is thought that iron deficiency and dopamine metabolism disorders are intertwined with each other and responsible for the general picture.

## TREATMENT

RLS treatment is divided into two as non-pharmacological and pharmacological treatments. There is no definitive treatment for the disease and symptomatic treatment is given. Non-pharmacological treatment alone is not sufficiently effective, so this is combined with pharmacological treatment to try to obtain maximum effectiveness from the treatment. Non-pharmacological treatment includes exercise, sleep hygiene, infrared rays, electrical stimulation, vibrational stimulation, transcranial magnetic stimulation, yoga, and acupuncture.

In pharmacological treatment, systemic iron deficiency should be investigated first, and it should not be forgotten that the symptoms may regress with iron supplementation.

- Oral iron preparation should be given if serum ferritin is ≤ 75 µg/L or transferrin saturation is less than 20%.
- Dopamine agonists are the most effective group of drugs in the treatment of RLS. In this context, pramipexole, ropinirole and rotigotin are the supplements that can be used. Dopamine agonists should be taken 1-3 hours before the symptoms begin. Calcium channel $\alpha2\delta$ ligands, such as gabapentin and pregabalin, can be combined with treatment in the case of augmentation and tolerance development.
- Pramipexole: Initial dose 0.125 mg
  Maximum daily dose 0.75 mg.
- Ropinirol: Initial dose 0.25 mg
  Maximum daily dose 4 mg.
- Rotigotine patch: Initial dose 1 mg
  Maximum daily dose 3 mg.
- Levodopa/carbidopa and levodopa/benserazide combinations have not received FDA approval and are used in treatment at low doses. They are not as effective as dopamine agonists.

Although the α2δ ligands gabapentin and pregabalin were not approved by the FDA, gabapentin enacarbil was approved by the FDA. It is used alone or as a combination in treatment. Disadvantages include drug interactions, addictive effects and the need for close monitoring for dose adjustment.

Opioids can be used in patients with severe pain. Benzodiazepines can also be used in cases of anxiety, depressive mood, and sleep disorder.

## Conclusion

RLS is a neurological disease with typical symptoms showing circadian characteristics. Most of the patients are diagnosed late and cannot get the appropriate treatment in the optimal time. Sleep disturbance is an inevitable end, as RLS symptoms are especially aggravated at night. This both affects the sleep quality of the patients and makes it a disease that interrupts their daily work.

RLS is diagnosed with typical anamnesis findings, and no extra examination is required for diagnosis. It should be kept in mind that RLS can be seen due to a primary or secondary cause, but it should be known that there is no change in diagnosis and treatment.

Currently, it is not possible to eliminate the disease with treatment, and non-pharmacological treatment should be added to symptomatic treatment. Systemic iron deficiency should be investigated and if necessary, must be replaced.

## References

Ahmad, A., & Didia, S. C. (2020). Effects of Sleep Duration on Cardiovascular Events. *Current cardiology reports*, *22*(4), 1-5.

Allen, R. P., Picchietti, D. L., Garcia-Borreguero, D., Ondo, W. G., Walters, A. S., Winkelman, J. W., ... & International Restless Legs Syndrome Study Group. (2014). Restless legs syndrome/Willis–Ekbom disease diagnostic criteria: updated International Restless Legs Syndrome Study Group (IRLSSG) consensus criteria–history, rationale, description, and significance. *Sleep medicine*, *15*(8), 860-873.

American Academy of Sleep Medicine. (2005). International classification of sleep disorders. *Diagnostic and coding manual*, 51-55.

Berger, K., Luedemann, J., Trenkwalder, C., John, U., & Kessler, C. (2004). Sex and the risk of restless legs syndrome in the general population. *Archives of internal medicine*, *164*(2), 196-202.

Bliwise, D. L., Zhang, R. H., & Kutner, N. G. (2014). Medications associated with restless legs syndrome: a case–control study in the US Renal Data System (USRDS). *Sleep medicine*, *15*(10), 1241-1245.

Connor, J. R., Patton, S. M., Oexle, K., & Allen, R. P. (2017). Iron and restless legs syndrome: treatment, genetics and pathophysiology. *Sleep medicine*, *31*, 61-70.

Didato, G., Di Giacomo, R., Rosa, G. J., Dominese, A., de Curtis, M., & Lanteri, P. (2020). Restless legs syndrome across the lifespan: Symptoms, pathophysiology, management and daily life impact of the different patterns of disease presentation. *International Journal of Environmental Research and Public Health*, *17*(10), 3658.

Earley, C. J., Barker, P. B., Horská, A., & Allen, R. P. (2006). MRI-determined regional brain iron concentrations in early-and late-onset restless legs syndrome. *Sleep medicine*, *7*(5), 458-461.

Ferri, R., Manconi, M., Plazzi, G., Bruni, O., Cosentino, F. I., Ferini-Strambi, L., & Zucconi, M. (2012). Leg movements during wakefulness in restless legs syndrome: time structure and relationships with periodic leg movements during sleep. *Sleep medicine*, *13*(5), 529-535.

Garcia-Borreguero, D., Silber, M. H., Winkelman, J. W., Högl, B., Bainbridge, J., Buchfuhrer, M., ... & Allen, R. P. (2016). Guidelines for the first-line treatment of restless legs syndrome/Willis–Ekbom disease, prevention and treatment of dopaminergic augmentation: a combined task force of the IRLSSG, EURLSSG, and the RLS-foundation. *Sleep medicine*, *21*, 1-11.

Hening, W. A., Allen, R. P., Washburn, M., Lesage, S. R., & Earley, C. J. (2009). The four diagnostic criteria for Restless Legs Syndrome are unable to exclude confounding conditions ("mimics"). *Sleep medicine*, *10*(9), 976-981.

Kendzerska, T., Kamra, M., Murray, B. J., & Boulos, M. I. (2017). Incident cardiovascular events and death in individuals with restless legs syndrome or periodic limb movements in sleep: a systematic review. *Sleep*, *40*(3), zsx013.

Kolla, B. P., Mansukhani, M. P., & Bostwick, J. M. (2018). The influence of antidepressants on restless legs syndrome and periodic limb movements: a systematic review. *Sleep medicine reviews*, *38*, 131-140.

Lubetkin, E. I., & Jia, H. (2018). Burden of disease due to sleep duration and sleep problems in the elderly. *Sleep health*, *4*(2), 182-187.

Merlino, G., Serafini, A., Robiony, F., Valente, M., & Gigli, G. L. (2009). Restless legs syndrome: differential diagnosis and management with rotigotine. *Neuropsychiatric disease and treatment*, *5*, 67.

Padula, W. V., Phelps, C. E., Moran, D., & Earley, C. (2017). Allocating provider resources to diagnose and treat restless legs syndrome: a cost-utility analysis. *Sleep medicine*, *38*, 44-49.

Picchietti, D. L., Hensley, J. G., Bainbridge, J. L., Lee, K. A., Manconi, M., McGregor, J. A., ... & International Restless Legs Syndrome Study Group. (2015). Consensus clinical practice guidelines for the diagnosis and treatment of restless legs syndrome/Willis-Ekbom disease during pregnancy and lactation. *Sleep medicine reviews*, *22*, 64-77. Prosperetti, C., & Manconi, M. (2015). Restless legs syndrome/Willis-Ekbom disease and pregnancy. *Sleep medicine clinics*, *10*(3), 323-329.

Provini, F., Vetrugno, R., Meletti, S., Plazzi, G., Solieri, L., Lugaresi, E., ... & Montagna, A. P. (2001). Motor pattern of periodic limb movements during sleep. *Neurology*, *57*(2), 300-304.

Rinaldi, F., Galbiati, A., Marelli, S., Cusmai, M., Gasperi, A., Oldani, A., ... & Strambi, L. F. (2016). Defining the phenotype of restless legs syndrome/Willis–Ekbom disease (RLS/WED): A clinical and polysomnographic study. *Journal of neurology*, *263*(2), 396-402.

Trenkwalder, C., Allen, R., Högl, B., Clemens, S., Patton, S., Schormair, B., & Winkelmann, J. (2018). Comorbidities, treatment, and pathophysiology in restless legs syndrome. *The Lancet Neurology*, *17*(11), 994-1005.

Wijemanne, S., & Ondo, W. (2017). Restless Legs Syndrome: clinical features, diagnosis and a practical approach to management. *Practical neurology*, *17*(6), 444-452.

Winkelmann, J., Allen, R. P., Högl, B., Inoue, Y., Oertel, W., Salminen, A. V., ... & Sampaio, C. (2018). Treatment of restless legs syndrome: Evidence-based review and implications for clinical practice (Revised 2017) §. *Movement Disorders*, *33*(7), 1077-1091.

Xu, X. M., Liu, Y., Jia, S. Y., Dong, M. X., Cao, D., & Wei, Y. D. (2018). Complementary and alternative therapies for restless legs syndrome: an evidence-based systematic review. *Sleep medicine reviews*, *38*, 158-167.

In: Musculoskeletal Pain (Common Clinical Presentations) ISBN: 978-1-68507-410-4
Editors: Mehmet Cenk Turgut and Serdar Toy 

*Chapter 11*

# GONARTHROSIS

***Fahri Erdi Malkoç*, MD***
Department of Orthopedics and Traumatology,
Haydarpasa Numune Training and Research Hospital, Istanbul, Turkey

## ABSTRACT

One of the most common joint diseases in the world is osteoarthritis (OA) (Felson, 1988). Knee osteoarthritis is a common chronic joint disease, which causes limitation of movement and pain (Page, Hinman & Bennell, 2011). Regional cartilage damage, such as fibrillation and thinning, is observed in OA (Kerin, Patwari, Kuettner, Cole, & Grodzinsky, 2002). All joint tissues such as the synovium, subchondral bone, and joint ligaments but especially cartilage tissue are affected (Berenbaum, 2013). OA can be classified as primary and secondary (Altman et al., 1986). Trauma, infection and biochemical and inflammatory processes are the main causes of secondary OA. The exact cause of primary osteoarthritis is unknown. Age, ethnicity, physical characteristics and genetics are thought to play a role in the development of primary osteoarthritis (Johnson & Hunter, 2014).

All three compartments of the knee can be affected by arthrosis to varying degrees. OA can affect only one compartment, or it can affect three parts of the joint with varying severity (Ledingham, Regan, Jones, & Doherty, 1993). The medial compartment is predominantly affected in about half of the patients (Willis-Owen, Brust, Alsop, Miraldo, & Cobb, 2009).

* Corresponding Author's E-mail: malkocerdi@gmail.com.

## INTRODUCTION

The complaints of patients with knee OA are stiffness, pain and swelling. Patients have decreased passive and active range of motion (ROM) in the knee joint and crepitus occurs during movement. Symptoms of patients with OA increase with daily activity. They decrease with rest. Symptoms progressively increase when OA spreads to the three compartments of the knee. They are not relieved by rest and patients complain of pain at night (Hussain, Neilly, Baliga, Patil, & Meek, 2016).

On physical examination, a knee effusion may be found. Generally, range of motion is decreased. All areas of the joint should be palpated and tenderness should be evaluated at different points. The presence of crepitus (cracking or popping sounds and sensations with joint movement) should be observed. The mobility of the knee joint should be evaluated. The tenderness of the soft tissues associated with the joint should be checked. Also, the passive and active range of motion of the knee should be determined (Lespasio et al., 2017).

In the physical examination, the patient's gait with the passive and active ROM should also be evaluated. The patient's gait should be analyzed in both the sagittal plane and the coronal plane. Knee instability should be evaluated in both standing and supine positions. Stress tests for instability should be done. A detected possible antalgic gait can show us the flexion deformity of the knee. Overall, it should be investigated whether there is an inward or outward slippage of the knee during walking. Extremity alignment should be observed in the patient in both planes. Varus or valgus deformity can be found. These deformities show the location of involvement, the medial or lateral compartment of the knee. Knee pain may also appear as referred pain as a result of pathologies in other regions. Therefore, the patient's spine and hip joints should be examined (Hussain et al., 2016).

Radiography is the most commonly used imaging modality in the diagnosis of OA. It provides a visualization of osteophytes, subchondral sclerosis and cysts that indicate the involvement of OA. It is still the gold standard imaging method. Radiography is also used to evaluate joint space width (JSW). The severity of OA can be evaluated radiographically. Kellgren and Lawrence (KL) scoring is a generally accepted rating system. It is based on osteophyte and joint space narrowing seen on the radiograph (Hayashi, Roemer, Jarraya, & Guermazi, 2013) (Kellgren & Lawrence, 1957).

MRI is used to visualize soft tissues such as articular cartilage, menisci, and synovium, as well as fluid collection and problems in the bone marrow. The advantage of MRI over radiography is showing these pathologies. However, it is not routinely used due to its high cost (Kellgren & Lawrence, 1957) (Alizai et al., 2015).

## NON-SURGICAL TREATMENT

Patient education, exercise and weight control can provide a significant regression of symptoms in the early period. These should definitely be considered before pharmacological treatment (Kan et al., 2019).

The association of being obese or overweight with OA is well defined. It was determined that this situation increased the incidence of OA by 2.5 to 4.6 times. A proportional relationship was found between the body mass index and the frequency of OA, and it was shown that there was a one-third increase with an increase of 5 $kg/m^2$ (Zheng & Chen, 2015). The importance of body weight control is clearly demonstrated. It has been proven that OA symptoms can be reduced by half with weight control (Kan et al., 2019) (Felson, Zhang, Anthony, Naimark, & Anderson, 1992).

There are many types of exercises. Aerobic, strength and isokinetic exercises are some of them. With any of these, patients' symptoms can be greatly regressed. Meanwhile, patients can regain some of their lost mobility with exercise (Dong et al., 2018). It has been proven that after exercise therapy applied to patients with OA knee, pain decreases, and in addition quality of life and physical functions increase (Fransen et al., 2015).

It has been shown that paracetamol has not been very successful in relieving the symptoms of knee OA patients. Therefore, it is no longer the first pharmacological agent recommended for the pain of patients with OA (Bannuru, Dasi, & McAlindon, 2010). Nonsteroidal anti-inflammatory drugs (NSAIDs) are often used to control the symptoms of patients with knee OA. Among them, diclofenac has been shown to be the most effective agent in reducing pain and improving function (150 mg/day). However, it should be kept in mind that side effects can be observed in the long-term or high-dose use of these drugs (Lespasio et al., 2017).

Another group of pharmacological agents in patients with knee OA, is molecules administered to the knee. Many physicians practice knee injections in the clinic. Studies have shown that methylprednisolone applied to the knee joint is successful in reducing the symptoms of patients with OA (Tian, Cheng, Zhang, & Chen, 2018). The effect of methylprednisolone can last up to 1.5 to 2 months (Jüni et al., 2015).

Another group of molecules applied to the knee joint is hyaluronic acid (HA) derivatives. Hyaluronic acid, which has been in the practice of physicians for a long time, is applied intra-articularly and supports the synovial fluid. Methylprednisolone and HA derivative drugs have similar effects in this patient group. They are successful in reducing the symptoms of patients with OA. When the side effects of both groups of pharmacological agents were examined in the long term, no significant difference was observed (Ran, Yang, Ren, Wang, & Dong, 2018). Studies have shown that single-dose and multiple-dose HA treatment has achieved similar success in relieving the symptoms of patients (Vincent, 2019).

Platelet-rich plasma (PRP) administered intra-articularly is another treatment option in patients with knee OA (Turgut, Okay, Tuncer, & Yıldırım, 2020). PRP is obtained from whole blood. It contains a high amount of growth factors. In some studies, it has been shown that PRP treatment is more effective in the short term compared to placebo and HA (Chen et al., 2019).

Another option that is applied intra-articularly is mesenchymal stem cell therapy. Studies show that this treatment option can alleviate symptoms in patients with knee OA in the short term and it is safe (Ma et al., 2020) (Kim et al., 2020). However, there are not enough RCT studies to know the effect of mesenchymal stem cell therapy in patients with knee OA. Also, there is insufficient evidence that MSC treatment improves cartilage in the knee joint (Kim et al., 2019).

## SURGICAL TREATMENT

Some patients with mild and moderate OA are treated with arthroscopic surgery. The characteristics of patients who benefit from arthroscopic surgery are young age, mechanical symptoms, medial joint line tenderness and unstable degenerative meniscal tear (Hussain et al., 2016) (Moseley et al., 2002) (Kirkley et al., 2008) (Dervin, Stiell, Rody, & Grabowski, 2003).

Surgical treatment options for non-advanced medial compartment arthrosis include unicompartmental knee arthroplasty (UKA) and high tibial osteotomy. HTO and UKA indications are similar: 55-65 years old, not being obese, mild varus deformity, absence of instability, unrestricted ROM, and moderate degree medial compartment arthrosis. It has been shown that HTO surgery performed in patients younger than 65 years of age is more successful than in patients older than 65 years. Both surgical techniques have been shown to have satisfactory results in selected patient groups. It has been shown that the range of motion in patients who underwent HTO was superior to those who underwent UKA. For patients with a more active life, HTO may be a more appropriate surgical option. The treatment to be applied should be selected according to the patient's age, BMI, OA degree and activity level (Trieb et al., 2006) (Cao, Mai, Wang, Feng, & Huang, 2018) (Dettoni et al., 2010).

TKA is preferred to improve symptoms and restore function in patients with end-stage OA. Pain is significantly reduced in 95% of patients who underwent TKA, and it is a safe and cost-effective treatment option with a complication rate of 1-2% (Roos & Arden, 2016) (Lespasio et al., 2017).

## Conclusion

The survival of the knee replacement implant is up to 15 years (Duffy, Trousdale, & Stuart, 1998). Considering the findings, the patient should be evaluated from all aspects and appropriate treatment should be preferred. Patient education, weight control and exercise should be considered in first line therapy, and arthroplasty should be the last option (Hussain et al., 2016).

## References

Alizai, H., Roemer, F. W., Hayashi, D., Crema, M. D., Felson, D. T., & Guermazi, A. (2015). An update on risk factors for cartilage loss in knee osteoarthritis assessed using MRI-based semiquantitative grading methods. *European Radiology,* 25(3), 883-893.

Altman, R., Asch, E., Bloch, D., Bole, G., Borenstein, D., Brandt, K., Hochberg, M. (1986). Development of criteria for the classification and reporting of osteoarthritis: classification of osteoarthritis of the knee. *Arthritis & Rheumatism: Official Journal of the American College of Rheumatology,* 29(8), 1039-1049.

Bannuru, R., Dasi, U., & McAlindon, T. (2010). 558 Reassessing the Role of Acetaminophen in Osteoarthritis: Systematic Review and Meta-Analysis. *Osteoarthritis and Cartilage,* 18, S250.

Berenbaum, F. (2013). Osteoarthritis as an inflammatory disease (osteoarthritis is not osteoarthrosis!). *Osteoarthritis and Cartilage,* 21(1), 16-21.

Cao, Z., Mai, X., Wang, J., Feng, E., & Huang, Y. (2018). Unicompartmental knee arthroplasty vs high tibial osteotomy for knee osteoarthritis: a systematic review and meta-analysis. *The Journal of Arthroplasty,* 33(3), 952-959.

Chen, P., Huang, L., Ma, Y., Zhang, D., Zhang, X., Zhou, J., Wang, Q. (2019). Intra-articular platelet-rich plasma injection for knee osteoarthritis: a summary of meta-analyses. *Journal of Orthopaedic Surgery and Research,* 14(1), 1-11.

Dervin, G. F., Stiell, I. G., Rody, K., & Grabowski, J. (2003). Effect of arthroscopic debridement for osteoarthritis of the knee on health-related quality of life. *JBJS,* 85(1), 10-19.

Dettoni, F., Bonasia, D. E., Castoldi, F., Bruzzone, M., Blonna, D., & Rossi, R. (2010). High tibial osteotomy versus unicompartmental knee arthroplasty for medial compartment arthrosis of the knee: a review of the literature. *The Iowa Orthopaedic Journal,* 30, 131.

Dong, R., Wu, Y., Xu, S., Zhang, L., Ying, J., Jin, H., Tong, P. (2018). Is aquatic exercise more effective than land-based exercise for knee osteoarthritis? *Medicine,* 97(52).

Duffy, G. P., Trousdale, R. T., & Stuart, M. J. (1998). Total knee arthroplasty in patients 55 years old or younger: 10-to 17-year results. *Clinical Orthopaedics and Related Research (1976-2007),* 356, 22-27.

Felson, D. T. (1988). Epidemiology of hip and knee osteoarthritis. *Epidemiologic Reviews,* 10, 1-28.

Felson, D. T., Zhang, Y., Anthony, J. M., Naimark, A., & Anderson, J. J. (1992). Weight loss reduces the risk for symptomatic knee osteoarthritis in women: the Framingham Study. *Annals of Internal Medicine,* 116(7), 535-539.

Fransen, M., McConnell, S., Harmer, A. R., Van der Esch, M., Simic, M., & Bennell, K. L. (2015). Exercise for osteoarthritis of the knee: a Cochrane systematic review. *British Journal of Sports Medicine,* 49(24), 1554-1557.

Hayashi, D., Roemer, F. W., Jarraya, M., & Guermazi, A. (2013). Imaging of osteoarthritis. *Geriatric Imaging*, 93-121.

Hussain, S., Neilly, D., Baliga, S., Patil, S., & Meek, R. (2016). Knee osteoarthritis: a review of management options. *Scottish Medical Journal,* 61(1), 7-16.

Johnson, V. L., & Hunter, D. J. (2014). The epidemiology of osteoarthritis. *Best Practice & Research Clinical Rheumatology,* 28(1), 5-15.

Jüni, P., Hari, R., Rutjes, A. W., Fischer, R., Silletta, M. G., Reichenbach, S., & da Costa, B. R. (2015). Intra-articular corticosteroid for knee osteoarthritis. *Cochrane Database of Systematic Reviews* (10).

Kan, H., Chan, P., Yan, C., Chiu, P., Yeung, S., Ng, Y., Ho, T. (2019). Non-surgical treatment of knee osteoarthritis. *Hong Kong Medical Journal.*

Kellgren, J., & Lawrence, J. (1957). Radiological assessment of osteo-arthrosis. *Annals of the Rheumatic Diseases,* 16(4), 494.

Kerin, A., Patwari, P., Kuettner, K., Cole, A., & Grodzinsky, A. (2002). Molecular basis of osteoarthritis: biomechanical aspects. *Cellular and Molecular Life Sciences CMLS,* 59(1), 27-35.

Kim, S. H., Djaja, Y. P., Park, Y.-B., Park, J. G., Ko, Y. B., & Ha, C. W. (2020). Intra-articular injection of culture-expanded mesenchymal stem cells without adjuvant surgery in knee osteoarthritis: a systematic review and meta-analysis. *The American Journal of Sports Medicine,* 48(11), 2839-2849.

Kim, S. H., Ha, C. W., Park, Y. B., Nam, E., Lee, J. E., & Lee, H. J. (2019). Intra-articular injection of mesenchymal stem cells for clinical outcomes and cartilage repair in osteoarthritis of the knee: a meta-analysis of randomized controlled trials. *Archives of Orthopaedic and Trauma Surgery,* 139(7), 971-980.

Kirkley, A., Birmingham, T. B., Litchfield, R. B., Giffin, J. R., Willits, K. R., Wong, C. J., D'Ascanio, L. M. (2008). A randomized trial of arthroscopic surgery for osteoarthritis of the knee. *New England Journal of Medicine,* 359(11), 1097-1107.

Ledingham, J., Regan, M., Jones, A., & Doherty, M. (1993). Radiographic patterns and associations of osteoarthritis of the knee in patients referred to hospital. *Annals of the Rheumatic Diseases,* 52(7), 520-526.

Lespasio, M. J., Piuzzi, N. S., Husni, M. E., Muschler, G. F., Guarino, A., & Mont, M. A. (2017). Knee osteoarthritis: a primer. *The Permanente Journal,* 21.

Ma, W., Liu, C., Wang, S., Xu, H., Sun, H., & Fan, X. (2020). Efficacy and safety of intra-articular injection of mesenchymal stem cells in the treatment of knee osteoarthritis: A systematic review and meta-analysis. *Medicine,* 99(49).

Moseley, J. B., O'Malley, K., Petersen, N. J., Menke, T. J., Brody, B. A., Kuykendall, D. H., Wray, N. P. (2002). A controlled trial of arthroscopic surgery for osteoarthritis of the knee. *New England Journal of Medicine,* 347(2), 81-88.

Page, C. J., Hinman, R. S., & Bennell, K. L. (2011). Physiotherapy management of knee osteoarthritis. *International Journal of Rheumatic Diseases,* 14(2), 145-151.

Ran, J., Yang, X., Ren, Z., Wang, J., & Dong, H. (2018). Comparison of intra-articular hyaluronic acid and methylprednisolone for pain management in knee osteoarthritis: A meta-analysis of randomized controlled trials. *International Journal of Surgery,* 53, 103-110.

Roos, E. M., & Arden, N. K. (2016). Strategies for the prevention of knee osteoarthritis. *Nature Reviews Rheumatology,* 12(2), 92.

Tian, K., Cheng, H., Zhang, J., & Chen, K. (2018). Intra-articular injection of methylprednisolone for reducing pain in knee osteoarthritis: a systematic review and meta-analysis. *Medicine,* 97(15).

Trieb, K., Grohs, J., Hanslik-Schnabel, B., Stulnig, T., Panotopoulos, J., & Wanivenhaus, A. (2006). Age predicts outcome of high-tibial osteotomy. *Knee Surgery, Sports Traumatology, Arthroscopy,* 14(2), 149-152.

Turgut, M., Okay, E., Tuncer, K., & Yıldırım, Ö. S. (2020). Clinical outcomes of intraarticular PRP and corticosteroid combination in advanced osteoarthritis. *Ann. Clin. Anal. Med.,* 11(Suppl 3), S233-238.

Vincent, P. (2019). Intra-articular hyaluronic acid in the symptomatic treatment of knee osteoarthritis: A meta-analysis of single-injection products. *Current Therapeutic Research,* 90, 39-51.

Willis-Owen, C. A., Brust, K., Alsop, H., Miraldo, M., & Cobb, J. P. (2009). Unicondylar knee arthroplasty in the UK National Health Service: an analysis of candidacy, outcome and cost efficacy. *The Knee,* 16(6), 473-478.

Zheng, H., & Chen, C. (2015). Body mass index and risk of knee osteoarthritis: systematic review and meta-analysis of prospective studies. *BMJ Open,* 5(12).

In: Musculoskeletal Pain (Common Clinical Presentations) ISBN: 978-1-68507-410-4
Editors: Mehmet Cenk Turgut and Serdar Toy 

*Chapter 12*

# MENISCOPATHY

***Murat Bakır*, MD***
Department of Orthopedics and Traumatology,
Sultan 2nd Abdulhamid Han Training and Research Hospital,
Istanbul, Turkey

## ABSTRACT

Meniscopathy is a broad concept that encompasses all pathologies of the meniscus. Meniscopathy can be treated with conservative or arthroscopic surgery. It has been determined that the meniscus prevents the formation of arthrosis and has a role in normal knee function. For this reason, in the current treatments of all diseases of the meniscus, there is an attempt to protect the meniscus.

## INTRODUCTION

The meniscus is a double crescent-shaped, asymmetrical fibrocartilage structure. It is for load distribution, proprioception, joint adaptation, stabilization and lubrication in the knee joint (Chirichella et al. 2019). Meniscopathy contains all pathologies of the meniscus in general terms. In this section, meniscus tears, degenerative meniscus, parameniscal cyst and discoid meniscus pathologies will be discussed.

* Corresponding Author's E-mail: dr.murat.bakir1991@gmail.com.

## Anatomy

There are two menisci in the knee: medial and lateral. The lateral meniscus is smaller and more rounded than the medial meniscus. The menisci are attached to the tibial plateau by meniscotibial ligaments from the anterior and posterior horns.

The body of the lateral meniscus has no connection to the capsule, so it is more mobile and more resistant to meniscus tears than the medial meniscus (Markes et al. 2020). Mostly, it has a complex fibrillar structure of type 1 collagen. Most of the fibrillar structure consists of circumferential fibers that resist compression stress. Radial array fibers sit between the circumferential fibers and resist the occurrence of tears (Arnoczky, S.P., Warren, R.F. and J.M. 1988).

The menisci are fed by blood flow from the perimeniscal capillary plexus formed by the superior medial and lateral geniculate arteries. The peripheral 10%-30% of each menisci is vascularized, and their remaining parts are fed by synovial fluid (Figure 1). This situation has led to the division of the meniscus into zones according to their vascularization from the periphery to the center. These have been defined as red-red, red-white and white-white zones from the periphery to the center (Arnoczky, S.P., Warren, R.F. and J.M. 1988).

## Meniscal Tears

We encounter acute meniscus tears after knee trauma that often happens during sports activities with specific symptoms.

Patients generally define this as their knees being rotated and sharp pain with a popping/tearing sound. After the first symptoms are alleviated, swelling and exacerbation of pain may be experienced in repetitive movements. Having pain along the joint line should be suspected in terms of a meniscus tear with McMurray and Apley tests in the physical examination. Mechanical locking may be seen in the bucket-handle or flap type of meniscus tears.

Patients with a chronic meniscus tear generally complain about knee pain, intermittent swelling and mechanical symptoms during knee movements. For the male gender, risk factors for degenerative tears are advanced age and having a profession needing knee movements, such as climbing or crouching (Snoeker et al. 2013).

Meniscus tears are classified according to where they occur, their depth and form of occurrence in magnetic resonance (MR) imaging or during arthroscopy (Figure 2). The tear classification (grade) is done by sagittal MR imaging. Confirmable tears in the arthroscopy include Grade 0, normal meniscus; Grade I, intrasubstance, globular-appearing signal not extending to the articular surface; Grade II, linear increased signal not extending to the articular surface; and Grade III, superior and/or inferior increased signal extending to the articular surface (Fox et al. 2015).

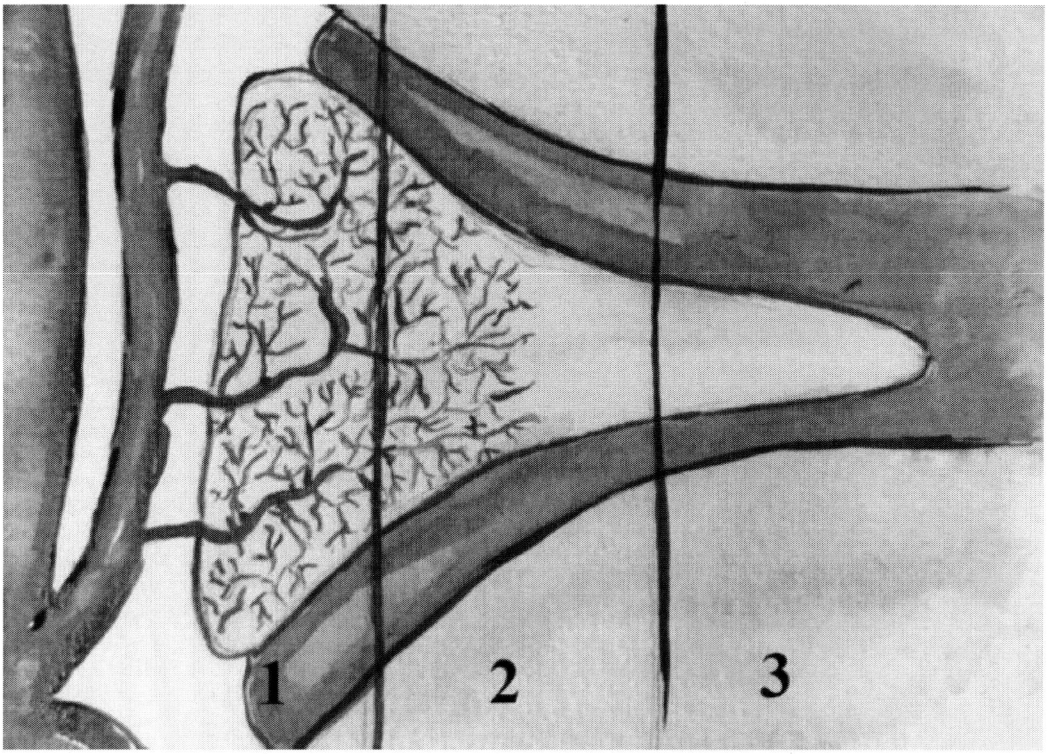


Figure 1. (1) red-red (RR), (2) red-white (RW), and (3) white-white (WW) zones.

Longitudinal tears occur in the surface radial collagen fibers between the circumferential collagen fibers. When a big rupture occurs, a torn meniscus may shift to the intercondylar notch and this situation is described as a "bucket-handle" tear (Nguyen et al. 2014). Longitudinal tears are more commonly related to trauma and can be typically seen in the red-white and white-white zones. The longitudinal tears seen in the capsular junction of the medial meniscus posterior horn are called ramp lesions (Terzidis et al. 2006).

Horizontal tears are mostly asymptomatic and they divide the meniscus into 2 pieces without breaking the circumferential fibers. Radial meniscus tears are seen most commonly in the lateral meniscus. They occur as a result of the tearing of circumferential fibers, so they cause "hoop stress" to be lost. Oblique radial tears may cause mechanical symptoms by forming flap-type tears. Complex or degenerative tears typically contain several tear configurations and these are the most common meniscus lesions in patients of middle and advanced age. Degenerative and radial tears are related to cartilage loss with higher rates (Fox et al. 2015).

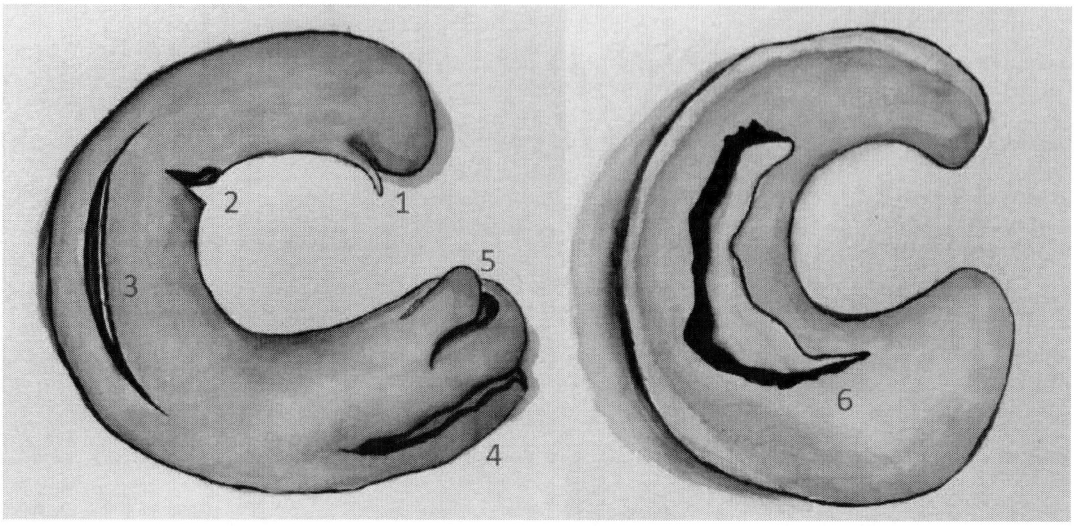


Figure 2. Illustration of meniscal tears (1) Vertical flap; (2) Radial; (3) Longitudinal; (4) Horizontal; (5) Horizontal flap; and (6) Displaced longitudinal tear (bucket-handle).

Since there are no defined symptoms that are examination specific to meniscus root tears, it can be difficult to make a clinical diagnosis. It has been shown that this type of tear may be finely diagnosed in MR imaging. A "ghost sign" is characteristic of a meniscus tear (Figure 3). If the posterior horn of the medial meniscus is not just medial to the posterior cruciate ligament in arthroscopy, a root tear should be suspected. In meniscus root tears, "hoop stress" is lost as in radial tears (Kennedy et al. 2020).

The treatment of meniscus tears varies according to the clinic that admits the patient. Patients with an acute meniscus tear without decreased range of motion, locking and instability can be treated conservatively. The RICE (rest, ice, compression, elevation) treatment should be applied in the acute stage. Not burdening the affected extremity may relieve the patient. However, a tolerated amount of weight load is permissible. Symptoms can be improved in 6 weeks with physiotherapy.

Early-stage physiotherapy should aim to ensure joint range of motion and knee swelling are under control. In the late period, the aim should be to prevent the shortening of the quadriceps and hamstring muscles and increase proprioception (Chirichella et al. 2019). In a study, in patients with a degenerative meniscus tear between the ages of 38 and 58, an improvement in quality-of-life scores and an increase in quadriceps strength were found with KOOS (knee injury and osteoarthritis outcome score) after 12 weeks of physiotherapy. No additional surgical intervention was required during the 1-year follow-up of patients (Stensrud et al. 2012).

In meniscus tears, surgical treatment is generally recommended for patients who continue to complain of locking, tripping and pain in spite of conservative treatment. The most common surgical treatment is arthroscopic partial meniscectomy. In studies, physiotherapy after partial meniscectomy has been shown to reduce pain and increase function. However, no randomized studies suggest partial meniscectomy has an advantage over conservative treatment. In randomized controlled trials conducted in patients with a degenerative meniscus tear, the advantages of arthroscopic partial meniscectomy over conservative treatment were not determined.

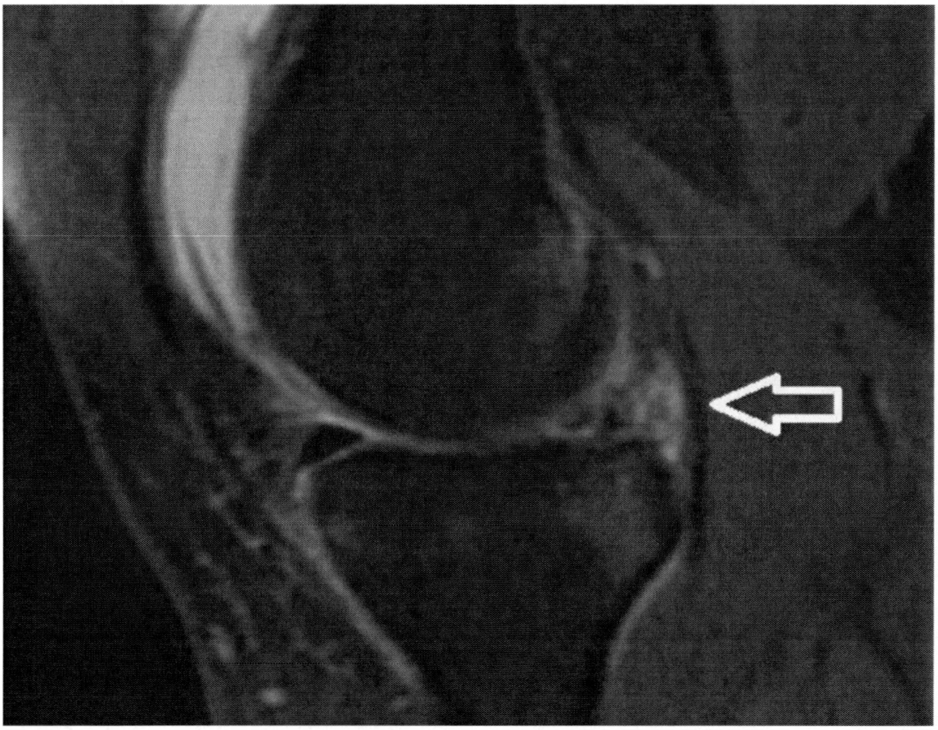

Figure 3. A "ghost sign" on MR imaging suggests a meniscal root tear.

As the importance of the meniscus knee functions became clear, maintaining and repairing the meniscus became popular. The meniscus should be protected as much as possible to reduce the risk of osteoarthritis and maintain knee functions. Arthroscopic repair has a higher chance of success with tears that are larger than 1 cm and smaller than 4 cm in the acute, vertical, red-red zone in patients younger than 40 years of age. The repair of horizontal tears has achieved similar success to other types of tears with new techniques (Kurzweil et al. 2014). Trephination, rasping and the use of the fibrin clot in meniscus tears increase the recovery rate. Meniscus repair performed with anterior cruciate ligament reconstruction has a higher chance of success. Meniscus repair is described as outside-in, inside-out and all-inside according to the direction of insertion of the sutures. In addition to the inside-out stitching which is accepted as the gold standard, the all-inside stitching technique has improved and achieved similar results. It also performs well for tears in the posterior horn (Chirichella et al. 2019).

Better IKDC (International Knee Documentation Committee) and Lysholm scores were found in patients who underwent meniscal repair in meniscal root tears than in those who underwent meniscectomy. It also prevents joint space narrowing and the development of osteoarthritis. The transtibial pull-out technique is used to repair meniscus root tears (Kennedy et al. 2020).

## Parameniscal Cysts

Parameniscal cysts are caused by a meniscus tear in the meniscus periphery. Intra-articular mucoid materials from the canal formed along the tear cause mucoid degeneration in the meniscus. If this degeneration progresses to the periphery of the joint, a parameniscal cyst is formed. This is generally accompanied by a horizontal tear. However, this may also be seen with other types of tears. In the treatment, cyst decompression and a proper meniscus tear repair should be performed (Nguyen et al. 2014).

## Discoid Meniscus

A discoid meniscus is defined as a half-moon rather than a crescent. It is more common in the lateral meniscus. Watanabe made a discoid meniscus classification in 1969.

Generally, the discoid meniscus is asymptomatic, presenting clinically when a tear occurs. Disorganized collagen, lack of vascularization and mucoid degeneration predispose tearing in the discoid meniscus. Discoid menisci are more common than bucket-handle and complex tears (Kocher et al. 2017).

The discoid meniscus should be suspected if there is a band extending from anterior to posterior with a thickness of >5mm in the middle of the meniscus in a row of 3 planes, the bowtie shape is seen in the sagittal plane, the sizes of the anterior and posterior horns differ, the whole meniscus is seen in all coronal planes from front to back, and the transversus length is >15mm (Saavedra et al. 2020).

Observation alone is recommended as a treatment for incidentally detected patients with a discoid meniscus. In patients with a symptomatic discoid meniscus, meniscus saucerization should be performed by diagnostic arthroscopy. During this procedure, at least 6-8 mm of the peripheral meniscus should be left. If there is a meniscus tear, it should be repaired, and if not, a partial meniscectomy should be performed. Fixation should be done if instability is present (Kim et al. 2016).

## CONCLUSION

Menisci are important structures with a capability of healing after injury. Doctors should evaluate many parameters in the treatment of meniscus tears. Meniscus protection has gained considerable awareness in recent years. In order to prevent the development of gonarthrosis and to maintain a healthy knee function, the treatment method should be determined according to the patient and the tear pattern. If surgical treatment is to be performed, as much of the meniscus should be preserved as possible.

## REFERENCES

Arnoczky, S. P., Warren, R. F. S. and J. M. (1988). Meniscal repair using an exogenous fibrin clot. *An experimental study in dogs.*

Chirichella, P. S., Jow, S., Iacono, S., Wey, H. E. and Malanga, G. A. (2019). Treatment of knee meniscus pathology: Rehabilitation, surgery, and orthobiologics. *PM & R,* 11(3), 292 - 308. https://doi.org/ 10.1016/j.pmrj.2018.08.384.

Fox, A. J. S., Wanivenhaus, F., Burge, A. J., Warren, R. F. and Rodeo, S. A. (2015). The human meniscus: A review of anatomy, function, injury, and advances in treatment. In *Clinical Anatomy*, (Vol. 28, Issue 2, pp. 269 - 287). John Wiley & Sons, Inc. https://doi.org/10.1002/ ca.22456.

Kennedy, M. I., Strauss, M. and LaPrade, R. F. (2020). Injury of the Meniscus Root. In *Clinics in Sports Medicine,* (Vol. 39, Issue 1, pp. 57 - 68). W.B. Saunders. https://doi.org/10.1016/j.csm.2019.08.009.

Kim, J.-G., Han, S.-W. and Lee, D.-H. (2016). Diagnosis and Treatment of Discoid Meniscus. *Knee Surgery and Related Research*, 28(4), 255 - 262. https://doi.org/10.5792/ksrr.16.050.

Kocher, M. S., Logan, C. A. and Kramer, D. E. (2017). Discoid lateral meniscus in children: Diagnosis, management, and outcomes. In *Journal of the American Academy of Orthopaedic Surgeons*, (Vol. 25, Issue 11, pp. 736 - 743). Lippincott Williams & Wilkins. https:// doi.org/10.5435/JAAOS-D-15-00491.

Kurzweil, P. R., Lynch, N. M., Coleman, S. and Kearney, B. (2014). Repair of horizontal meniscus tears: A systematic review. In *Arthroscopy - Journal of Arthroscopic and Related Surgery*, (Vol. 30, Issue 11, pp. 1513 - 1519). W.B. Saunders. https://doi.org/10.1016/ j.arthro.2014.05.038.

Markes, A. R., Hodax, J. D. and Ma, C. B. (2020). Meniscus Form and Function. In *Clinics in Sports Medicine*, (Vol. 39, Issue 1, pp. 1 - 12). W.B. Saunders. https://doi.org/10.1016/j.csm.2019.08.007.

Nguyen, J. C., De Smet, A. A., Graf, B. K. and Rosas, H. G. (2014). MR imaging-based diagnosis and classification of meniscal tears. *Radiographics,* 34(4), 981 - 999. https://doi.org/10.1148/ rg.344125202.

Saavedra, M., Sepúlveda, M., Tuca, M. J. and Birrer, E. (2020). Discoid meniscus: Current concepts. *EFORT Open Reviews*, 5(7), 371 - 379. https://doi.org/ 10.1302/2058-5241.5.190023.

Snoeker, B. A. M., Bakker, E. W. P., Kegel, C. A. T. and Lucas, C. (2013). Risk factors for meniscal tears: A systematic review including meta-analysis. In *Journal of Orthopaedic and Sports Physical Therapy*, (Vol. 43, Issue 6, pp. 352 - 367). Movement Science Media. https:// doi.org/10.2519/jospt.2013.4295.

Stensrud, S., Roos, E. M. and Risberg, M. A. (2012). A 12-week exercise therapy program in middle-aged patients with degenerative meniscus tears: A case series with 1-year follow-up. *Journal of Orthopaedic and Sports Physical Therapy,* 42(11), 919 - 931. https://doi.org/10.2519/ jospt.2012.4165.

Terzidis, I. P., Christodoulou, A., Ploumis, A., Givissis, P., Natsis, K. and Koimtzis, M. (2006). Meniscal tear characteristics in young athletes with a stable knee: Arthroscopic evaluation. *American Journal of Sports Medicine,* 34(7), 1170 - 1175. https://doi.org/10.1177/ 0363546506287939.

In: Musculoskeletal Pain (Common Clinical Presentations) ISBN: 978-1-68507-410-4
Editors: Mehmet Cenk Turgut and Serdar Toy 

*Chapter 13*

# ROTATOR CUFF TEARS

***Ferhan Bozkurt**, MD***
Department of Orthopedics and Traumatology
Keçiören Training and Research Hospital, Ankara, Turkey

## ABSTRACT

Rotator cuff tears are a broad-spectrum disease group that can cause disability with different clinical manifestations, ranging from clinically silent lesions that occur with age against a traumatic or degenerative background to massive retracted tears. The ultimate goal is to prevent disability. At this point, patient- and lesion-specific treatments are needed. Age, tear type, smoking, and the presence of retraction and fatty degeneration affect the treatment results. The aim of this chapter is to evaluate the clinic and treatment of rotator cuff tears in the light of current information.

## INTRODUCTION

While human beings use their lower extremities for walking, posture, gross movement and weight-bearing, their upper extremities are used for finer motor movements. The main functional task of the shoulder and elbow joint complex is to carry and support the hand at the level of fine skill to the desired coordinates in 3-dimensional space. In addition to the performance of independent, basic daily life activities, increased life expectancy, individuality and the need to work until old age in societies have increased the importance of having a healthy shoulder joint complex for hand use.

*Corresponding Author's E-mail: ferhanbozkurt@gmail.com.

## ANATOMY

The rotator cuff is a dynamic structure consisting of four muscles that have a role in the balanced movements of the upper extremities, surrounding the humeral head. It is also involved in shoulder joint stabilization by pushing the head of the humerus into the glenoid cavity through the "concavity compression" (Matsen et al., 1991) pathway.

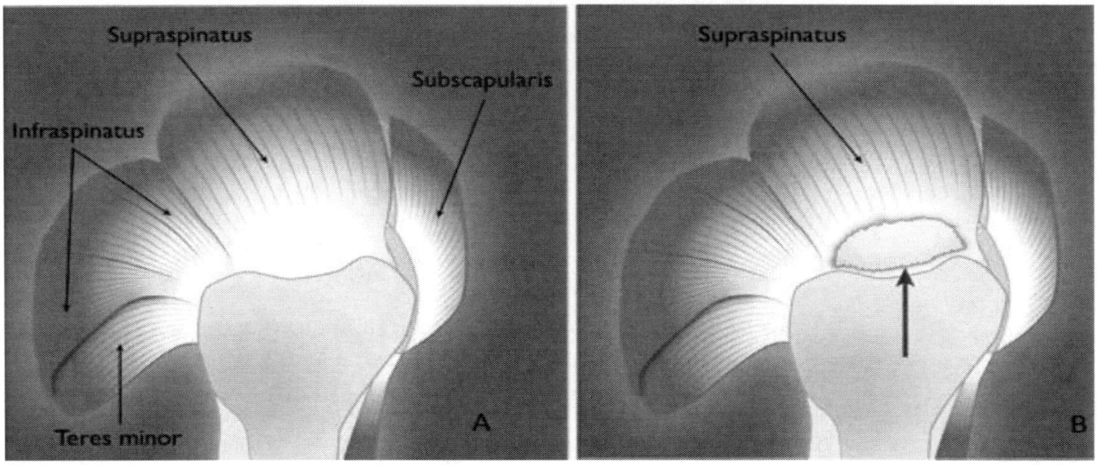


Figure 1. Rotator cuff tendons (A), Supraspinatus tear (B).
https://commons.wikimedia.org/wiki/File:Full_thickness_tear.jpg)

### Supraspinatus

This innervates from the n.suprascapularis (C5, C6, superior truncus). It is supplied from the suprascapular artery. It begins from the supraspinatus fossa on the superior of spine scapula and ends in the footprint that exists in the superior of the humerus greater tubercle facet. It assists the deltoid muscle by performing abduction of the shoulder joint.

### Infraspinatus

This innervates from the n.suprascapularis (C5, C6, superior truncus). It is supplied from the subscapular and scapular circumflex arteries. It is attached from the inferior of the spine scapula body of the scapula posterior to the middle of the humerus greater tubercle. It is the primary external rotator of the shoulder joint.

### Subscapularis

This innervates from the upper and lower subscapular nerve (C5, C6, C7, posterior cord). It is supplied by the subscapular artery. The body of the scapula, by taking the origin from the subscapular fossa ends humerus lesser tubercle. It performs adduction and internal rotation to the humerus.

### TeresMinor

This innervates from the n.axillaris (C5-C6 posterior cord). It is supplied from the subscapular and circumflexarteries. It attaches to the humerus greater tubercle sub-layer from its origin at the scapula margo lateralis. It performs external rotation to the head of the humerus.

## HISTOLOGY

The main task of tendons is to transfer the forces produced by the muscles to the bone, provide flexibility against impact, and proprioception. They consist of tenoblasts, tenocytes, and fibroblasts. Tenocytes produce anaerobic energy and because of their hypoxia and necrosis resistance, their recovery time takes longer. The main tendon structure is made of 60% collagen. 95% of the collagen in tendons is type 1 collagen. Essential glycoproteins in the tendon structure are also fibronectin and tenascin-C. While fibronectin has a function in recovery, tenascin-C has a role in stabilization (Vogel&Heinegard, 1985). The tendons attach to the lamellar bone through fibrous cartilage. While nociceptors function as pain receptors, mechanoreceptors (Golgi organ) are in the muscle tendon junction and relay pressure tension changes to the nervous system.

The rotator cuff is composed of 5 histological layers (Clark, J.M.&Harryman, D.T. 1992). The superficial first layer is composed of coracohumeral ligament extensions with a thickness of 1 mm. The second layer is 3-5 mm thick and contains parallel fibers of the main tendon. The third layer is 3mm thick and composed of an oblique course at 0-45 degrees of the main tendon fibers. The fourth layer composes loose ligament tissue and deep fibers of the coracohumeral ligament along with thick collagen fibers. The fifth layer composes the joint capsule. Most tears occur on the articular face. This is because the resistance of the rotator cuff's articular surface layers is half of the bursal surface layer.

## Epidemiology and Risk Factors

Many extrinsic and intrinsic factors have been identified that increase rotator cuff pathologies. The extrinsic factors are acromion morphology, acromioclavicular joint disorders, subacromial and subcoracoid impingement, coracoacromial ligament hypertrophy, overuse, repetitive micro-trauma and overhead activity, while age, smoking, hyperlipidemia, genetics, and activity level can be considered as intrinsic factors.

### Age

Rotator cuff tears are sometimes asymptomatic, and some people do not feel the need for treatment, even though they have symptoms. This situation causes the population incidence to be underestimated more than anticipated. The frequency of pathology observed in the cuff increases with older age. Asymptomatic tears become symptomatic within 2-3 years at a rate of 50%. Community ultrasonography scans showed cuff tears in a 13% incidence in the age range of 50-59 years, a 20% incidence in the age rangeof 60-69 years, a 31% incidence in the range 70-79 years, and a 51% incidence in those over 80 years (Tempelhof et al., 1999).

### Smoke

Tissue perfusion and oxygenation are impaired because of the vasoconstriction effect of nicotine on the arteries. While this causes an increase in the number of structural apoptotic cells and proliferative activity, it also causes a decrease in the number of tenocytes (Lundgreen et al., 2014). Significant fat accumulation and fibrogenesis were observed in smokers because of increased inflammation in the rotator cuff (Kim, J.Y. et al., 2019).

### Hypercholesterolemia

An accumulation of the lipid structure in the tendons increases the risk of a tear. There is a high connection between the total cholesterol, triglyceride levels and rotator cuff pathologies (Abboud, J., Dec, A., &Kim, J.S., 2010).

### Genetic Predisposition

Many studies have shown that genetic factors may have a role in the development of rotator cuff pathology. People with a rotator cuff tear have a significantly increased risk in comparison to the normal population from their 3rd-degree genetic relatives (Tachdjian et al., 2009). Though there are many unclear points in the relation between a rotator cuff tear and a genetic predisposition, there are differences in the expression of genes that have a role in apoptosis, structural stress, cell metabolism, perfusion, genes in the collagen and extracellular matrix regulation (Longo et al., 2019).

## Pathophysiology

Depending on etiological reasons, there may be situations from tendinitis to a full thickness tear in the process (Neer, C.S., 1983). Also, depending on etiological reasons, disorders of the collagen structure begin with inflammation and continue with a tendinitis situation. A tendinitis response is positive to the anti-inflammatory drugs. If the process continues chronically, changes develop in the tendon collagen architecture. While type 1 collagen decreases, type 3 collagen begins to increase (Khan et al., 1999). The tendinosis situation involves thickness in the tendon structure, proteoglycan increase, separation in collagen ligaments, and an increase in pathological vascularity. In the radiological imaging methods, a structurally thicker tendon may be observed in tendinosis; however, this structure is unstable. Anti-inflammatory drugs lose their efficiency in this situation. With the continuation of the load on the tendon, the process progresses to a micro tear and then to a macro tear.

## Clinical Evaluation

The first stage of the evaluation is to get a clear anamnesis. Differential diagnoses are eliminated with anamnesis. Generally, the main complaints of patients are pain, weakness, limitation of movement and crepitation. Cervical discopathy, syringomyelia, angina, reflecting pain to the visceral organ, thoracic outlet syndrome and brachial neuropathy can be observed in the differential diagnosis.

In the human musculoskeletal system, shoulder pain is the most common after back and knee pain. The most common cause of shoulder pain is rotator cuff pathologies (Urwin et al., 1998). Pain is mostly felt in the anterolateral, posterior of the shoulder. While cervical pathology pain has relief with overhead movements, rotator cuff pain increases with overhead and shoulder flexion movements.

Muscle weakness may sometimes be the only symptom. In particular, abduction weakness is observed. A pseudoparalysis situation that occurs without nerve damage is observed in severe tear cases.

The type of limitation of movement indicates the pathology. A shoulder joint which is actively and passively restricted in all directions indicates a frozen shoulder, the limitation of internal rotation indicates impingement syndrome, and the limitation of abduction indicates a rotator cuff tear.

## Physical Examination

Examination of the patient begins with a comparative inspection with both shoulders open. Arm swings are observed during walking. There is an evaluation as to whether there is a scapular or spinal deformity. Deltoid muscle atrophy suggests axillary nerve damage. Posterior scapula atrophy is seen in cuff atrophy as well as in suprascapular nerve pathologies.

In palpation, especially the acromioclavicular joint and bicipital groove tuberculum majus and minus, as well as the presence of an axillary mass, lymphadenopathy and sensitivities should be examined.

In addition to vascular and sensory examinations, triceps and biceps deep tendon reflexes should be compared, neurologically.

The shoulder joint movement range is provided from the glenohumeral joint and the scapulothoracic joint. The average range of movement of the shoulder joint complex is 183 degrees of abduction, 75 degrees of adduction, 70 degrees of internal rotation, 104 degrees of external rotation, 62 degrees of extension, and 170 degrees of elevation (abduction + forward flexion). It can be difficult to make a specific diagnosis of the complex anatomy of the region and there are a number of differential diagnoses. A personalized approach from the general to the specific is essential. For an accurate diagnosis, special tests are required.

## Neer Impingement Finding and Test

The patient's scapula is fixed and the arm is passively moved along the shoulder flexion arc. Pain under the acromion in the range of 60-120 rum indicates that the finding is positive. In the Neer impingement test, 10 cc of 1% lidocaine is applied locally to the subacromial region. The movement axis is examined again. Loss of pain means that the test is positive. It should be considered that the test may be negative for shoulder instability.

## Hawkins-Kennedy Test

After 90º of passive flexion of the shoulder and elbow has been taken, the shoulder joint is passively forced into internal rotation. The compression caused by the tuberculum majus getting under the acromion and the coracoacromial ligament is investigated. The impingement and test are positive in the case of pain (Figure2A).

## Jobe's Test

Supraspinatus tendon pathology is investigated. The patient's shoulder joint is abducted 90° and elevated 30° forward in the horizontal plane. The patient is asked to internally rotate the shoulder joint with the thumb pointing at the ground. In this position, the patient is asked to resist the resistance applied towards the ground. The test is positive in the case of weakness or pain (Figure2B).

## Drop Arm Test

The supraspinatus tendon in the patient's shoulder joint is passively abducted to 90° and released. The patient is asked to slowly bring their arm to adduction. A sudden fall in the arm during the movement axis indicates a supraspinatus tendon tear.

## External Rotation Lag Test

The infraspinatus tendon is evaluated. Passively, the elbow is placed at 90° of flexion, the shoulder at 20º of elevation and maximum external rotation. The patient is asked to maintain the position. The test is positive if the arm is neutral from external rotation (Figures2C, 2D).

## Hornblower's Test

The teres minor tendon is evaluated. While the patient's elbow joint is at 90° of flexion, the shoulder joint is placed at 90° of flexion and external rotation. The test is positive if the patient is unable to maintain the position and the shoulder joint falls to internal rotation (Figures2E, 2F).

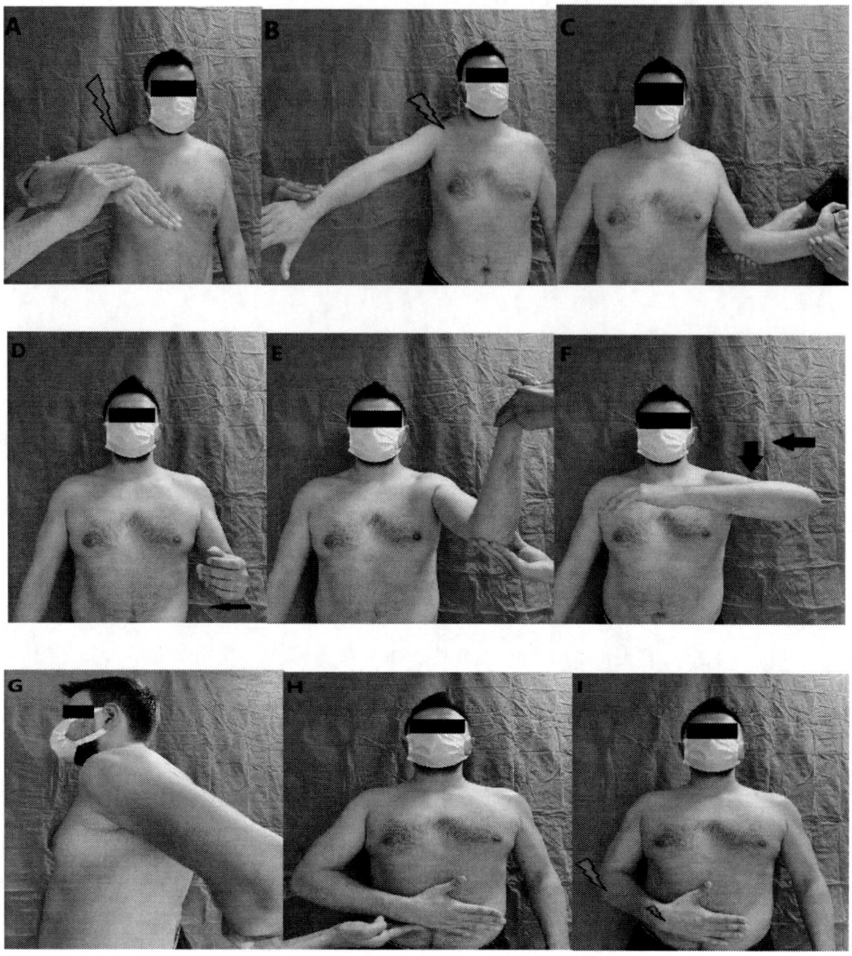


Figure 2. (A) Hawkins-Kennedy Test, (B) Jobe's Test, (C,D) External Rotation Lag Test, (E, F)Hornblower's test, (G) Lift-off Test, (H,I) Belly-press Test (from the author's archive).

## Internal Rotation Lag Test

The subscapularis tendon is evaluated. The patient's hand is brought passively to the thoracic region in the dorsal region and is asked to hold their hand here. The test is positive if the patient cannot hold their hand and lowers it to the lumbar region.

## Lift-Off Test

The subscapularis sub-ligaments are evaluated. The patient's hand is passively taken to the dorsal lumbar region. The patient is asked to remove their hand from their body along with their forearm. If the patient cannot do this, the test is positive (Figure2G).

## Belly Press Test

The subscapularis tendon upper ligaments are evaluated. The patient is asked to press their hand against their abdomen while the shoulder is in adduction. The test is positive if the elbow moves to the posterior and the wrist moves to flexion during compression (Figure 1H, 1I).

## Imaging Methods

After a detailed physical examination, radiological examinations are used for diagnosis. Arthrography, magnetic resonance imaging, and ultrasonography may be requested in some cases to contribute to the diagnosis and treatment stages according to the suspected pathology (Robertson et al., 1995).

## Direct Roentgenogram

A radiological evaluation of the shoulder begins with a roentgenogram. This gives information about the bone structure of the joint. It allows differential diagnoses to be identified such as neoplasia, glenohumeral arthrosis, and calcific tendinitis. Recommended direct radiographs are anteroposterior (AP), True AP, 15-30° caudal angle, scapula Y, axillary and supraspinatus outlet graphs.

Acromioclavicular degeneration and spur, cystic changes in the tuberculum majus, and calcific tendinitis are evaluated in True AP and AP graphs. The subacromial space is the distance between the upper border of the humeral head and the lower border of the acromion. This distance is 7-14 mm under normal conditions (Nove-Josserand et al., 1996). Superior migration of the humerus head and tuberculum majus deformities are observed in massive tears.

Acromion morphology is seen in the scapula Y graph and supraspinatus outlet graph. Acromial shapes have been described as type 1; flap, type 2; curved, andtype 3; hooked (Bigliani et al., 1986). The osacromiale is best seen in the axillary graph.

## Ultrasonography

USG is a low-cost, non-invasive, dynamic, fast, and non-radioactive imaging method. It can be reliably used in the diagnosis of rotator cuff tear and the evaluation of the treatment. USG magnetic resonance imaging allows diagnosis in patients who cannot use MRI. Muscles are seen as hypoechoic and the biceps tendon is seen as hyperechoic. The association of joint effusion with fluid accumulation in the subdeltoid and subacromial bursa has been reported to have high specificity and a high predictive value for rotator cuff tears (Hollister et al., 1995).

## Magnetic Resonance Imaging

Soft tissue around the shoulder is the most specific and sensitive examination to show the anatomy. Though it is a non-invasive method, it is not the first chosen radiological method. It is important to support the findings of the physical examination and to help the surgeon in patients who are scheduled for surgery. A normal rotator cuff MRI has a low intensity inall sequences (McMonagle& Vinson, 2012). Most pathology is observed in the supraspinatus tendon. In the presence of tendinopathy, intermediate signal changes and thickening of the tendon can be observed. Partial tears in the supraspinatus can be in the form of a bursal surface, articular surface and interstitial (delamination) (Murrell & Walton, 2001). Articular surface tears of the supraspinatus tendon footprint, called PASTA, require a special approach. In suspicious cases, MR arthrography is taken in the abduction external rotation position to ensure it can be distinguished from tendinosis. Full thickness rotator cuff tears are observed along with all layers of the tendon in MRI. Retraction, atrophy in the muscle mass and fatty degeneration can be seen in the late-diagnosed cases. Atrophy is evaluated in the sequences of sagittal MRI. All sizes of all cuff musclesare almost the same, asymmetric mass loss is interpreted in favor of atrophy and it is reversible. Fatty degeneration is evaluated according to the Goutallier classification (Goutallier et al., 1994). While there is no fatty infiltration in stage 0, there are fatty streaks in stage 1. There is a greater amount of muscle than fat in stage 2, and the amount of muscle is equal to fat in stage 3. There is more fat than muscle in stage 4, and it is a poor prognostic factor for primary repair surgery. It should be considered that similar atrophy and fatty degeneration may develop the cause of suprascapular nerve compression. Full thickness tears are classified as small <1cm, medium 1-3 cm, large 3-5 cm, and massive >5 cm according to the amount of retraction (McMonagle& Vinson 2012). Large and massive tears may be accompanied by an infraspinatus or subscapularis tear as well as a supraspinatus tendon tear. Subscapularis tears are less common, but they are associated with biceps tendon subluxation or dislocation.

# CLINICAL TREATMENT

Subjective and objective scoring systems of the physician are used to evaluate the success of clinical treatment.Though there are many scoring scales, the most commonly used scoring scales are the Constant-Murley (Constant &Murley, 1987) and Western Ontario rotator cuff index (WORC) (Kirkley et al., 2003).

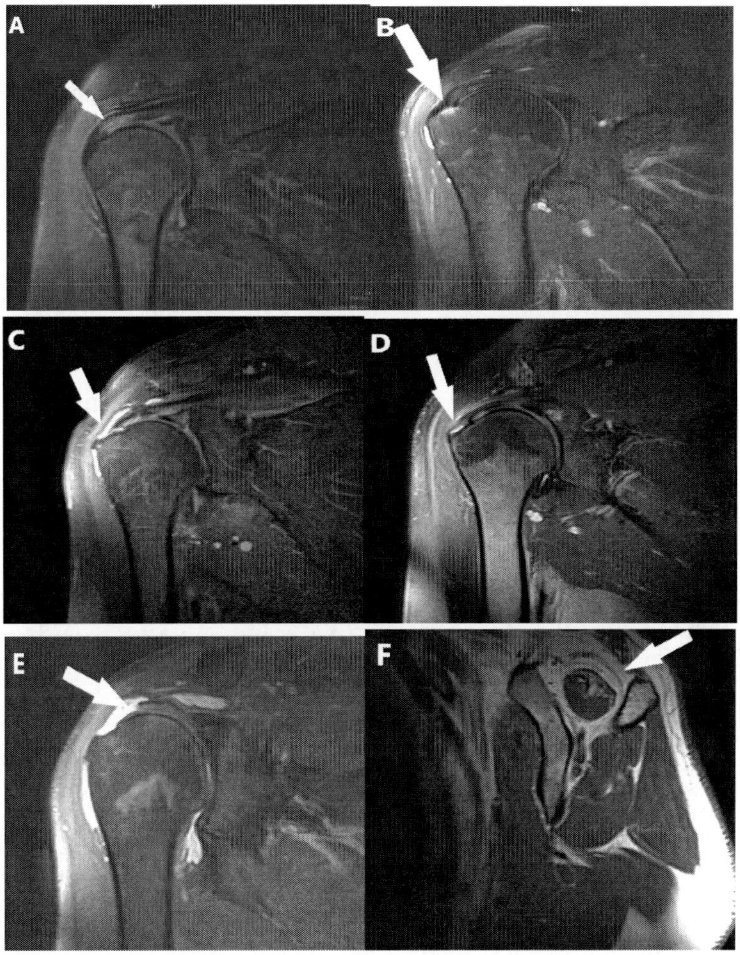


Figure3. (A) Supraspinatus tendinosis, (B) PASTA lesion, (C) Supraspinatus bursal surface partial tear, (D) Supraspinatus interstitial tear, (E) Supraspinatus retracted full thickness tear, (F) Supraspinatus Goutallier Stage 2 fatty degeneration (from the author's archive).

Considering the increasing incidence of rotator cuff tears with aging, it can be predicted that the current tear will grow over time. The opinion that torn tendons cannot heal on their own in the process is agreed. An increase in type 3 collagen levels, an increase in proteoglycan, a decrease in the number of tenocytes, and an increase in pathological vascularity make the tendon unstable, causing micro tears and then macro tears and full thickness tears in partial tears. When the natural course of asymptomatic or untreated cases is followed, it has been shown that 23% of them become symptomatic within two years (Yamaguci et al., 2006), accompanied by atrophy and fatty degeneration in the muscle mass. In the arthropathy of a rotator cuff tear, the development of glenohumeral arthritis is seen because the balance of forces on the humeral head is disturbed in the continuation of the process (Jensen et al., 1999). There is a strong correlation between pain and the progression of the partial tear to the full thickness tear. The tear mostly begins from the most stressed anterior section of the supraspinatus. It should be considered that 50% of the anterior part of the supraspinatus footprint is formed by the capsule in surgical treatment planning. Partial tears that exceed 50% of the tendon are repaired with surgical treatment as a rule (Fukuda, H., 2003). Some publications have shown that the tear can begin in the infraspinatus (Kim et al., 2010).

Partial rotator cuff tears may show different clinical cases. They can be asymptomatic as well as painful enough to limit daily life activities. The pain is usually more severe than in full thickness tears. The reason for this is that the amount of stress in the remaining healthy tendon increases. It was found that when patients with partial tears were followed up for 2 years in some studies, 66% of patients continued to live asymptomatically and their tears did not progress to full thickness tears (Mall et al., 2010). If symptomatic partial rotator cuff tears are less than 50%, it is recommended to follow conservative treatment methods for 6 months without a surgical decision (Finnan, R.P., & Crosby, L.A., 2010).

The main aim of conservative treatment methods is to relieve the pain and ensure the functional joint range of movement. For the pain, non-steroidal anti-inflammatory drugs, subacromial steroid and hyaluronic acid injections in selective cases and physical therapy can be applied.

Physical therapy is determined specifically for the clinical condition of the patient. The first stage of the treatment is educating the patient. Lifestyle modifications, anxiety control, avoidance of overhead activities, relaxation exercises and avoidance of tobacco products are discussed in the education. Pain management, training of the periscapular muscles and strengthening of the rotator muscles are the aims. Cold application, analgesic and regenerative mode TENS, interference, ESWT, HIL-therapy, ultrasound, HVPC and Kinesio taping, and magnetotherapy can be applied for pain control.

Though applications of platelet-rich plasma and mesenchymal stem cells are promising, their clinical use is limited. Adhesion and joint stiffness can occur after platelet-rich plasma applications (Jo et al., 2011).

Surgical treatment indications include an acute traumatic tear in the young, subacromial impingement syndrome and partial cuff tears that do not respond to conservative treatment, partial cuff tears of 50% or more, and full thickness tears with Goutallierstage 1,2, and 3 fatty degeneration. Many studies show that the results of surgical treatment are more promising than those of conservative treatment (Namdari et al., 2014).

The aim of surgical treatment is to ensure the tendon is concentrically attached to its own footprint. The surgical method can be open, mini-open or arthroscopic. Depending on the type of tear and size, a single-row repair, double-row repair, transesophageal echocardiogram (TOE) repair or double-layer repair can be applied (Turgutet al. 2021).

Acromioplasty can be performed according to the acromion type and coracoacromial ligament hypertrophy during surgery.

The age and type of fatty degeneration are the most important factors that affect the results of surgical treatment. The success of treatment after surgery will be lower than expected, especially because fatty degeneration based on infraspinatus tear will disrupt the joint strength balance and biomechanics, unlike supraspinatus tears (Gladstone, J.N. et al., 2007). Similarly, early surgical repair is recommended for subscapularis tendon tears. Smoking, obesity, osteoporosis, diabetes, tear size and duration are the main factors affecting the results of surgical treatment.

## Conclusion

The age and type of fatty degeneration are the most important factors that determine the prognosis of rotator cuff tears. In addition to these, the tear effect on the tendon structure and the condition of the patient's symptoms should be considered when planning the treatment of the patients. It is recommended to apply conservative treatment for 3-6 months before deciding on surgery in patients with partial tears. Surgical treatment should not be delayed in patients who do not benefit from conservative treatment and qualified full thickness tears.

## References

Abboud J.A., Kim J.S. The effect pf hypercholesterolemia on rotator cuff disease. *Clin Orthop Relat Res* 2010; 468:1493-7.

Bigliani L., Morrison D., April E. The morphology of the acromion and its relationship to rotator cuff tears. *Orthop Trans* 1986; 10: 216.

Clark J.M., Harryman D.T. (1992) Tendons, Ligaments, and capsule of the rotator cuff. Gross and microscopic anatomy. *J Bone Joint Am* 1992 Jun;74(5): 713-25.

Constant C.R., Murley A.H., A clinical method of functional assessment of the shoulder.*ClinOrthopRelat*1987; 214160-4.

Finnan R.P., Crosby L.A. Partial thickness rotator cuff tears. *J Shoulder Elbow Surg 2010*; 19:609-16.

Fukuda H. The management of partial-thickness tears of the rotator cuff. *J Bone Joint Surg Br* 2003; 85:3-11.

Gladstone J.N., Bishop J.Y., Lo I.K., Flatow E.L. Fatty infiltration and atrophy of the rotator cuff do not improve after rotator cuff repair and correlate with poor functional outcome. *Am J Sports Med* 2007; 35:719-28.

Goutallier D., Postel J.M., Bernageau J., Lavau L., Voisin M.C. Fatty muscle degeneration in cuff ruptures. Pre - and post-operative evaluation by CT SCAN sa. *Clinorthop Relat Res* 1994; 304:78-83.

Hollister M.S., Macl L.A., Patten R.M., WinterT.C. 3rd, Matsen F.A 3rd., Veith R.R., Association of sonographically detected subacromial/subdeltoid bursal effusion and intraartricular fluid with rotator cuff tear. *AJR Am J Roentgenol* 1995; 165:605-8.

Jensen K.L., Williams G.R Jr, Russell I.J., Rockwood C.A Jr., Rotator cuff tear arthropathy. *J Bone Joint Surg* 1999; 81:1312-24.

Jo C.H., Kim J.E., Yoon K.S., Lee J.H., Kang S.B. et al., Does platelet rich plasma accelerate recovery after rotatro cuff repair? A prospective cohort study. *Am J Sports Med* 2011; 39:2082-90.

Khan K.M., Cook J.L., Bonar F., Harcourt P., Astrom M., Histopatho-logy of common tendinopathies. Update and implication for clinical management. *Sport Med* 1999; 27: 393-408.

Kim H.M., Dahiya N., Teefey P.A., Middleton W.D., Stobbs G., Steger-May K. Et al., Location and initiation of degenerative rotator cuff tears: an analysis of the three hundred and sixty shoulders. *J Bone and Joint Surgery Am* 2010; 92:1088-96.

Kirkley A., Alvarez C., Griffin P., The development and evaluation of the disease-specific quality-of-the-life questionnaire for disorders of the rotator cuff: The Western Ontario Rotator Cuff Index. *Clin J Sport Med* 2003; 13:84-92.

Kirsten L., Lian O.B., Scott A.P. Nassap, Fearon A.,Engebretsen L. Rotator cuff tear degeneration and cell apoptosis in smokers versus nonsmokers. *Arthroscopy* 2014 Aug;30(8): 936-41.

Lee Y.S., Kim J.Y., Ki S.Y., Chung S.W. Effects of smoking on the expression of genes and proteins related fat infiltration, inflammation and fibrosis in the rotator cuff muscles of patients with chronic rotator cuff tears: a pilot study. *Arthroscopy* 2019 Dec;35 (12): 3181-3191.

Longo G.U., Candela V., Berton A., Salvatore G., Guarnieri A., DeAngelis J., Nazarian A., Denaro V. Genetic basis of rotator cuff injury: a systematic rewiew. *BMC Medical Genetics* 2019 Sep 2;20(1): 149.

Mall N.A., Kim H.M., Keener J.D., Steger-May K., Teefey P.A., Middleton W.D. et al.,. Symptomatic progress of asymptomatic rotator cuff tear: a prospective study of clinical and sonographic variables. *J Bone Joint Surg Am* 2010; 92:2623-33.

Matsen, F.A., Harryman, D.T. and Sidles, J.A. (1991) Mechanics of Glenohumeral instability. *Clinics in sport medicine Oct;* 10 (4):783-8.

McMonagle P., Vinson E.N., MRI of the shoulder: Rotator Cuff. *Appl Radiol* 2012; 41:20-8.

Murrel G.A., Walton J.R., Diagnosis of rotator cuff tears. *The Lancet* 2001; 357:769-70.

Namdari S. Donegan R.P., Chamberlain A.M., Galatz L.M., Yamaguchi K., Keener. D. Factor affecting outcome after structural failure of repaired rotator cuff tears. *J Bone Joint Surg Am* 2014;96:99-105.

Neer C.S. 2nd. Impingement lesions. *Clin Orthop Relat Res* 1983 Mar; (173): 70-7.

Nove-Josserand L., Levigne C., Noel E., Walch G. The acromio-humeral interval. A study of the factors influencing its height. *Rev Chir Orthop Reparatrice Appar Mot* 1996; 82:379-85.

Robertson P.L., Schweitzer M.E., Mitchell D.G., Schlesinger F., Epstein R.E., Frieman B.G., Rotator cuff disorders: interobserver and intraobserver variation in diagnosis with MR imaging. *Radiology* 1995; 194:831-5.

Tashjian R.Z., Farnham J.M., Albright F.S., Teerlink C.C., Cannon-Albright L.A., For an inherited predisposition contributing to the risk for rotator cuff disease. *J Bone Joint Surg Am.* 2009;91(5):1136-42.

Tempelhof S., Rupp P., Seil R. Age-related prevalence of rotator cuff tears in asymptomatic *shoulders. J Shoulder Elbow Surgery* 1999; 8:296-9.

Turgut M.C., Toy, S., Mehmet, K., &Engin, M.Ç., Clinical and Functional Outcomes of Using Double-Row Transosseous Fixation Material in Advanced Age Treatment of Rotator Cuff Tears: Treatment of Rotator Cuff Tears. *Arch Curr Med Res*. 2021;2(2), 57-63.

Urwin M., Symmons D., Allison T., Brammah T., Busby H., Roxby M., Estimating the burden of musculoskeletal disorders in the community: The comparative prevalence of symptoms at different anatomical sites, and the relationship to social deprivation. *Annals of the Rheumatic Diseases* 1998;57:649-55.

Vogel K.G., Heinegard D. (1985) Characterization of preteoglykans from adult bovine tendon. *J BiolChem*1985; 260:9298-306.

Yamaguchi K., Ditsios K., Middleton W.D., Hildebolt C.F., Galatz L.M., Teefey P.A., The demographic and morphological features of rotator cuff disease. A composition of asymptomatic and symptomatic shoulders. *J Bone Joint Surg Am* 2006; 88:1699-704.

In: Musculoskeletal Pain (Common Clinical Presentations) ISBN: 978-1-68507-410-4
Editors: Mehmet Cenk Turgut and Serdar Toy 

*Chapter 14*

# SHOULDER IMPINGEMENT SYNDROME

***Erdem Sahin**, *MD***

Department of Orthopedics and Traumatology, Health Sciences University Erzurum Regional Training and Research Hospital, Erzurum, Turkey

## ABSTRACT

Impingement syndrome is mechanical compression of the rotator cuff tendons under the antero-inferior part of the acromion and in the flexion and internal rotation position of the shoulder. Two mechanical theories have been proposed as to the cause of the space narrowing in SIS. These can be defined as "intrinsic degeneration" and "extrinsic compression." SIS is diagnosed with anamnesis, physical examination and complementary imaging methods. There are 2 options in the treatment of SIS: conservative and surgical. A personal treatment plan is edited for each patient according to pain, functional status and accompanying pathologies.

**Keywords:** shoulder, subacromial, impingement syndrome

* Corresponding Author's E-mail: dr.erdemsahin@gmail.com.

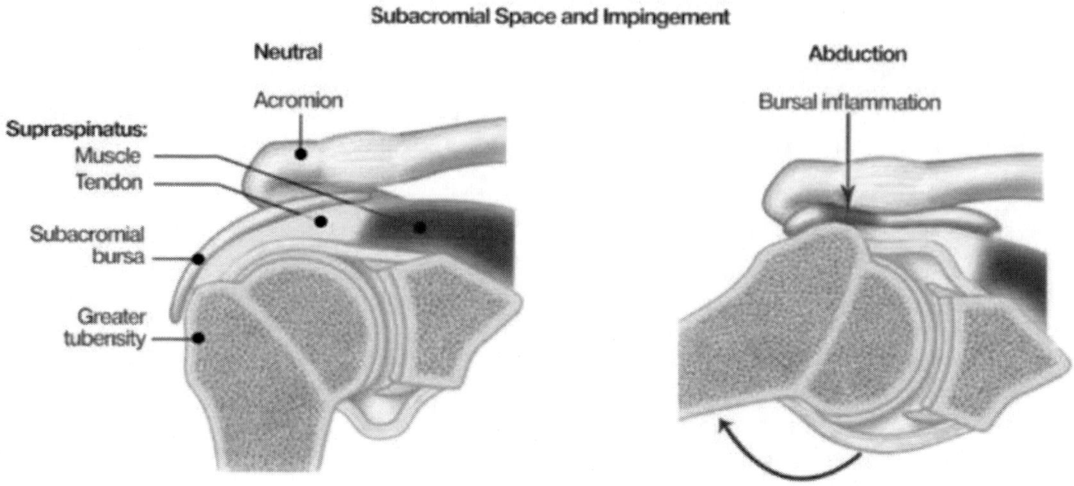


Source: From the author's individual archives.

Figure 1. Subacromial Space.

## INTRODUCTION

Impingement syndrome was described by Neer in 1972 as the mechanical compression of the rotator cuff tendons under the antero-inferior part of the acromion and in the flexion and internal rotation position of the shoulder (Neer, 1972).

The subacromial space is the region bounded by the humeral head and tuberculum majus inferiorly, the anterior third of the acromion, the coracoacromial ligament, the coracoid protrusion and the acromioclavicular joint and the acromioclavicular ligament in the superior (Neer, 1972). Within the space are the supraspinatus tendon, the subacromial bursa, the long head of the biceps brachii tendon and the capsule of the shoulder joint (Figure 1).

Shoulder impingement syndrome (SIS) can present in many forms, ranging from inflammation to degeneration of the bursa and rotator cuff tendons as a result of the narrowing of the subacromial space (Michener et al., 2003).

## ETIOLOGY

Two mechanical theories have been proposed as to the cause of the space narrowing in SIS. These can be defined as "intrinsic degeneration" and "extrinsic compression."

Intrinsic degeneration is partial or full thickness tendon tears because of the degenerative process that occurs with overuse, tension overload or trauma of the tendons

(Budoff et al., 1998). The main reason is the blood supply decreases in the rotator cuff tendons.

Extrinsic compression is inflammation and degeneration of the tendon because of mechanical compression by some external structures to the tendon. These are altered scapular or glenohumeral kinematics, posterior capsular tightness and acromial or coracoacromial arch pathology (Neer, 1972).

There is no consensus on the etiology in the literature, but it is probably caused by the combination of extrinsic compression and intrinsic degeneration.

## DIAGNOSIS

SIS is diagnosed with anamnesis, physical examination and complementary imaging methods.

SIS is the most common cause of shoulder pain and dysfunction; patients usually present with complaints of pain in overhead movements and an inability to lie on the affected shoulder at night.

In physical examination, first of all, the range of motion of the shoulder and the strength of the rotator cuff are evaluated. Especially the cervical spine should be included in the examination in terms of differential diagnosis other than the patient's shoulder.

Specific defined tests that provoke symptoms are valuable physical examination methods in the diagnosis of SIS. The Neer sign and the Hawkins test, which are frequently used, provoke symptoms by narrowing the subacromial distance.

In the Neer sign, the scapula is stabilized by the hand of the examiner and the shoulder is passively brought to maximum flexion (Figure 2). Feeling pain indicates a positive test (Neer, 1983). In the Hawkins test, the presence of pain is questioned by performing maximum internal rotation after the shoulder is passively flexioned by 90° forward (Figure 3). Some studies (Pappas et al., 2006; Roberts et al., 2002) have shown that the Hawkins test causes more narrowing in the subacromial area compared to the Neer sign.

The Neer impingement test is characterized by decreases of pain in provocative tests performed after approximately 10 ml of local anesthetic is administered to the subacromysal area (Neer, 1983).

Many tendon pathologies can accompany SIS, and specific tests have been described to reveal them.

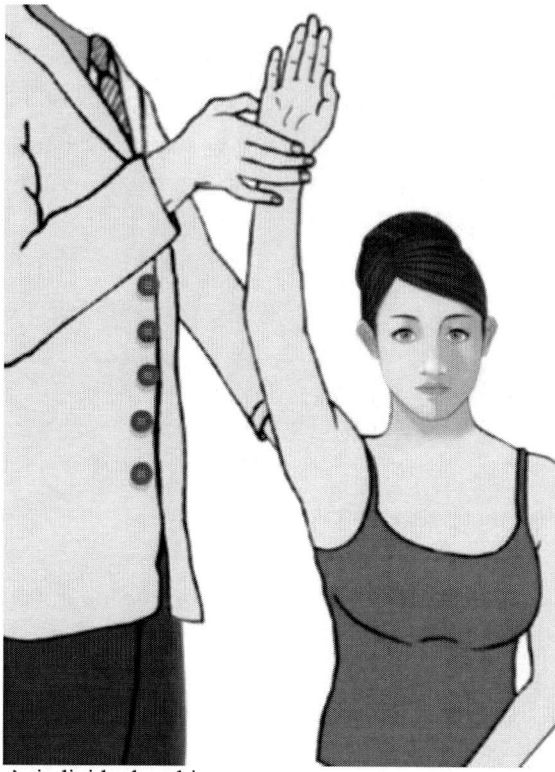

Source: From the author's individual archives.

Figure 2. Neer sign.

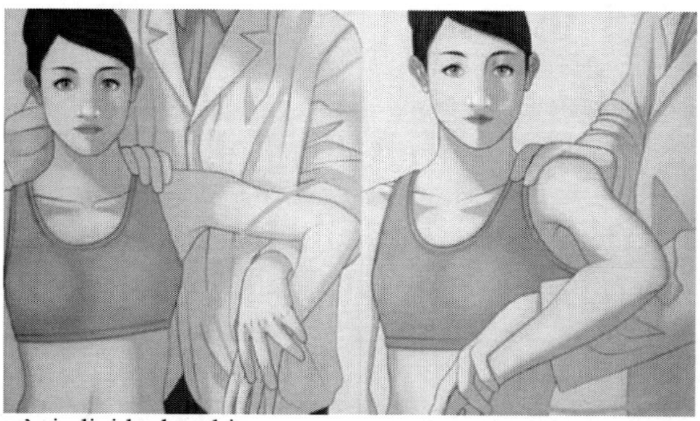

Source: From the author's individual archives.

Figure 3. Hawkins test.

Firstly, radiographs are preferred in the imaging methods. It is aimed to evaluate the glenohumeral joint, acromion and acromioclavicular joint in radiographs. These include antero-posterior views in internal and external rotation, an axillary view and a supraspinatus outlet view (Figure 4). A high-riding humeral head with a narrowed subacromial space (<7 mm) suggests a rotator cuff tear. Subchondral cysts and sclerosis in the tuberculum majus, and sclerosis and spur formation in the anterior of the acromion are also important findings on AP radiography. A curved or beaked anterior acromion, as seen on the outlet view, is often associated with impingement. An axillary view may show an os acromiale. Bigliani et al. classified acromial morphology and correlated it with rotator cuff tears in 1986 (Bigliani et al., 1986). They described three types of acromion: flat (type I), curved (type II) and hooked (type III) (Figure 5). In addition, West Point axillary and Streyker notch views are useful in evaluating glenoid rim and Hill-Sachs lesions.

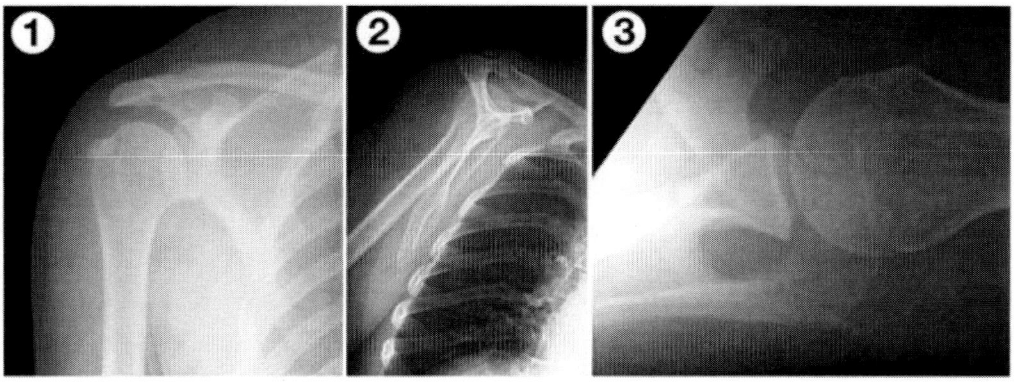


Source: From the author's individual archives. 1. Anteroposterior view 2. Supraspinatus Outlet view 3. Axillary view.

Figure 4. Shoulder X-Ray Views.

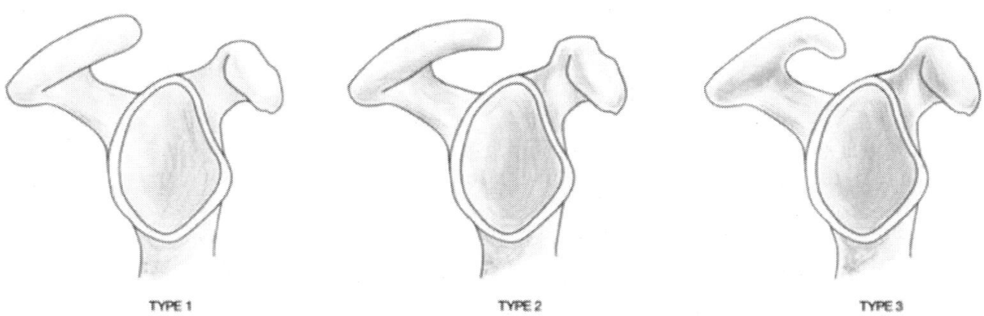


Source: From the author's individual archives. Type 1 (flat), Type 2 (curved), Type 3 (hooked).

Figure 5. Bigliani classification [7].

When a patient is thought to have a rotator cuff tear, various imaging studies may be performed to confirm the diagnosis. Although ultrasonography has emerged as a useful tool because of its ability to obtain dynamic images, the utility of ultrasound depends heavily on the experience of the radiologist.

Magnetic resonance imaging (MRI) is an advantageous method because it has a non-invasive method and does not contain radiation. Tendinitis, bursitis, biceps tendon pathologies, muscle atrophy, acromioclavicular joint pathologies and the acromion type are seen in MRI. It is especially helpful in demonstrating the presence of a partial or full thickness tear in the rotator cuff.

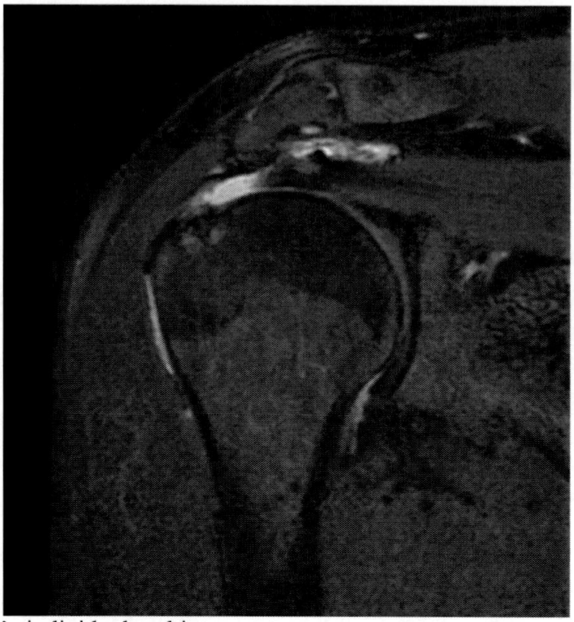

Source: From the author's individual archives.

Figure 6. Rotator cuff tear with subacromial impingement.

## Treatment

There are 2 options in the treatment of SIS: conservative and surgical. A personal treatment plan is edited for each patient according to pain, functional status and accompanying pathologies.

The frequently preferred conservative treatment is non-steroidal anti-inflammatory drugs, steroid injections into the subacromial space and physiotherapy. Surgical treatment is open or arthrocopic subacromial decompression.

Kromer et al. (Kromer et al., 2009) and Dorrestijin et al. (Dorrestijin et al., 2009) show that there is no statistically significant difference between physiotherapy and surgical treatment, so they recommend physiotherapy for each patient first.

The rehabilitation program aims to prevent pain in the patient, regression of inflammation, muscle atrophy, recovery of a painless range of motion (ROM) and normalization of shoulder arthrokinematics in the acute phase. In this phase, active periodic rest and avoiding activities that increase pain are desired, while pendular shoulder exercises, to strengthen the inner and outer shoulder rotator muscles, biceps, deltoids and scapular stabilizing muscles are recommended. If success is achieved in the acute phase, the recovery rehabilitation phase is passed and at this phase, it is aimed to fully recover the ROM, return to a symptom-free daily life and develop neuromuscular power.

Steroid injection with local anesthetic into the subacromial space can be used in both diagnosis and treatment. The study by Codsi (Codsi, 2007) showed that steroid injection alone was never a SIS treatment, and it should be applied to patients who did not succeed in changing the level of pain after six weeks of physiotherapy, or to reduce the pain threshold in the first physiotherapy.

Surgical treatment is generally recommended for patients whose complaints do not heal despite conservative treatment for 3-6 months. It has been shown that surgical treatment will be more successful in patients who do not have limitation of movement in the shoulder, who have reduced pain after lidocaine injection, who have Type 3 acromion and who have changes in the rotator cuff on MRI (Chang, 2004).

In the comparative study conducted by Odenbring (Yamamoto et al., 2010), it was stated that arthroscopic decompression was clinically superior in long-term follow-up against open surgery. It has been shown in recent patient series that arthroscopic subacromial decompression continues to have an effect on long-term follow-up and has been successful (Lunsjö et al., 2011). Although this surgical method is successful in the middle and advanced age group, it has been shown to be more successful in patients in the advanced age group (57 years and over) compared to physiotherapy (Biberthaler, 2013).

A shoulder immobilizer can be provided to feel comfortable in the early period after subacromial decompression. Afterwards, it should be removed as soon as possible and active passive ROMs should be started as learned in previous rehabilitation phases. The patients can usually return to normal activities after 3-4 months and to an active sports life.

## CONCLUSION

SIS is a common disorder of shoulder pain and dysfunction. Evidence suggests that extrinsic, intrinsic and combinations of biomechanical mechanisms play a role. SIS is diagnosed with anamnesis, physical examination and complementary imaging methods. Conservative treatment methods are first tried in treatment, and surgical treatment is recommended for patients who do not benefit from them. In the literature, many surgical interventions that include debridement and open or arthroscopic acromioplasty have been shown to be successful. However, there is a need for further clinical studies on the diagnosis and treatment of SIS.

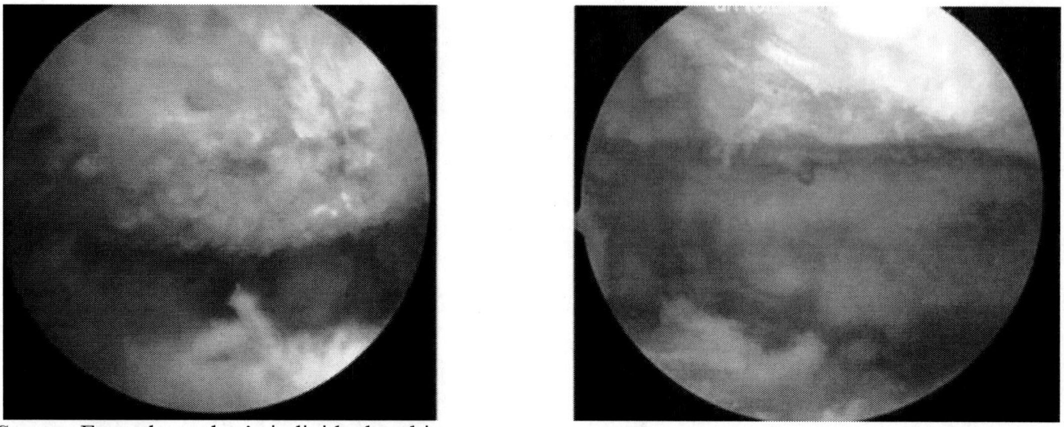

Source: From the author's individual archives.

Figure 7. Arthroscopic acromioplasty with burr impingement.

## References

Biberthaler, P., Beirer, M., Kirchhoff, S., Braunstein, V., Wiedemann, E., & Kirchhoff, C. (2013). Significant benefit for older patients after arthroscopic subacromial decompression: a long-term follow-up study. *International Orthopaedics*, 37(3), 457-462. https://doi.org/10. 1007/s00264-012-1760-x.

Bigliani, L. U., Morrison, D. S., April, E. W. (1986). The morphology of the acromion and its relationship to rotator cuff tears. *Ortho. Trans*. 10,228.

Budoff, J. E., Nirschl, R. P., & Guidi, E. J. (1998). Débridement of partial-thickness tears of the rotator cuff without acromioplasty. Long-term follow-up and review of the literature. *The Journal of Bone and Joint Surgery. American volume*, 80(5), 733-748. https://doi.org/10. 2106/00004623-199805000-00016.

Chang, W. K. (2004). Shoulder impingement syndrome. *Physical Medicine and Rehabilitation Clinics of North America*, 15(2), 493-510. https:// doi.org/10.1016/ j.pmr.2003.12.006.

Codsi, M. J. (2007). The painful shoulder: when to inject and when to refer. *Cleveland Clinic Journal of Medicine*, 74(7), https://doi.org/10. 3949/ccjm.74.7.473.

Dorrestijn, O., Stevens, M., Winters, J. C., van der Meer, K., & Diercks, R. L. (2009). Conservative or surgical treatment for subacromial impingement syndrome? A systematic review. *Journal of Shoulder and Elbow Surgery*, 18(4), 652-660. https://doi.org/10.1016/j.jse. 2009.01.010.

Kromer, T. O., Tautenhahn, U. G., de Bie, R. A., Staal, J. B., & Bastiaenen, C. H. (2009). Effects of physiotherapy in patients with shoulder impingement syndrome: a systematic review of the literature. *Journal of Rehabilitation Medicine*, 41(11), 870-880. https://doi.org/ 10.2340/16501977-0453.

Lunsjö, K., Bengtsson, M., Nordqvist, A., & Abu-Zidan, F. M. (2011). Patients with shoulder impingement remain satisfied 6 years after arthroscopic subacromial decompression: a prospective study of 46 patients. *Acta Orthopaedica*, 82(6), 711-713. https://doi.org/10.3109/ 17453674.2011.623571.

Michener, L. A., McClure, P. W., & Karduna, A. R. (2003). Anatomical and biomechanical mechanisms of subacromial impingement syndrome. *Clinical Biomechanics (Bristol, Avon)*, 18(5), 369-379. https://doi.org/10.1016/s0268-0033(03)00047-0.

Neer. C. S., 2nd (1972). Anterior acromioplasty for the chronic impingement syndrome in the shoulder: a preliminary report. *The Journal of Bone and Joint Surgery. American volume*, 54(1), 41-50.

Neer. C. S., 2nd (1983). Impingement lesions. *Clinical Orthopaedics and Related Research*, (173), 70-77.

Pappas, G. P., Blemker, S. S., Beaulieu, C. F., McAdams, T. R., Whalen, S. T., & Gold, G. E. (2006). *In vivo* anatomy of the Neer and Hawkins sign positions for shoulder impingement. *Journal of Shoulder and Elbow Surgery*, 15(1), 40-49. https://doi.org/ 10.1016/j.jse.2005.04. 007.

Roberts, C. S., Davila, J. N., Hushek, S. G., Tillett, E. D., & Corrigan, T. M. (2002). Magnetic resonance imaging analysis of the subacromial space in the impingement sign positions. *Journal of Shoulder and Elbow Surgery*, 11(6), 595-599. https://doi.org/10.1067/mse.2002. 127095.

Yamamoto, N., Muraki, T., Sperling, J. W., Steinmann, S. P., Itoi, E., Cofield, R. H., & An, K. N. (2010). Contact between the coracoacromial arch and the rotator cuff tendons in nonpathologic situations: a cadaveric study. *Journal of Shoulder and Elbow Surgery*, 19(5), 681-687. https://doi.org/10.1016/j.jse.2009.12.006.

In: Musculoskeletal Pain (Common Clinical Presentations) ISBN: 978-1-68507-410-4
Editors: Mehmet Cenk Turgut and Serdar Toy 

*Chapter 15*

# BICEPS TENDINOPATHY

***Emel Güler*, MD***
Department of Physical Therapy and Rehabilitation,
Division of Algology, University of Sivas Cumhuriyet, Sivas, Turkey

## ABSTRACT

Biceps tendinopathy is a relatively common ailment that typically presents as pain, tenderness, and weakness in the tendon of the long head of the biceps brachii. Pathologies occurring in the insertio part of the muscle shouldn't be hope for. A thorough patient history, physical examination and radiographic evaluation are necessary for diagnosis. Nonsurgical management including rest, nonsteroidal anti-inflamatuvar drugs, physical therapy and injection is approached first in patients with mild disease. Surgical management is indicated for refractory pain or severe disease.

## INTRODUCTION

The shoulder is the joint of the body with the widest range of motion. One of the anatomical formations providing the continuity of the movement and stabilization of this joint, also called the glenohumeral, is the long head of the biceps brachii muscle tendon. It has a vital role in joint stabilization. Shoulder pain is one of the most common musculoskeletal pathologies, and biceps tendinopathy is one of these pain sources. Meyer first described it in 1936 (Meyer, 1937).

Its etiology is divided into primary and secondary causes:

* Corresponding Author's E-mail: emelguler@cumhuriyet.edu.tr.

- Primary; This is an isolated tendon injury in the bicipital groove without any shoulder pathology. It constitutes 5% of biceps tendinopathies. It is seen due to mechanical stress in young athletes and sports people or bicipital groove anomalies.
- Secondary; This is seen due to shoulder pathologies such as rotator cuff lesion, superior labrum anteroposterior lesion (SLAP), or impingement syndrome (Churgay, 2009; Hassan & Patel, 2019; Longo et al., 2011).

When considering biceps tendon pathologies, the focus is often on proximal biceps tendon lesions, but distal biceps tendon pathologies are also not uncommon. An annual distal tendon partial or complete rupture has an incidence of 1.2 per 100,000 (Frank, Cotter, Strauss, Jazrawi, & Romeo, 2018).

When diagnosing biceps tendinopathy, which is common in clinical practice and adversely affects upper extremity functions and quality of life, it is necessary to have good knowledge of the anatomical structure.

## ANATOMY

The biceps brachii, of Latin origin, means the two heads of the arm, and it is one of the three muscles of the anterior compartment of the upper arm. It consists of two parts called the caput longum and the caput breve. The nervus musculocutaneous innervates it (originating from the fasciculus lateralis (C5-6-7) of the plexus brachialis). The caput longum originates from the scapula tuberculum supraglenoidale and the caput breve from the processus coracoideus end of the scapula. The caput longum part is about 9 cm long, and its intense sensory sympathetic fiber innervation explains its role in the etiology of anterior shoulder pain. The capsuloligamentous complex, called the bicipital pulley (composed of the coracohumeral and superior glenohumeral ligament), stabilizes the caput longum tendon. The tendon of the long head crosses over the caput humeri within the joint capsule and emerges from the joint, wrapped in a synovial sheath (Figure 1).

It proceeds to the proximal one-third of the humerus within the synovial sheath. Besides, a membrane called the *Vinculum* is located in the synovial sheath and develops from the long head running in the humeral groove. It has superior localization during rotation and provides vascular feeding of the tendon. It is thought that this structure protects from the *Popeye deformity* seen as a result of the long head total lesion.

The distal tendons of the muscle cross the elbow joint and terminate on the posterior surface of the tuberositas radii and in the fascia profunda on the inner side of the forearm with a band called the aponeurosis bicipitalis. At the distal biceps musculotendinous junction, the bicipital aponeurosis (also called the lacertus fibrosus) originates from the distal bicipital tendon and is located on the radial tuberosity and proximal ulna. This structure prevents retraction of the tendon in biceps tendon injury (Schwantes & Byerly, 2021). The function of the muscle is flexion of the arm and flexion and supination of the forearm. How does tendinopathy develop in the biceps muscle, whose anatomical structure is examined in detail?

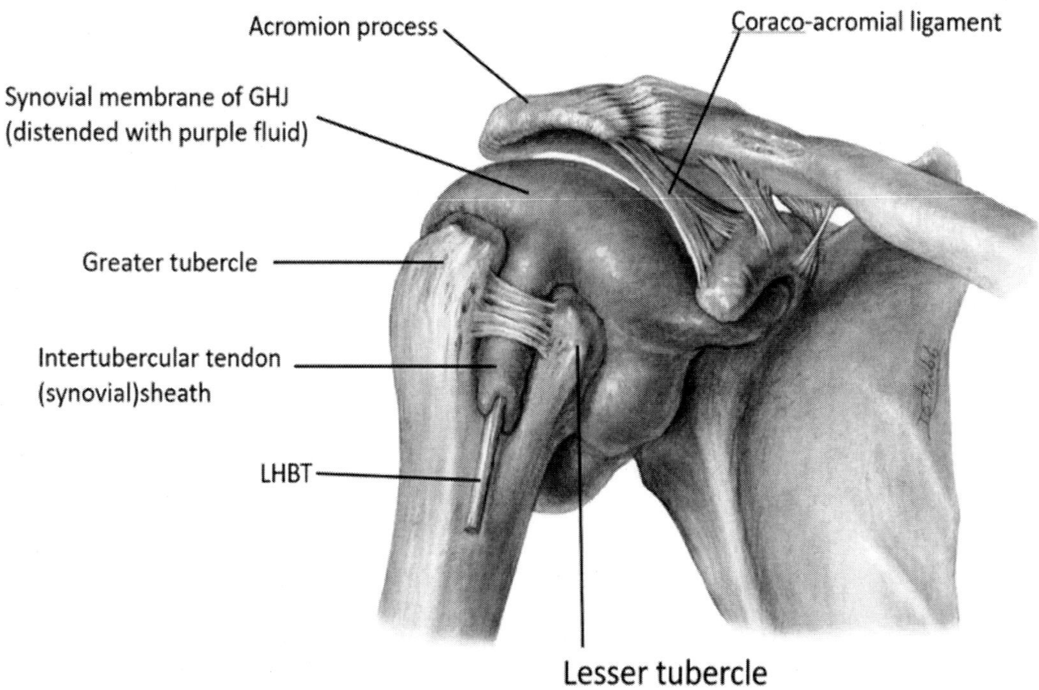


Figure 1. Anatomy of M. Biceps Brachii (Gofeld, Hurdle, & Agur, 2019).

## Tendinopathy Formation Mechanisms

By definition, this is the clinical designation of the tendon and surrounding tissues without defining a specific pathology. Therefore, this definition includes tendinitis, tendinosis, paratenonitis, and tendon ruptures. While tendinitis describes an inflammatory pathology, tendinosis denotes a degenerative tendon clinic not necessarily accompanied by inflammation, and paratenonitis is defined as tissue inflammation around the tendon. Tendinopathy is characterized by loss of function, localized swelling, and progressive morning stiffness. Crepitation may be detected during palpation due to fibrin precipitation in the fibrinogen-rich fluid around the tendon. Since it is a general definition, anamnesis, physical examination, and imaging methods are used in etiology (Raney, Thankam, Dilisio, & Agrawal, 2017).

Nowadays, four theories are put forward in etiology;

- Mechanical,
- Vascular,
- Apoptosis, and
- Neural.

We examine these theories in detail;

### *Mechanical Theory*

This is explained as tendon fatigue and failure due to repetitive loading on the tendon in everyday physiological stress. This theory is defined for the degenerative clinic. It occurs by repetitive microscopic damage accumulating over time. It cannot explain why certain tendon areas are affected or the mechanism of pain formation (Jomaa et al., 2020; Mosca et al., 2018).

### *Vascular Theory*

The tendon needs vascular nutrition to meet its metabolic needs. Certain areas of some tendons are more prone to vascular malnutrition than others. A hypovascular area is very open to degenerative changes (Ohberg & Alfredson, 2004).

### *Apoptosis Theory*

In this theory, the result of deterioration seen in tendinopathy is increased intracellular stress followed by programmed cell death. Increased cell death and increased friction between the collagen fibers cause the fibers to break down and make the tendon susceptible to tearing.

### *Neural Theory*

In neural theory, also called neurogenic theory, it is suggested that nerve endings and mast cells function as modulators of tendon homeostasis and mediators of adaptive response to mechanical load. Overstimulation of nerve endings and mast cells causes pathologies in the tendon matrix due to changes in neuronal homeostasis. Although it explains the mechanism of pain formation, not every tendinopathy is painful (Challoumas, Biddle, & Millar, 2020).

All the theories mentioned above should be considered as a whole and evaluated to explain the clinical findings.

Other factors that are blamed can be listed as;

- Genetic predisposition,
- Medicines: steroids, fluoroquinolones, and statins, and
- Environmental factors: smoking, metabolic dysfunction (e.g., diabetes, hyperlipidemia) (Challoumas et al., 2020).

## Physical Examination

During anamnesis, the patient complains of deep throbbing pain in the anterior shoulder, localized in the bicipital groove. The pain increases, especially at night or after physical activity. In addition, the patient's occupation, comorbidities, and medications must be questioned. During the inspection, the presence of redness, ecchymosis, and swelling in the anatomical localization of the biceps brachii muscle should be checked. Popeye's sign may be seen. Popeye's sign is a prominent muscle swelling distal to the biceps brachii muscle. It is clinically seen as a result of the long head of the biceps muscle translocating to the distal due to total tendon rupture (Lim, Lee, & Liew, 2020).

Both shoulder and elbow joints are evaluated for joint range of motion. The function of the muscle is forearm supination and elbow flexion. Some special tests are used in the physical examination. These are as follows;

### Speed's Test

Shoulder flexion is performed by applying resistance to the wrist while the shoulder is in 90 degrees of elevation or the arm is drooping to the side, the forearm is supinated, and the elbow is extended. The presence of pain suggests bicipital tendon pathology (Hanchard, Lenza, Handoll, & Takwoingi, 2013).

### Yergason's Test

With the elbow flexed to 90 degrees and the forearm pronated, one hand fixes the patient's elbow, and the other hand holds the patient's wrist. Counterforce is applied as the patient brings his arm to external rotation and forearm to supination. In this case, if the long biceps head is unstable, it slides to the groove lateral, and the patient feels pain (Hanchard et al., 2013).

### Hook Test

This is used for diagnostic purposes in distal biceps tendon pathology. While the patient's elbow is in active supination at 90 degrees of flexion, the index finger is placed lateral to the biceps tendon in the antecubital fossa. The finger can palpate the hook-shaped tendon. However, in distal tendon rupture, the finger cannot find a hook-shaped tendon to grasp (O'Driscoll, Goncalves, & Dietz, 2007).

Tenderness and pain may be seen in the bicipital groove or at the distal tendon attachment site during palpation.

## Imaging Methods

### Radiography and Computed Tomography

This is used to evaluate both the proximal and distal parts of the biceps brachii muscle. The distance between the acromion and the humeral head should be 7-14 mm in the anteroposterior view for the glenohumeral joint. Osteophyte, fracture, and calcification can be detected.

### Ultrasound (US)

This is a fast and effective method. Its advantages are being economical and noninvasive. Tendon thickening, synovial sheath tenosynovitis/ hypertrophy, and fluid increment around the tendon in the bicipital groove can be evaluated. It has high sensitivity and specificity (Zappia et al., 2019).

### Magnetic Resonance Imaging and Arthrography

Obtaining a multiplanar image and high soft-tissue resolution provides great advantages. Effusion within the tendon sheath, and thickening of the tendon, tear, or dislocation may be viewed. In magnetic resonance arthrography, both intra-articular and extra-articular structures are displayed in detail. However, its invasiveness is its most significant disadvantage.

### Arthroscopy

This is the most effective method in the evaluation of the intra-articular part of the biceps. It is an invasive method and has 100% diagnostic value.

## TREATMENT

Conservative treatment methods take the first place. However, the clinician should first evaluate the tendinopathy risk factors like repetitive trauma, drugs used by the patient, family history of inflammatory rheumatological disease or comorbid diabetes and hyperlipidemia, and establish a treatment protocol.

Nonsteroidal anti-inflammatory agents (NSAI) are the first choice in medical treatment. However, paracetamol may be preferred in cases where NSAI side effects should be avoided. Long-term use of the arm at head level should be avoided, and cold therapy, splint use, and rest are recommended in the acute period. Apart from this, physical therapy modalities like iontophoresis, ESWT (extracorporeal shock wave therapy), therapeutic ultrasound, and low-level laser therapy can be used. In local injection treatment, steroids and PRP (platelet-rich plasma) can be used. Surgical treatment is recommended for patients not responding to conservative treatment. Let us consider the treatment methods used in a little more detail.

### Physical Therapy Modalities

#### *Iontophoresis Treatment*

This is a physical therapy modality allowing different substances to pass through the skin using electric current. The galvanic current ionizes the substances and allows the ions to pass through the skin. Thus, the drugs penetrate the tissue. The most commonly used medical agent is corticosteroids (Gurcay, Unlu, Gurcay, Tuncay, & Cakci, 2012).

#### *Therapeutic Ultrasound (US)*

The different permeability of US sound waves in each tissue forms the basis of its therapeutic effectiveness. Its principal effects are increased blood flow, increased tissue metabolism, change in axonal function, increased connective tissue elasticity, and increased permeability of biological membranes.

#### *Low-Level Laser Therapy*

This creates reactive vasodilation by reducing the pain perception of sensory nerves and spasms in muscle arterioles with its photochemical effects. In the synovial membrane, regeneration by protein synthesis increases collagen synthesis by accelerating fibroblast activity and has analgesic and anti-inflammatory effects by increasing β-endorphins (Farivar, Malekshahabi, & Shiari, 2014).

### *ESWT (Extracorporeal Shock Wave Therapy)*

Overstimulation of the treated area (hyperstimulation) provides analgesia by reducing the transmission of pain signals to the brainstem, and is thus effective on pain. It also affects pain transmission by acting on substance P and calcitonin gene-related peptide expression (van der Worp, van den Akker-Scheek, van Schie, & Zwerver, 2013; Wang, 2012).

## Injection

### *Steroid Injection*

Steroid injection into the tendon sheath or peritendinous tissue has been used for many years and is currently performed with imaging methods (such as ultrasound or fluoroscopy) (Yiannakopoulos, Megaloikonomos, Foufa, & Gliatis, 2020).

### *PRP (Platelet-Rich Plasma) Injection*

Since tendinopathies are now generally considered to be a degenerative process rather than an inflammatory process, PRP usage to stimulate tendon healing has significantly increased (Barker, Bell, Connell, & Coghlan, 2015). Chemokines, cytokines, and growth factors released from platelets induce protein production in target cells responsible for collagen synthesis and cellular proliferation. The protein content of PRP functions as cell adhesion molecules and promotes fibroblast migration. It is suggested that activation of these cells accelerates tendon healing (Le, Enweze, DeBaun, & Dragoo, 2018). Studies on PRP applications rich in leukocytes (neutrophils) and poor in leukocytes (neutrophils) increase. However, there are no definite answers about which type will be used in which pathologies (Lana et al., 2019).

### *Mesenchymal Stem Cell Therapy*

This appears to be promising in tendon repair and regeneration. The most commonly used mesenchymal stem cell types are those derived from bone marrow and adipose tissue.

Although the mechanism of action is still not fully explained, it provides the release of paracrine factors in the target tissue, and regulates the immune response in the local microenvironment, as well as tissue regeneration (Challoumas et al., 2020; Qazi, Mooney, Duda, & Geissler, 2017).

## Surgical Treatment

This is applied in cases that do not respond to conservative treatment, have symptoms longer than three months, and require definitive surgery in imaging methods. The most commonly used surgical methods are reconstructive technique, tenotomy, and tenodesis.

### *Tenotomy*

This should be preferred when there is no cosmetic concern and simultaneous rotator cuff surgical repair is required (We, Vinanti, Rossato, Arnaldi, & Aldegheri, 2012).

### Advantages

- Technically easy, low cost,
- Rehabilitation is simple and short-term,
- It does not require immobilization.

### Disadvantages

- Deformity (Popeye deformity),
- Cramp persists for several months (especially in patients under 40 years of age),
- Weakness in the form of elbow flexion weakness.

### *Tenodesis*

The intra-articular part of the tendon is resected, and the remaining tendon is fixed from its proximal part to the proximal part of the humerus. Tenodesis is required in the following conditions:

- To restore resting muscle length, thus maintaining the relationship of muscle length and tension,
- To prevent muscle atrophy,
- To provide elbow flexion and forearm supination strength,
- To prevent cosmetic deformity.

The type of surgery to be applied to the patient should be chosen according to the patient's age, cosmetic concerns, changes in adjacent anatomical structures, and the need to intervene in these structures during surgery (Biz et al., 2012).

***Surgical Treatment Complications***

The most common complications are as follows (Friedman et al., 2015; Varacallo & Mair, 2021);

**Biceps Tenotomy**

- Cosmetics: Popeye (Popeis) deformity: 10-70%
- Muscle spasm/cramp: 15-25%
- Biceps pain: 10-20%.

**Biceps Tenodesis**

- Groove pain: 0-25%
- Cosmetic ("Popeye") deformity: 10-15%
- Muscle spasm/cramp: 5-10%
- Biceps pain: 5-10%.
- Humerus shaft fracture: In recent case reports, spiral humerus fractures have been observed in surgical procedures using an 8 mm intervention screw. In particular, increased fracture susceptibility with stretching the humerus with torsional load is worrisome (Sears, Spencer, & Getz, 2011).

After surgery, patients should be included in the rehabilitation program.

## Conclusion

Tendon of biceps brachii pathology is recognized as one of the causes of pain in shoulder and elbow diseases. Besides the physical examination, several imaging protocols have been proposed for the diagnosis of biceps tendinopathies. It should not be forgotten that there are many treatment options after diagnosis and resistant cases should be evaluated surgically.

## References

Barker, S. L., Bell, S. N., Connell, D., & Coghlan, J. A. (2015). Ultrasound-guided platelet-rich plasma injection for distal biceps tendinopathy. *Shoulder Elbow,* 7(2), 110-114. doi:10.1177/ 1758573214567558.

Biz, C., Vinanti, G. B., Rossato, A., Arnaldi, E., & Aldegheri, R. (2012). Prospective study of three surgical procedures for long head biceps tendinopathy associated with rotator cuff tears. *Muscles Ligaments Tendons J.*, 2(2), 133-136.

Challoumas, D., Biddle, M., & Millar, N. L. (2020). Recent advances in tendinopathy. *Fac. Rev.*, 9, 16. doi:10.12703/b/9-16.

Churgay, C. A. (2009). Diagnosis and treatment of biceps tendinitis and tendinosis. *Am. Fam. Physician,* 80(5), 470-476.

Farivar, S., Malekshahabi, T., & Shiari, R. (2014). Biological effects of low level laser therapy. *Journal of Lasers in Medical Sciences,* 5(2), 58.

Frank, R. M., Cotter, E. J., Strauss, E. J., Jazrawi, L. M., & Romeo, A. A. (2018). Management of Biceps Tendon Pathology: From the Glenoid to the Radial Tuberosity. *J. Am. Acad. Orthop. Surg.,* 26(4), e77-e89. doi:10.5435/JAAOS-D-17-00085.

Friedman, J. L., FitzPatrick, J. L., Rylander, L. S., Bennett, C., Vidal, A. F., & McCarty, E. C. (2015). Biceps Tenotomy versus Tenodesis in Active Patients Younger Than 55 Years: Is There a Difference in Strength and Outcomes? *Orthop. J. Sports Med.,* 3(2), 2325967115570848. doi:10.1177/2325967115570848.

Gofeld, M., Hurdle, M. F., & Agur, A. (2019). Biceps Tendon Sheath Injection: An Anatomical Conundrum. *Pain Med.,* 20(1), 138-142. doi:10.1093/pm/pny051.

Gurcay, E., Unlu, E., Gurcay, A. G., Tuncay, R., & Cakci, A. (2012). Assessment of phonophoresis and iontophoresis in the treatment of carpal tunnel syndrome: a randomized controlled trial. *Rheumatol. Int.,* 32(3), 717-722. doi:10.1007/s00296-010-1706-9.

Hanchard, N. C., Lenza, M., Handoll, H. H., & Takwoingi, Y. (2013). Physical tests for shoulder impingements and local lesions of bursa, tendon or labrum that may accompany impingement. *Cochrane Database Syst. Rev.* (4), CD007427. doi:10.1002/14651858. CD007427.pub2.

Hassan, S., & Patel, V. (2019). Biceps tenodesis versus biceps tenotomy for biceps tendinitis without rotator cuff tears. *J. Clin. Orthop. Trauma,* 10(2), 248-256. doi:10.1016/j.jcot.2018.12.013.

Jomaa, G., Kwan, C. K., Fu, S. C., Ling, S. K., Chan, K. M., Yung, P. S., & Rolf, C. (2020). A systematic review of inflammatory cells and markers in human tendinopathy. *BMC Musculoskelet. Disord.,* 21(1), 78. doi:10.1186/s12891-020-3094-y.

Lana, J. F., Huber, S. C., Purita, J., Tambeli, C. H., Santos, G. S., Paulus, C., & Annichino-Bizzacchi, J. M. (2019). Leukocyte-rich PRP versus leukocyte-poor PRP - The role of monocyte/macrophage function in the healing cascade. *J. Clin. Orthop. Trauma,* 10(Suppl 1), S7-S12. doi:10.1016/j.jcot.2019.05.008.

Le, A. D. K., Enweze, L., DeBaun, M. R., & Dragoo, J. L. (2018). Current Clinical Recommendations for Use of Platelet-Rich Plasma. *Curr. Rev. Musculoskelet. Med.,* 11(4), 624-634. doi:10.1007/s12178-018-9527-7.

Lim, C. H., Lee, K. A., & Liew, J. W. (2020). Popeye's sign: biceps tendon rupture. *BMJ Case Rep.,* 13(2). doi:10.1136/bcr-2019-234205.

Longo, U. G., Loppini, M., Marineo, G., Khan, W. S., Maffulli, N., & Denaro, V. (2011). Tendinopathy of the tendon of the long head of the biceps. *Sports Med. Arthrosc. Rev.,* 19(4), 321-332. doi:10.1097/JSA. 0b013e3182393e23.

Meyer, A. (1937). Chronic functional lesions of the shoulder. *Archives of Surgery,* 35(4), 646-674.

Mosca, M. J., Rashid, M. S., Snelling, S. J., Kirtley, S., Carr, A. J., & Dakin, S. G. (2018). Trends in the theory that inflammation plays a causal role in tendinopathy: a systematic review and quantitative analysis of published reviews. *BMJ Open Sport Exerc. Med.,* 4(1), e000332. doi:10.1136/bmjsem-2017-000332.

O'Driscoll, S. W., Goncalves, L. B., & Dietz, P. (2007). The hook test for distal biceps tendon avulsion. *Am. J. Sports Med.,* 35(11), 1865-1869. doi:10.1177/0363546507305016.

Ohberg, L., & Alfredson, H. (2004). Effects on neovascularisation behind the good results with eccentric training in chronic mid-portion Achilles tendinosis? *Knee Surg. Sports Traumatol. Arthrosc.,* 12(5), 465-470. doi:10.1007/s00167-004-0494-8.

Qazi, T. H., Mooney, D. J., Duda, G. N., & Geissler, S. (2017). Biomaterials that promote cell-cell interactions enhance the paracrine function of MSCs. *Biomaterials,* 140, 103-114. doi:10.1016/j. biomaterials.2017.06.019.

Raney, E. B., Thankam, F. G., Dilisio, M. F., & Agrawal, D. K. (2017). Pain and the pathogenesis of biceps tendinopathy. *Am. J. Transl. Res.,* 9(6), 2668-2683.

Schwantes, J., & Byerly, D. W. (2021). Biceps Tendon Sheath Injection *StatPearls*. Treasure Island (FL).

Sears, B. W., Spencer, E. E., & Getz, C. L. (2011). Humeral fracture following subpectoral biceps tenodesis in 2 active, healthy patients. *J. Shoulder Elbow Surg.,* 20(6), e7-11. doi:10.1016/j.jse.2011.02.020.

van der Worp, H., van den Akker-Scheek, I., van Schie, H., & Zwerver, J. (2013). ESWT for tendinopathy: technology and clinical implications. *Knee Surg. Sports Traumatol. Arthrosc.,* 21(6), 1451-1458. doi:10. 1007/s00167-012-2009-3.

Varacallo, M., & Mair, S. D. (2021). Proximal Biceps Tendinitis and Tendinopathy *StatPearls*. Treasure Island (FL).

Wang, C. J. (2012). Extracorporeal shockwave therapy in musculoskeletal disorders. *J. Orthop. Surg. Res.,* 7, 11. doi:10.1186/1749-799X-7-11.

Yiannakopoulos, C. K., Megaloikonomos, P. D., Foufa, K., & Gliatis, J. (2020). Ultrasound-guided versus palpation-guided corticosteroid injections for tendinosis of the long head of the biceps: A randomized comparative study. *Skeletal Radiology,* 49(4), 585-591.

Zappia, M., Chianca, V., Di Pietto, F., Reginelli, A., Natella, R., Maggialetti, N., Faletti, C. (2019). Imaging of long head biceps tendon. A multimodality pictorial essay. *Acta Biomed.,* 90(5-S), 84-94. doi:10.23750/abm.v90i5-S.8351.

In: Musculoskeletal Pain (Common Clinical Presentations) ISBN: 978-1-68507-410-4
Editors: Mehmet Cenk Turgut and Serdar Toy 

*Chapter 16*

# CUBITAL TUNNEL SYNDROME

***Mehmet Eren**, *MD***
Department of Hand Surgery, Başakşehir Çam and Sakura City Hospital, Istanbul, Turkey

## ABSTRACT

Cubital tunnel syndrome is the most common compression neuropathy in the upper extremity after carpal tunnel syndrome (Boone, Gelberman & Calfee, 2015). The most common site of compression of the ulnar nerve is the elbow, and this is known as cubital tunnel syndrome (Karatas, Apaydin, Uz, Tubbs, Loukas, & Gezen, 2009). Entrapment of the ulnar nerve in the cubital tunnel can occur in the acute or chronic process. Risk factors include female gender, advanced age, systemic neuropathy (such as diabetes), occupations requiring repetitive or challenging elbow flexion, and sleeping with elbow flexion (Davidge & Mackinnon, 2015). Conservative treatment that is applied for 2-4 months can be started in many patients with mild cubital tunnel syndrome. At least 3 months of conservative treatment can be preferred in patients with a motor conduction velocity of more than 40 m/sec along the elbow with electrodiagnostic tests (MacKinnon & Novak, 2017). In patients with chronic symptoms and muscle atrophy, surgical treatment is often required in patients with failed conservative treatment (Palmer & Hughes, 2010). Surgical options include in situ decompression, subcutaneous transposition, intramuscular transposition, submuscular transposition, and medial epicondyectomy (Novak & Mackinnon, 2009).

* Corresponding Author's E-mail: drmehmeteren@hotmail.com.

## INTRODUCTION

Cubital tunnel syndrome is the most common compression neuropathy in the upper extremity after carpal tunnel syndrome (Boone, Gelberman, Calfee, 2015). The ulnar nerve can be entrapped at many different points along its course. However, the most compressed region is the elbow and this case is known as cubital tunnel syndrome (Karatas, Apaydin, Uz, Tubbs, Loukas & Gezen, 2009).

There are 4 regions where the ulnar nerve can be trapped around the elbow. From proximal to distal, these regions can be organized as the arcade of Struthers, the medial intermuscular septum, the medial condyle gutter and the Osborne arcuate ligament (Figure 1).

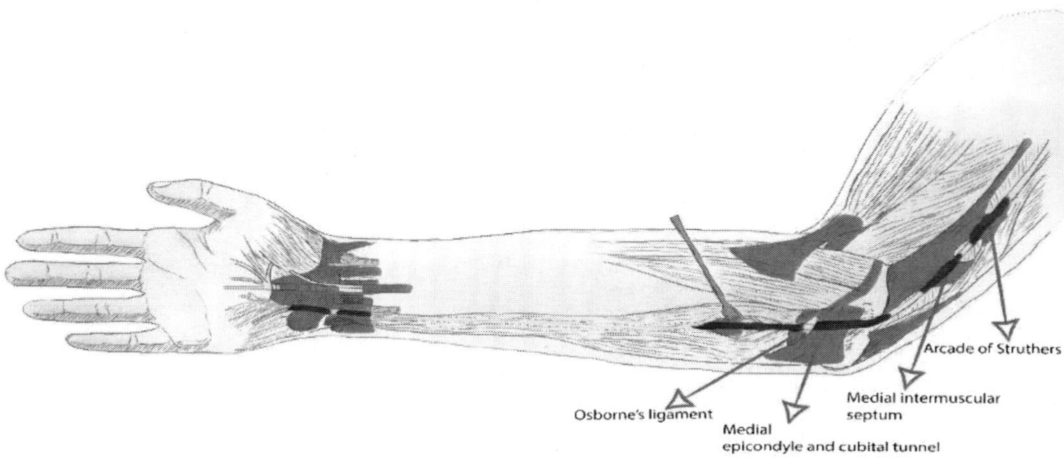


Figure 1. Possible trap regions of the ulnar nerve at the elbow level.

Entrapment of the ulnar nerve in the cubital tunnel can occur in the acute or chronic process. Neuronal ischemia, repetitive activities requiring elbow flexion, and scar tissues that develop as a result of trauma can have a role as an etiological factor in the chronic compression. Acute trauma to the ulnar nerve during elbow fractures and surgical procedures, and with above-elbow plaster may have a role as an etiological factor in ulnar nerve entrapment in the acute process (MacKinnon & Novak, 2017). In addition, subluxation of the ulnar nerve may lead to the development of cubital tunnel syndrome (Novak, Mehdian & von Schroeder, 2012). Female gender, advanced age, systemic neuropathy (such as diabetes), occupations requiring repetitive or challenging elbow flexion, and sleeping with elbow flexion are included in the other risk factors (Davidge & Mackinnon, 2015). Biomechanical studies have shown that the cubital tunnel area is reduced by 55% by elbow flexion (Apefelberg & Larson, 1973). This reduction will increase the pressure on the ulnar nerve and cause the symptoms of ulnar nerve entrapment. Pechan and Julis defined increased pressure in the cubital tunnel from elbow flexion and noted that the pressure can reach even more dangerous levels with wrist extension or shoulder abduction (or both) (Pechan & Julis, 1975).

It is hard to diagnose cubital tunnel syndrome because mostly patients do not notice till the symptoms are severe and the nerve is damaged (Andrews, Rowland, Pranjal & Ebraheim, 2018). Mostly, patients admit with symptoms of both sensory and motor disorders. The degree of sensory and motor disorders is important in making the treatment decision that can range from conservative to surgical treatment. It is crucial that the anatomy and pathophysiology of each case of cubital tunnel syndrome are understood for accurate diagnosis and treatment (Andrews et al., 2018).

## ANATOMY

The ulnar nerve originates from the C8-T1 nerve roots and continues as a terminal branch of the medial cord. In the upper part of the arm, the ulnar nerve is located posteromedial of the brachial artery, posterior of the intermuscular septum, and anterior of the medial head of the triceps muscle in the upper part of the arm. The arcade of Struthers is a deep brachial fascial band covering the ulnar nerve about 8 cm proximal to the medial epicondyle (MacKinnon & Novak, 2017). At the elbow, the ulnar nerve passes through the structures that form the cubital tunnel. The ligament of Osborne forms the roof of the cubital tunnel. The Osborne ligament, also known as the cubital retinaculum, is a ligament that extends from the medial epicondyle to the olecranon bursitis and continues with the humeral and ulnar fascial connection of the flexor carpi ulnaris (FCU) (Granger, Sardi & Iwanaga, 2017). While the floor of the cubital tunnel consists of the medial collateral ligament (MCL) and the elbow joint capsule, the medial epicondyle and olecranon act as walls on both sides (Huang, Samadani & Zager, 2004). While the elbow is at 135° flexion, it is shown that the height and width of the area of the tunnel decrease and the ulnar nerve is entrapped between the Osborne ligament and the MCL in a max level (James, Sutton, Werner, Basu, Allison & Palmer, 1988). After passing through the cubital tunnel, the ulnar nerve runs deep into the forearm between the ulnar and humeral heads of the flexor carpi ulnaris muscle.

## CLINICAL PRESENTATION

Cubital tunnel syndrome may occur with both sensory and motor disorders resulting in temporary or permanent loss of function (Norkus & Meyers, 1994). Complaints are usually paresthesia and numbness in the little finger and ring finger with pain in the inner side of the elbow and forearm. In delayed clinical admissions or untreated cases muscle weakness and atrophy can occur over time (Folberg, Weiss & Akelman, 1994; Bradshaw & Shefner, 1999). Because the elbow flexion entraps the cubital tunnel area and ulnar nerve, paresthesias generally become severe with elbow flexion activities such as usage of the phone or those requiring repetitive elbow movements (Bozentka, 1998; Robertson & Saratsiotis, 2005; Granger et al., 2017; Gelberman, Yamaguchi & Hollstien, 1998; Werner, Ohlin & Elmqvist, 1985). Patients may have difficulty with daily life activities such as opening jars or holding pens (Andrews et al., 2018). Eventually, the appearance of the hand may become a claw deformity because of intrinsic muscle failure and the opposite function of the FDP (Folberg et al., 1994).

Evaluation begins with inspection and palpation, as in every clinical examination. With careful inspection, muscle atrophy and claw hand deformity can be noticed; at the same time, a careful palpation examination can evaluate whether the ulnar nerve is subluxated at the medial epicondyle level (Norkus & Meyers, 1994). Patients with cubital tunnel syndrome have a 4-fold higher rate of admission with atrophy than patients with carpal tunnel syndrome (Mallette, Zhao, Zurakowski & Ring, 2007).

Provocative tests (the Tinel test, elbow flexion test, and scratch collapse test) are important, especially in the early diagnosis of cubital tunnel syndrome. The Tinel test is performed by gently tapping the nerve to be examined with the tip of the finger. The test is considered to be positive with the formation of paresthesia in the distribution area of the nerve. The elbow flexion test is a provocative test like the Tinel test. In the elbow flexion test, the shoulder is kept in slight abduction, and the elbow is fully flexed and held in this position. In this way, the cubital tunnel will narrow and the pressure on the ulnar nerve will increase. The test is considered to be positive if there is paresthesia and/or tingling in the distribution of the ulnar nerve in the forearm and hand (Posner, 2000). The scratch collapse test is another provocative test used in the diagnosis of cubital tunnel syndrome. In this test, while the patient forces both shoulders to externally rotate against resistance, the examiner draws the area suspected of nerve entrapment with their fingertip. The test is positive if a short-term loss of muscle resistance develops in the patient (Figure 2). The scratch collapse test contains an essentially higher affectability (69%) than the Tinel test (54%) and the elbow flexion test (46%), and has a common precision drawing nearer 90% for the conclusion of cubital tunnel syndrome (Cheng, Mackinnon-Patterson, Beck & Mackinnon, 2008).

Intrinsic muscle failure may develop after prolonged ulnar nerve entrapment. As a result of paralysis of both the lumbrical and interosseous muscles, the metacarpophalangeal joint of the ring finger and little finger develop hyperextension while flexion deformity develops in the proximal and distal interphalangeal joints. This deformity is named claw hand, intrinsic minus or Duchenne hand. The Masse sign occurs as a result of the flattening of the dorsal transverse metacarpal arch, and hand flattening. This fact is a result of hypothenar muscle paralysis. In hypothenar muscle paralysis, the normal flexion and supination of the fifth metacarpal are nonfunctional. Interosseous muscle insufficiency will lead to the appearance of Wartenberg's sign in cubital tunnel syndrome. Wartenberg's sign is characterized by adduction deficiency of the little finger and ulnar deviation. The little finger remains in abduction when the patient is asked to hold all of their fingers in adduction.

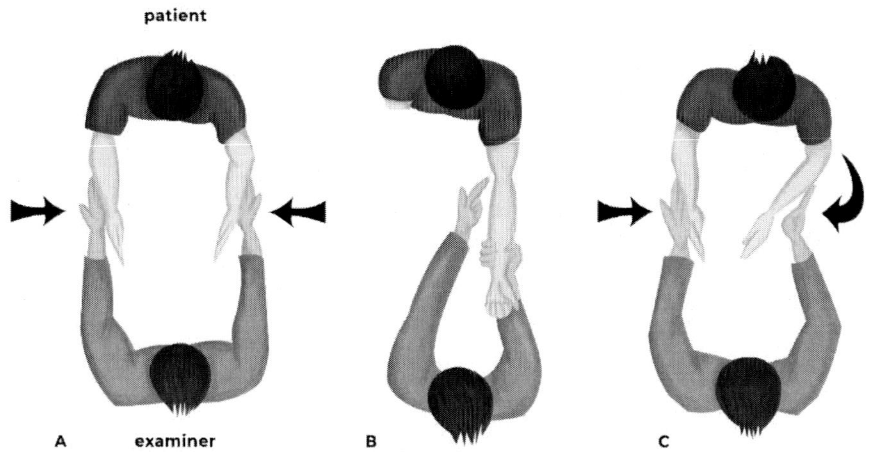


Figure 2. Scratch collapse test. A: The patient applies a forced external rotation of both shoulders against the resistance of the examiner. B: The examiner draws the nerve entrapment area with a fingertip. C: The test is positive if the patient has a loss of muscle resistance

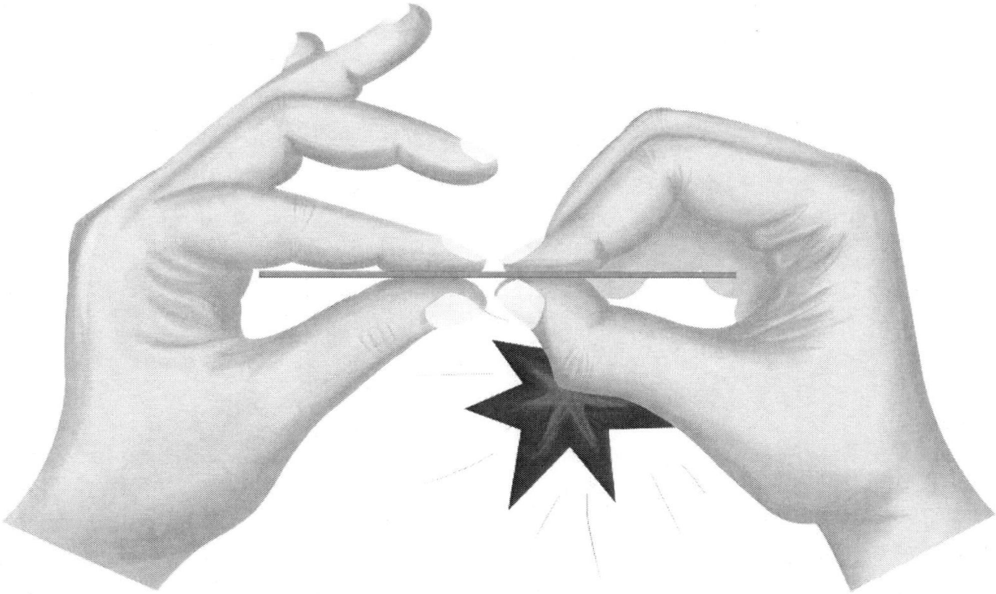

Figure 3. Froment's sign.

Patients with this symptom can also admit to the clinic with a difficulty in putting their hands in their trouser pockets (Palmer & Hughes, 2010; Rosenthal, 1996). When ulnar nerve entrapment causes adductor pollicis muscle weakness, thumb adduction become insufficient. To test this, the patient is requested to hold a piece of paper between the thumb and index finger. If thumb adduction is insufficient, the patient will use the flexor pollicis longus tendon to compensate for it and try to hold the paper by flexing the thumb interphalangeal joint (Folberg et al., 1994). This symptom is known as Froment's sign (Figure 3). Evaluation may be easier when done bilaterally.

## DIAGNOSTIC TESTS

Though clinical evaluation forms the basis of the diagnosis of cubital tunnel syndrome, diagnostic tests are also used. Elbow arthritis and the presence of osteophytes, bone deformities, and findings of previous trauma and soft tissue calcifications can be investigated with radiography (Palmer & Hughes, 2010; Bradshaw & Shefner, 1999; Ciccotti, Schwartz & Ciccotti, 2004). To eliminate the possibility of cervical radiculopathy and Pancoast tumor, radiographs of the cervical spine and chest should be analyzed. Electromyography (EMG) and nerve conduction studies may be done to help locate nerve entrapment (Andrews et al., 2018). In addition to determining other regions of compression in the electrodiagnostic studies, the diagnosis of other disease processes as upper motor neuron disease or peripheral neuropathy becomes possible. In patients with mild or moderate nerve entrapment, the electrodiagnostic tests can confirm or eliminate the diagnosis. In patients with severe symptoms, electrodiagnostic tests can be performed for prognosis and can help to predict expectations of nerve and muscle recovery (Palmer & Hughes, 2010). As many systemic and metabolic causes may lead to ulnar nerve entrapment, patients should also be screened for systemic and metabolic conditions (Bozentka, 1998; Norkus & Meyers, 1994 Posner, 2000).

## CONSERVATIVE TREATMENT

When cubital tunnel syndrome is diagnosed, the daily life activities of patient should be modified and guided. Patients should be informed that the phone should not be held against the ear for a long time and elbow flexion should be avoided during sleep. By giving assistive devices, the patient's compliance with the treatment can be increased. Static night splints for sleeping with the elbow extension position and soft elbow pads to protect the ulnar nerve from direct pressure can be used in conservative treatment. Conservative treatment applied for 2-4 months can be started in many patients with mild cubital tunnel syndrome. At least 3 months of conservative treatment may be preferred in patients with a motor conduction velocity of more than 40 m/sec along the elbow with electrodiagnostic tests (MacKinnon & Novak, 2017). In patients with chronic symptoms and muscle atrophy, surgical treatment is often required in patients when conservative treatment has failed (Palmer & Hughes, 2010).

## SURGICAL TREATMENT

There are many options in the surgical treatment of cubital tunnel syndrome and much controversy over which of these options is the most appropriate surgical treatment (MacKinnon & Novak, 2017). The aim in surgical treatment is the decompression of the ulnar nerve along the entire cubital tunnel. Surgical options include in situ decompression, subcutaneous transposition, intramuscular transposition, submuscular transposition, and medial epicondyectomy (Novak & Mackinnon, 2009). In a meta-analysis to compare results following the in situ decompression and submuscular transposition of the ulnar nerve, data from 10 studies were combined, and the authors found no statistical difference between procedures (Macadam, Gandhi & Bezuhly, 2014).

### In Situ Decompression

The ulnar nerve is reached by making a 6-10 cm incision between the medial epicondyle and the olecranon. Care should be taken to not damage the medial antebrachial cutaneous nerve. The ulnar nerve should be sufficiently decompressed to distal and proximal. Additionally, there is a need to perform neurolysis. Mobilization of the ulnar nerve is evaluated by moving the elbow joint during the operation. Anterior transposition or medial epicondylectomy should be considered if the ulnar nerve subluxes to the anterior of the medial epicondyle during flexion (MacKinnon & Novak, 2017). The literature shows that in situ decompression is a low failure rate treatment and anterior transposition can be the performed treatment for patients with repetitive symptoms (Goldfarb, Sutter, Martens & Manske, 2009).

### Subcutaneous Anterior Transposition

Considering the submuscular position of the ulnar nerve above and below the cubital tunnel, a wide proximal and distal approach is required to locate the nerve subcutaneously and avoid proximal or distal bending. Approximately, a 15 cm long incision is performed. The motor branches of the ulnar nerve to the FCU and flexor digitorum profundus (FDP) should be preserved. The ulnar nerve is located anteriorly and subcutaneously by preserving vascular support (MacKinnon & Novak, 2017). In a study prospectively comparing in situ decompression and subcutaneous anterior transposition, there was no statistically significant difference between the two methods in terms of pain, sensory and motor deficits, and nerve conduction velocities.

## Intramuscular Transposition

The ulnar nerve is considered to be more sheltered in intramuscular transposition than in subcutaneous transposition. However, intramuscular dissection also has a greater risk of scarring. The process is similar to subcutaneous transposition, not including the gutter dissected in the flexor-pronator group muscle in line with the position of the ulnar nerve in the transposed position (MacKinnon & Novak, 2017; Henry, 2006).

## Submuscular Transposition

Though submuscular transposition is a preferred method for treating previously unsuccessful cubital tunnel syndrome surgeries, it is a surgical method that has limitations such as wide dissection, recompression of the nerve under the muscle mass, and the risk of heterotopic ossification. The flexor-pronator muscle mass is gradually cut 1-2 cm distal to the medial epicondyle to allow fractional lengthening of the muscle. The ulnar collateral ligament and the median nerve should be identified and protected during the procedure (MacKinnon & Novak, 2017). In a study comparing retrospectively the clinical results of subcutaneous and submuscular transposition, there was no statistically significant difference between the two methods (Charles, Coulet, Rouzaud, Daures & Chammas, 2009).

## Medial Epicondylectomy

This technique's potential complication is medial elbow instability that may occur with excessive resection of the epicondyle. O'Driscoll et al., showed that only 20% of the epicondyle depth can be removed without damaging the anterior of the medial collateral ligament and described a safer removal plane to obscure the anteroinferior origin of the ligament from the epicondyle (O'Driscoll, Jaloszynski & Morrey, 1992). During osteotomy, care should be taken to not enter the elbow joint and not to separate the ulnar collateral ligament (MacKinnon & Novak, 2017). In patients with cubital tunnel syndrome treated with partial medial epicondylectomy, it is shown that symptoms are relieved without the development of elbow instability; however, medial elbow pain was observed in 45% of patients at the 6-month follow-up (Efstathopoulos, Themistocleous, Papagelopoulos, Choros, Gerostathopoulos & Soucacos, 2006).

## Conclusion

Cubital tunnel syndrome is the most common compression neuropathy in the upper extremity after carpal tunnel syndrome (Boone, Gelberman & Calfee, 2015). It is hard to diagnose cubital tunnel syndrome, mostly because patients do not notice till the symptoms are severe and the nerve is damaged (Andrews, Rowland, Pranjal & Ebraheim, 2018). Mostly, patients admit with symptoms of both sensory and motor disorders. The degree of sensory and motor disorders is important in making the treatment decision that can range from conservative to surgical treatment (Andrews et al., 2018). There are many options in the surgical treatment of cubital tunnel syndrome and controversy still reigns over which of these options is the most appropriate surgical treatment (MacKinnon & Novak, 2017). The aim in surgical treatment is the decompression of the ulnar nerve along the entire cubital tunnel. It should not be forgotten that the motor branches of the ulnar nerve should be protected while providing adequate decompression. It is crucial that the anatomy and pathophysiology of each case of cubital tunnel syndrome are understood for accurate diagnosis and treatment (Andrews et al., 2018).

## References

Andrews, K., Rowland, A., Pranjal, A., Ebraheim, N. (2018). Cubital tunnel syndrome: Anatomy, clinical presentation, and management. *Journal of Orthopaedics*, 15,832-836. https://doi.org/10.1016/j.jor. 2018.08.010.

Apefelberg, D B., Larson, S J. (1973). Dynamic anatomy of the ulnar nerve at the elbow. *Plastic and Reconstructive Surgery*, 51(1), 76–81.

Boone, S., Gelberman, R H., Calfee, R P. (2015). The management of cubital tunnel syndrome. *Journal of Hand Surgery*, 40(9), 1897–1904. https://doi.org/10.1016/j.jhsa.2015.03.011.

Bozentka, D J. (1998). Cubital tunnel syndrome pathophysiology. *Clinical Orthopaedics and Related Research*, (351), 90–94. http://www.ncbi. nlm.nih.gov/pubmed/9646751

Bradshaw, D Y., Shefner, J M. (1999). Ulnar neuropathy at the elbow. *Neurologic Clinics*, 17(3), 447–461 v-vi. https://doi.org/10.1016/ s0733-8619(05)70147-x.

Charles, Y P., Coulet, B., Rouzaud, J C., Daures, J P., Chammas, M. (2009). Comparative clinical outcomes of submuscular and subcutaneous transposition of the ulnar nerve for cubital tunnel syndrome. *Journal of Hand Surgery*, 34A,866–874. https://doi. org/10.1016/j.jhsa. 2009.01.008.

Cheng, C J., Mackinnon-Patterson, B., Beck, JL., Mackinnon, SE. (2008). Scratch collapse test for evaluation of carpal and cubital tunnel syndromes. *Journal of Hand Surgery,* 33A, 1518–1524. https:// doi.org/ 10.1016/j.jhsa.2008.05.022.

Ciccotti, M C., Schwartz, M A., Ciccotti, M G. (2004). Diagnosis and treatment of medial epicondylitis of the elbow. *Clinics in Sports Medicine*, 23(4), 693–705 xi. https://doi.org/10.1016/j.csm.2004.04. 011.

Davidge, K M., Mackinnon, S E. (2015). Nerve compressions. In: Farhadieh R, Bulstrode N, Cugno S, eds. *Plastic and Reconstructive Surgery: Approaches and Techniques.* Chichester, Wiley, 813–837.

Efstathopoulos, D G., Themistocleous, G S., Papagelopoulos, P J., Choros, G D., Gerostathopoulos, N E., Soucacos, P N. (2006). Outcome of partial medial epicondylectomy for cubital tunnel syndrome. *Clinical Orthopaedics and Related Research*, 444,134 –139. https://doi.org/ 10.1097/01.blo.0000201153.36948.29.

Folberg, C R., Weiss, A P., Akelman, E. (1994). Cubital tunnel syndrome. Part I: presentation and diagnosis. *Orthopaedic Review*, 23(2), 136–144. http://www.ncbi. nlm.nih.gov/pubmed/8196972.

Gelberman, R H., Yamaguchi, K., Hollstien, S B., Winn, S S., Heidenreich, Jr F P., Bindra, R R., Hsieh, P., Silva, M J. (1998). Changes in interstitial pressure and cross-sectional area of the cubital tunnel and of the ulnar nerve with flexion of the elbow. An experimental study in human cadavera. *Journal of Bone and Joint Surgery American volume*, 80(4),492–501. https://doi.org/10.2106/ 00004623-199804000-00005.

Goldfarb, C A., Sutter, M M., Martens, E J., Manske, P R. (2009). Incidence of re-operation and subjective outcome following in situ decompression of the ulnar nerve at the cubital tunnel. *Journal of Hand Surgery*, 34B,379–383. https://doi.org/10.1177/ 1753193408101467.

Granger, A., Sardi, J P., Iwanaga, J., Wilson, T J., Yang, L., Loukas, M., Oskouian, R J., Tubbs, RS. (2017). Osborne's ligament: a review of its history, anatomy, and surgical importance. *Cureus*, 9(3),e1080. https:// doi.org/10.7759/ cureus.1080.

Henry, M. (2006). Modified intramuscular transposition of the ulnar nerve. *Journal of Hand Surgery*, 31A, 1535–1542. https://doi.org/10.1016/ j.jhsa.2006.04.016.

Huang, J H., Samadani, U., Zager, E L. (2004). Ulnar nerve entrapment neuropathy at the elbow: simple decompression. *Neurosurgery*, 55(5),1150–1153https://doi.org/ 10.1227/01.neu.0000140841.28007. f2.

James, J., Sutton, L G., Werner, F W., Basu, N., Allison, M A., Palmer, AK. (2011). Morphology of the cubital tunnel: an anatomical and biomechanical study with implications for treatment of ulnar nerve compression. *Journal of Hand Surgery*, 36(12),1988–1995 https:// doi.org/10.1016/j.jhsa.2011.09.014.

Karatas, A., Apaydin, N., Uz, A., Tubbs, R., Loukas, M., Gezen, F. (2009). Regional anatomic structures of the elbow that may potentially compress the ulnar nerve. *Journal of Shoulder Elbow Surgery*, 18(4),627–631. https://doi.org/10.1016 /j.jse.2009.03.004

Macadam, S A., Gandhi, R., Bezuhly, M., Lefaivre, K A. (2014). Simple decompression versus anterior subcutaneous and submuscular transposition of the ulnar nerve for cubital tunnel syndrome: a meta-analysis. *Journal of Hand Surgery*, 33A, 1314–1324. https://doi.org/ 10.1016/j.jhsa.2008.03.006.

MacKinnon, S., Novak, C. (2017). Compression neuropathies— cubital tunnel syndrome. In: Green D, Hotchkiss R, Wolfe S, Pederson W, eds. *Green's operative hand surgery*. 7th ed. New York: Elsevier, 940-947.

Mallette, P., Zhao, M., Zurakowski, D., Ring, D. (2007). Muscle atrophy at diagnosis of carpal and cubital tunnel syndrome. *Journal of Hand Surgery*, 32A, 855–858. https://doi.org/10.1016/j.jhsa.2007.03.009.

Nabhan, A., Ahlhelm, F., Kelm, J., Reith, W., Schwerdtfeger, K., Steudel, WI. (2005). Simple decompression or subcutaneous anterior transposition of the ulnar nerve for cubital tunnel syndrome. *Journal of Hand Surgery*, 30B, 521–524. https://doi.org/10. 1016/j.jhsb.2005. 05.011.

Norkus, S A., Meyers, M C. (1994). Ulnar neuropathy of the elbow. Sports Medicine, 17(3), 189–199. https://doi.org/10.2165/00007256-199417 030-00005.

Novak, C B., Mackinnon, SE. (2009). Selection of operative procedures for cubital tunnel syndrome. *Hand,* 4(1),50–54. https://doi.org/ 10.1007/s115 52-008-9133-z.

Novak, C B., Mehdian, H., von Schroeder, HP. (2012). Laxity of the ulnar nerve during elbow flexion and extension. *Journal of Hand Surgery*, 37A, 1163–1167. https://doi.org/10.1016/j.jhsa.2012.03.016.

O'Driscoll, S W., Jaloszynski, R., Morrey, B F., An, K N. (1992). Origin of the medial ulnar collateral ligament. *Journal of Hand Surgery*, 17A, 164–168. https://doi.org/10.1016/0363-5023 (92)90135-c.

Palmer, B A., Hughes, T B. (2010). Cubital tunnel syndrome. *Journal of Hand Surgery,* 35A, 153–163. https://doi.org/ 10.1016/j.jhsa.2009. 11.004.

Pechan, J., Julis, I. (1975). The pressure measurement in the ulnar nerve. A contribution to the pathophysiology of the cubital tunnel syndrome. *Journal of Biomechanics,* 8, 75–79. https://doi.org/10.1016/0021-9290 (75)90045-7.

Posner, M A. (2000). Compressive neuropathies of the ulnar nerve at the elbow and wrist. *Instructional Course Lectures*, 49, 305–317. http://www.ncbi.nlm.nih. gov/pubmed/10829185.

Robertson, C., Saratsiotis, J. (2005). A review of compressive ulnar neuropathy at the elbow. *Journal of Manipulative and Physiological Therapeutics*, 28(5), 345. https://doi.org/10.1016/j.jmpt.2005.04.005.

Rosenthal, E A. (1996). Examination of hand and forearm: claw hand deformity & thumb deformity with ulnar palsy. In: *Peimer CA, ed. Surgery of the hand and upper extremity*. New York: McGraw-Hill, 83– 87.

Werner, C O., Ohlin, P., Elmqvist, D. (1985). Pressures recorded in ulnar neuropathy. *Acta Orthopaedica Scandinavica.*

In: Musculoskeletal Pain (Common Clinical Presentations) ISBN: 978-1-68507-410-4
Editors: Mehmet Cenk Turgut and Serdar Toy 

*Chapter 17*

# CARPAL TUNNEL SYNDROME

***Oktay Polat*, MD***
Department of Orthopedics and Traumatology
Ağrı Training and Research Hospital, Ağrı, Turkey

## ABSTRACT

Carpal tunnel syndrome (CTS) represents the most frequently observed entrapment neuropathy of the upper limb. It is considered to be associated with increased intracarpal pressure and decreased circulation of the median nerve. The CTS pathophysiology generally originates from combined compression and traction mechanisms.

The diagnosis of carpal tunnel syndrome is based on electromyography and nerve conduction studies. The treatment of CTS depends on the patient's severity. Conservative treatments are given in mild cases of CTS. It is necessary to perform surgical treatment in advanced cases in which conservative treatment is not beneficial and for which conservative treatment is not first considered. Surgical treatment aims to cut the transverse carpal ligament and relieve the carpal tunnel.

## INTRODUCTION

Carpal tunnel syndrome (CTS) represents the most frequently observed entrapment neuropathy of the upper limb. It is predicted to occur in 3.8% of the general population and makes up approximately 90% of all nerve entrapment syndromes. Numbness, pain, and paresthesia are among the symptoms of carpal tunnel syndrome observed in the early period. The above-mentioned symptoms usually emerge with some variation in the

* Corresponding Auhor's E-mail: pltkrdslr@hotmail.com.

thumb, index finger, and middle finger, and the ring finger's radial half (thumb side). Moreover, the pain may spread to the affected arm. Reduced fine motor coordination, hand weakness, thenar atrophy, and clumsiness may emerge with further progression (Ibrahim, Khan, Goddard, & Smitham, 2012).

## Etiology

It is considered to be associated with increased intracarpal pressure and decreased circulation of the median nerve. The reason for an increase in canal pressure in idiopathic CTS is still uncertain. Nevertheless, an increased amount of connective tissue seems to occur in the carpal canal, and it is usually in the form of non-inflammatory synovial fibrosis.

There are etiological causes such as occupations with excessive use of the hand, sex (more common in women), the size of the carpal tunnel, the wrist ratio (subjects with a ratio of the anterior-posterior-transverse diameter of the wrist above 0.7 are at a higher risk of CTS), genetic predisposition, obesity, rheumatologic diseases and pregnancy (Bland, 2005).

## Epidemiology

CTS is predicted to occur in approximately 1-4% of the general population, and its incidence per year was reported as reaching 276/100,000. It was also reported to be more common in women as shown by the female/male distribution of two-thirds to one-third. While CTS can occur in all age groups, the peak is observed in the age group of 40-60 years. Despite the fact that good postoperative clinical and electrophysiological outcomes have been stated even in patients with advanced CTS, it is commonly accepted that surgery can be inefficient in patients having advanced CTS.

It has been reported that the CTS epidemiology differs by ethnic origin. CTS continues to be an idiopathic syndrome, despite its association with some risk factors. It is possible to divide medical risk factors into three groups: mechanical, anatomical, and physiological risk factors. The above-mentioned three types can occur at the same time and affect each other (Yunoki et al., 2016).

## PATHOPHYSIOLOGY

Carpal tunnel syndrome (CTS) is multifactorial and usually originates from many social, occupational, and environmental risk factors specific to patients. For example, it is not always possible to detect a single specific cause if there is no space-occupying lesion that can be attributed to the symptoms stated by the patient, which can be appreciated in selected medical conditions (such as gout). However, the said relatively simple clinical presentations are comparatively rare compared to the majority of CTS presentations.

The CTS pathophysiology generally originates from combined compression and traction mechanisms. The compressive element of the pathophysiology involves a harmful cycle of an increase in pressure, obstruction of the overall venous outflow, increased local edema, and impairment in the intraneural microcirculation of the median nerve. Nerve dysfunction is endangered, and the nerve's structural integrity increases the dysfunctional environment to a further extent, the myelin sheath and axon develop lesions, and inflammation occurs in the surrounding connective tissues, which lose their normal physiological, supportive and protective functions. Repetitive traction and wrist motion worsen the negative environment and lead to further damage of the nerve (Sevy & Varacallo, 2021).

## ANATOMY

The scaphoid and trapezium are on the lateral side of the CT and the hamate and pisiform bones are on the medial side of the CT, and the base of the arch formed by this structure is covered by the transverse carpal ligament (Bland, 2005; Ibrahim et al., 2012; Yunoki et al., 2016). The flexor retinaculum covers the transverse carpal ligament. Four deep flexors, four superficial flexors, the flexor pollicis longus (FPL) and the median nerve pass through this structure.

The median nerve is the structure in the most volar part of the CT. The motor branch travels distally toward the palm and innervates the 1st and 2nd lumbrical muscles. Furthermore, the median nerve gives off its recurrent thenar motor branch, which innervates the opponens pollicis, the abductor pollicis brevis, the superficial head of the flexor pollicis brevis, and most of the thenar region muscles. The median nerve sensory branch passing through the CT senses the medial of the thumb, and the lateral part of the index finger, middle finger and ring finger. The median nerve has three main structures at the wrist level. The first structure is the median nerve's palmar cutaneous branch. This branch separates from the median nerve prior to the transverse carpal ligament and innervates the thenar region of the hand. There are variations of the palmar cutaneous branch. The second structure is the median nerve's recurrent motor branch. This branch separates from the median nerve via many variations. The extraligamentously separated form represents the most frequently observed form. The main median nerve, which is the last structure, bifurcates into the lateral and medial trunks and forms the digital nerves that sense the volar and radial parts of the first, second, third, and fourth fingers (Kürklü, Türkkan, & Tüzün, 2015).

## DIAGNOSIS

The diagnosis of carpal tunnel syndrome is based on nerve conduction and electromyography studies. The diagnosis of carpal tunnel syndrome is not confirmed by other clinical or special examinations, but they assist with excluding other diagnoses.

At the first step of the clinical diagnosis of CTS, there is a tendency for a patient to wake up from sleep with a feeling of numbness or swelling in the hand without any remarkable swelling. Extreme pain can be felt from the wrist, which spreads to the shoulder with tingling in the hands and fingers, and this is called brachialgia paresthetica nocturna. In the majority of cases, the pain stops after the hand is shaken. However, the hand can become stiff afterwards. The second step of CTS in the patient is symptoms occurring during the day. These symptoms emerge when the subject carries out a repetitive activity that involves the hand or wrist or maintains a certain position for long periods of time. Patients notice that they drop objects while grasping them and they are clumsy. Atrophy or hypotrophy occurs in the thenar eminence at the final step of the development of CTS.

### Physical Examination Tests

Tinel's test produces a positive outcome in the case that tapping lightly along the carpal tunnel causes symptoms in the median nerve distribution.

In Phalen's maneuver, the patient's wrist is flexed to 90 degrees, and the test is considered to be positive in the case that flexing causes symptoms in the median nerve distribution.

Durkan's test is performed by the physician placing both thumbs on top of each other and applying 30 seconds of pressure to the patient's transverse carpal ligament.

While Phalen's test was reported as the most sensitive test, the hand diagram and Tinel's test were reported as the most specific tests.

In their study on patients with CTS, Gellman et al. found that CT pressure was 32 mmHg when the wrist was in the neutral position, 99 mmHg at 90° of flexion, and 110 mmHg at 90° of extension. In the control group, these values were found to be 25, 31, and

30 mmHg, respectively (Gelberman, Hergenroeder, Hargens, Lundborg & Akeson, 1981; Genova, Dix, Saefan, Thakur & Hassan, 2020; Kürklü et al., 2015).

### Differential Diagnosis

Some diseases may provide symptoms similar to CTS and, therefore, a robust diagnosis is required to reveal subjects' medical conditions. Diseases such as carpometacarpal arthritis, cervical radiculopathy, de Quervain's tendinopathy, peripheral neuropathy with a history of pronator syndrome, diabetes mellitus and Raynaud's syndrome may show similar findings (Genova et al., 2020).

## TREATMENT

### Conservative Treatment

The treatment of CTS depends on the patient's severity. Conservative treatments are given in mild cases of CTS. It has been demonstrated that a 6-week night splint application reduces the symptoms between 30 and 70%, increases grip strength and improves sensory findings. It has been demonstrated that local steroid injections into the carpal tunnel ensure good relief of CTS in the short term. It is not recommended to administer more than 2 injections. Half of those who undergo the mentioned treatment should undergo surgery within a year. Oral steroids are not recommended. Exercises and mobilization interventions, including forearm/wrist-stretching home exercise regimens, can have some benefits. However, such treatment has a weak evidence base. It is possible to reduce exposure or change the job. In their review on conservative treatments used in patients with mild and moderate CTS, Jimenez et al. indicated that these treatments and techniques were not superior to each other (Del Barrio et al., 2018). Treatments such as vitamin B6 (pyridoxine), oral diuretics, botulinum toxin injections, lasers, and iontophoresis are not suggested for CTS since there is insufficient or conflicting evidence regarding their efficacy.

In the majority of cases, there is a possibility for subjects to continue working in the course of conservative treatment. Surgery should be considered if a job change is impossible or if the subject's complaints persist in spite of conservative treatment (Franklin & Friedman, 2015).

## Surgical Treatment

Surgical treatment must be performed in advanced cases in which conservative treatment is not beneficial and for which conservative treatment is not first considered. Surgical treatment aims to cut the transverse carpal ligament and relieve the carpal tunnel.

There are three different surgical techniques. The first is the open technique, which is relatively simple to carry out and provides good symptomatic relief with a low rate of complications in most subjects. However, longer incisions may lead to a longer duration of recovery and increased scar sensitivity, which may reduce patient satisfaction. Therefore, mini-open techniques have been developed with special retractors. Less scar formation and a shorter duration of recovery with a 2 cm incision increase patient satisfaction. In the endoscopic technique, the incision line and incision-related pain are reduced. However, sometimes poor visibility, difficulty in understanding the variations related to the median nerve's motor branch, a risk of iatrogenic nerve damage, and incomplete release can be considered as the disadvantages of endoscopic CTS treatment.

It is observed that the mini-open technique is the most preferred method by surgeons. In the literature, there are many studies showing no clinical difference three months after surgery between endoscopic and open techniques. However, the number of studies reporting less pain post-operatively and a shorter time before a return to work with an endoscopic technique is also quite high. The open technique is recommended in recurrence cases and diabetic patients. Postoperatively, patients are recommended to restrict their wrist movements for two days and utilize a night splint for three weeks in a neutral position for pain control. Patients should be released for all activities after 6-8 weeks (Chammas et al., 2014; Franklin & Friedman, 2015; Genova et al., 2020; Kürklü et al., 2015; Turgut, Saglam, & Toy, 2021; Yunoki et al., 2016).

# Conclusion

Characteristic complaints constitute the basis for the diagnosis of carpal tunnel syndrome, which is confirmed by electrophysiological tests. The treatment of carpal tunnel syndrome can be surgical or conservative, depending on the degree of effect on the patient's daily functioning.

## REFERENCES


Bland, J. D. (2005). Carpal tunnel syndrome. *Curr. Opin. Neurol., 18*(5), 581-585. doi:10.1097/01.wco.0000173142.58068.5a.

Chammas, M., Boretto, J., Burmann, L. M., Ramos, R. M., Neto, F. S., & Silva, J. B. (2014). Carpal tunnel syndrome-Part II (treatment)☆,☆☆. *Rev Bras Ortop, 49*, 437-445.

Del Barrio, S. J., Gracia, E. B., García, C. H., de Miguel, E. E., Moreno, J. T., Marco, S. R., & Laita, L. C. (2018). Conservative treatment in patients with mild to moderate carpal tunnel syndrome: A systematic review. *Neurologia (Engl. Ed.). 33*(9), 590-601.

Franklin, G. M., & Friedman, A. S. (2015). Work-related carpal tunnel syndrome: diagnosis and treatment guideline. *Phys. Med. Rehabil. Clin. N. Am., 26*(3), 523-537.

Gelberman, R. H., Hergenroeder, P. T., Hargens, A. R., Lundborg, G. N., & Akeson, W. H. (1981). The carpal tunnel syndrome. A study of carpal canal pressures. *J. Bone Joint Surg. Am., 63*(3), 380-383.

Genova, A., Dix, O., Saefan, A., Thakur, M., & Hassan, A. (2020). Carpal tunnel syndrome: a review of literature. *Cureus, 12*(3).

Ibrahim, I., Khan, W., Goddard, N., & Smitham, P. (2012). Suppl 1: carpal tunnel syndrome: a review of the recent literature. *Open Orthop. J., 6*, 69.

Kürklü, M., Türkkan, S., & Tüzün, H. Y. (2015). Karpal tünel sendromu ve median sinirin diğer tuzak nöropatileri. *TOTBİD Dergisi, 14*, 566-571.

Sevy, J. O., & Varacallo, M. (2021). Carpal Tunnel Syndrome. In *StatPearls*. Treasure Island (FL): StatPearls Publishing Copyright © 2021, StatPearls Publishing LLC.

Turgut, M. C., Saglam, G., & Toy, S. (2021). Efficacy of extracorporeal shock wave therapy for pillar pain after open carpal tunnel release: a double-blind, randomized, sham-controlled study. *Korean J. Pain., 34*(3), 315-321. doi:10.3344/kjp.2021.34.3.315.

Yunoki, M., Kanda, T., Suzuki, K., Uneda, A., Hirashita, K., & Yoshino, K. (2016). Importance of recognizing carpal tunnel syndrome for neurosurgeons: A review. *Neurol. Med. Chir.*, ra. 2016-0225.

In: Musculoskeletal Pain (Common Clinical Presentations) ISBN: 978-1-68507-410-4
Editors: Mehmet Cenk Turgut and Serdar Toy 

*Chapter 18*

# De Quervain Disease

***Birkan Kibar*, MD***
Department of Orthopedics and Traumatology,
Haydarpaşa Numune Training and Research Hospital, Istanbul, Turkey

## Abstract

Painful stenosing tenosynovitis of the first extensor compartment of the wrist, involving the abductor pollicis longus and extensor pollicis brevis tendons, is called de Quervain's disease. The patient complains of pain and tenderness, usually localized at the radial styloid and aggravated by thumb motion. With a splint or casts that keep the wrist slightly extended with thumb abduction, symptoms may regress, but symptoms tend to recur when the triggering activities are resumed after the cast is removed. Corticosteroid injections together with lidocaine may benefit 50-80% of patients. First extensor compartment release is required if the complaints do not regress with conservative treatment.

## Introduction

Painful stenosing tenosynovitis of the first extensor compartment of the wrist, involving the abductor pollicis longus (APL) and extensor pollicis brevis (EPB) tendons is called de Quervain's disease (Ilyas et al., 2007).

Below the extensor retinaculum, there are six separate compartments. The first compartment is on the lateral surface of the distal radius and includes the APL and EPB tendons. The APL and EPB tendons pass beneath a tunnel formed by the septa between

* Corresponding Author's E-mail: birkankibar545454@gmail.com.

the retinaculum and the radius, which is formed in a shallow groove in the radial styloid process and this tunnel is approximately 3 cm long (Lee et al., 2017).

Fritz de Quervain described the compression of the APL and EPB tendons in the radial styloid process in 1895. This was associated with repetitive ulnar deviation of the wrist and thumb abduction. If the first compartment tension is continuous and repetitive, friction occurs in the rigid retinacular sheath, followed by swelling, thickening of the extensor retinaculum, and narrowing of the fibro-osseous canal. Tendon compression of the first extensor compartment causes significant functional impairment and pain in the hand and wrist.

The patient complains of pain and tenderness, usually localized at the radial styloid and aggravated by thumb motion, lasting for several weeks or months (Viegas, 1986). It is mostly seen in people of 30 to 50 years old, and the disease is seen 6 to 10 times more frequently in women (Weiss et al., 1994). The disease also peaks in postpartum and lactating women (Avci et al., 2002).

There is local tenderness and pain on the radial styloid after the thumb is taken into the palm and the wrist is taken into ulnar deviation (Eichhoff's maneuver), and the findings are helpful in diagnosing the disease (Wu et al., 2018). Harry Finkelstein later described the pathognomonic examination maneuver: there is pain in the radial styloid after flexing the patient's thumb and rapidly ulnar deviating the wrist (Finkelstein, 1930).

De Quervain's disease should be distinguished from intersection syndrome. In intersection syndrome, there is crepitus, pain and swelling that are more proximal over the second compartment tendons. It can also interfere with the trigger thumb. The EPB tendon can be pseudo-triggering with a separate fibro-osseous tunnel, which can be confused with de Quervain's disease.

## TREATMENT

### Nonoperative Treatment

With a splint or casts that keep the wrist slightly extended with thumb abduction, symptoms may regress, but symptoms tend to recur when triggering activities are resumed after the cast is removed. Corticosteroid injections together with lidocaine may benefit 50-80% of patients (Weiss et al., 1994). A response to nonoperative therapy in pregnancy and lactation is good, and after lactation the situation tends to resolve. Avci et al., prospectively examined 19 wrists of 18 pregnant or lactating patients; 9 patients received only CS injection, all had a resolution, 1 had a late recurrence, complete relief was not seen in any of the 9 patients who only underwent splinting, and spontaneous resolution was observed in 8 after lactation (Avci et al., 2002).

There are many CS preparations on the market with different durations of action and solubility. Less soluble preparations may cause local complications such as depigmentation, subcutaneous atrophy, and fat necrosis. In addition, APL and EPB tendon ruptures can be seen as a result of repeated injections (Nguyen and Jones, 2012). Local anesthetics such as lidocaine can also be used for the immediate and temporary relief of complaints (Liang and McElroy, 2013).

## Injection Technique

When the thumb is abducted and hyperextended, the tendons of the first dorsal compartment can be easily palpated, and fluid is injected 1 cm proximal to the radial styloid. There may also be a septum in the first compartment and some of the solution may be applied slightly dorsal to the first injection point (Leslie et al., 1990).

In a series of 19 patients in which radiopaque dye was injected with CS into the first dorsal compartment, it was confirmed that the dye was in the first extensor compartment in 16 of 19 cases. The EPB compartment was missed in 13 of 19 patients, because there was a separate compartment in a deep location. This may be the cause of failed injections, like surgery, when a separate EPB compartment is not adequately released (Zingas, 1998).

If symptoms do not improve with the first injection, it can be repeated 4-6 weeks later, but repeated injections should be avoided in terms of local complications.

## Surgical Treatment

Surgical treatment should be considered in patients who do not respond to prolonged conservative treatment. The procedure can be performed under local infiltration anesthesia and pneumatic tourniquet or with WALANT (wide awake local anesthesia no tourniquet). We do the procedure with WALANT in our clinic. In order to recognize the radial nerve sensory branch and anatomical variations, a bloodless operation field is a must. A transverse incision is made proximally to the radial styloid. The terminal part of the radial nerve sensory branch runs on the surface of the first dorsal component and should be explored and protected during surgery. A longitudinal incision can also be made to reduce the risk of injury to the radial nerve sensory branch. However, a longitudinal incision may pose a risk for scar adherence of the cutaneous nerves. After passing through the epidermis by sharp dissection, subcutaneous fat should be passed with blunt dissection. The annular ligament is exposed and incised close to its dorsal side (to prevent palmar subluxation of the tendons). All tendons are explored. At this level, the EPB tendon can be distinguished by the muscle fibers, as the APL does not have muscle fibers at this level. Tendons are lifted with a clamp, and the patient is told to move the thumb to ensure decompression (Figure 1). If the tendons are not retracted from the radial styloid with ease, all subsheaths, aberrant tendons, and septa are loosened, and if there is thick tenosynovial tissue, debulking is performed. If a pneumatic tourniquet is used, it is opened and hemostasis is provided. Only the skin is sutured, and a light pressure dressing is applied. After the operation, as much movement is allowed as the patient can tolerate, and heavy activities are allowed after 4-6 weeks.

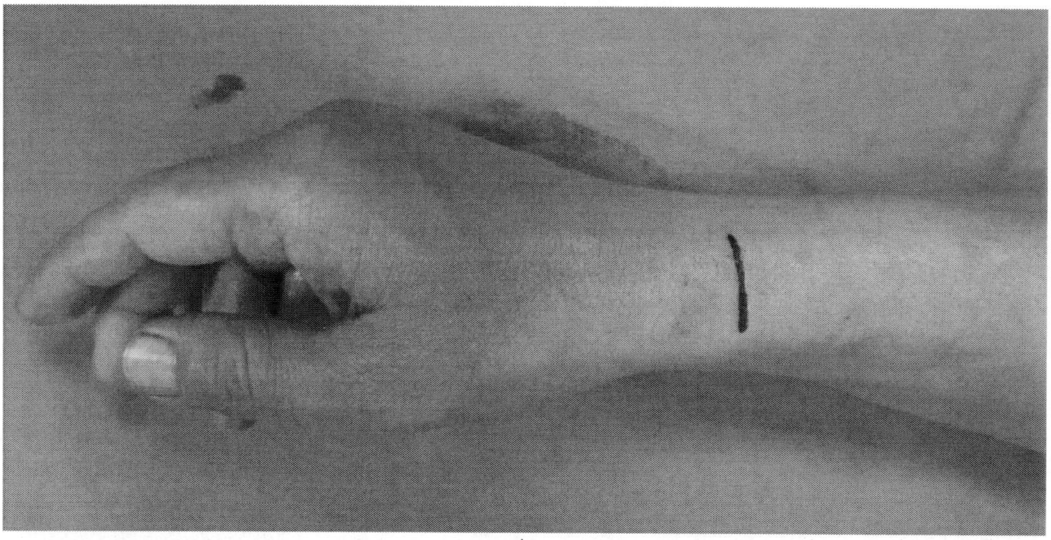

A

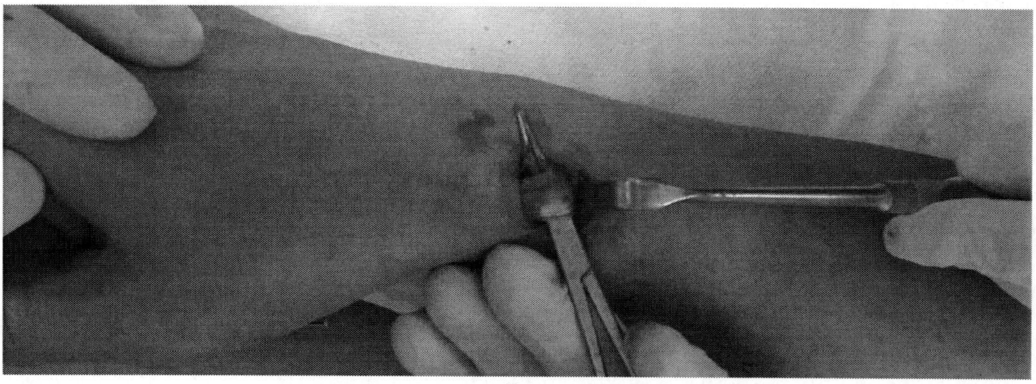

B

Figure 1. A: Transverse incision for de Quervain's disease surgery, B: first compartment tendons after release.

There are many variations in the first dorsal compartment of the wrist. Failing to recognize these variations and an insufficient release of the tendon sheaths may cause the continuation or recurrence of symptoms (Jackson et al., 1986).

## Complications

The most serious complication of surgery is iatrogenic radial nerve sensory branch injury and painful neuroma. Also, symptoms may persist after release, either due to insufficient release or inaccurate diagnosis. Hypertrophic and painful scars can be corrected with z-plasty. Palmar subluxation of tendons can be reconstructed with a brachioradialis tendon flap (McMahon et al., 1991).

## Conclusion

It is important to make the differential diagnosis of de Quervain's disease, which is painful tenosynovitis of the first wrist dorsal compartment, from other painful wrist conditions, and first extensor compartment release is required if complaints do not regress with conservative treatment.

## References

Avci S, Yilmaz C, Sayli U. (2002). Comparison of nonsurgical treatment measures for de Quervain's disease of pregnancy and lactation. *J. Hand Surg.* [Am], 27, 2, 322-4.

Finkelstein H. (1930). Stenosing tendovaginitis at the radial styloid process. *J. Bone Joint Surg. Am.*, 12, 509-40.

Ilyas A M, Ast M, Schaffer A A, Thoder J. (2007). De Quervain tenosynovitis of the wrist. *J. Am. Acad. Orthop. Surg.*, 15, 12,757–64.

Jackson W T, Viegas SF, Coon T M, Stimpson K D, Frogameni A D, Simpson J M. (1986). Anatomic variations in the first extensor compartment of the wirst. A clinical and anatomical study. *J. Bone Joint Surg. Am.*, 68, 6, 923-6.

Lee Z Y, Stranix J T, Anzai L, Sharma S. (2017). Surgical anatomy of the first extensor compartment: a systematic review and comparison of normal cadaver vs. De Quervain syndrome patients. *J. Plast Reconstr. Aesthet. Surg.*, 70, 1, 127-31.

Leslie B M, Ericson Jr W B, Morehead J R. (1990). Incidence of septum with the first dorsal compartman of the wirst. *J. Hand Surg. Am.,* 15, 1, 88-91.

Liang J, McElroy K. (2013). Hypopigmentation after triamnicolone injection for de Quervain tenosynovitis. *Am J Phys Med Rehabil*, 92, 7, 639.

McMahon M, Craig S M, Posner M A. (1991). Tendon subluxation after de Quervain's release: treatment by brachioradialis tendon flap. *J. Hand Surg. Am.*, 16, 1, 30-2.

Nguyen M L, Jones N F. (2012). Rupture of both the abductor pollicis longus and extensor pollicis brevis tendons after steroid injection for de quervain tenosynovitis. *Plast. Reconstr. Surg.*, 129, 5, 883-6.

Weiss A, Akelman E, Tabatai M. Treatment of de Quervain's disease. (1994). *J. Hand Surg.* [Am], 19, 4, 595-8.

Wu F, Rajpura A, Sandher D. (2018). Finkelstein's test is superior to Eichoff's test in the investigation of de Quervain's disease. *J. Hand Micrusurg.* 10, 2, 116-8.

Viegas S F. Trigger thumb of de Quervain's disease. (1986). *J. Hand Surg.* [Am], 11, 2, 235-7.

Zingas C, Failla J M, Holsbeeck M V. (1998). İnjection accuracy and clinical relief od de Quervain's tendinitis. *J. Hand Surg. Am.*, 23, 1, 89-96.

In: Musculoskeletal Pain (Common Clinical Presentations) ISBN: 978-1-68507-410-4
Editors: Mehmet Cenk Turgut and Serdar Toy 

*Chapter 19*

# LATERAL AND MEDIAL EPICONDYLITIS

***Merve Sekizkardeş Tütüncü*, MD***
Department of Physical Medicine and Rehabilitation,
Harakani State Hospital, Kars, Turkey

## ABSTRACT

Epicondylitis of the elbow is a widely encountered pathology seen both laterally and medially. Lateral epicondylitis, often referred to as "tennis elbow," is a very common problem of the extensor origin at the lateral epicondyle resulting from repetitive work- and/or athletic-related microtrauma. Typical symptoms include lateral elbow pain especially during extension of the wrist and decreased grip strength. Medial epicondylitis, also known as "golfer's elbow," is another common pathology, although less frequent when compared to lateral epicondylitis, which occurs due to repetitive valgus stress and common flexor tendon microtrauma. A typical patient complaint is pain on the medial aspect of the elbow, which is aggravated by daily activities and especially wrist flexion. A thorough history and a meticulous physical examination are essential for the epicondylitis diagnosis which is primarily clinical. Initially, imaging modalities are not indicated; however, recalcitrant cases, possible nerve entrapment syndromes, and inflammatory conditions may require imaging. Treatment methods include discontinuation of the exacerbating occupational and athletic activities, physical therapy modalities, exercises and injections. Patients who do not respond to conservative treatment modalities may be eligible for surgical interventions.

* Corresponding Author's E-mail: merve.sekizkardes@gmail.com.

# INTRODUCTION

Lateral epicondylitis, also known as "tennis elbow," is a very common tendinopathy of the lateral elbow often resulting from repetitive activities. The term "lawn tennis arm" was first used by Morris in 1883 to describe lateral arm injury due to playing lawn tennis (Morris, 1883). Lateral epicondylitis is reported to be encountered in up to 50% of tennis players, although this group comprises only 10% of the affected population (Priest et al., 1980). Occupational and athletic activities that lead to excessive repetitive stress on musculotendinous structures in the lateral aspect of the elbow can cause lateral epicondylitis. Inexperienced tennis players using incorrect backhand techniques and manual workers who use vibratory devices are especially at risk (De Smedt et al., 2007) (Shiri & Viikari-Juntura, 2011). The prevalence of lateral epicondylitis in the general population is reported to be between 1% and 3% with no associated gender predilection (Calfee et al., 2008). It is most commonly seen between the ages of 45 and 54. Age is a crucial factor in pathophysiology, and lateral epicondylitis is thus rarely seen below 30 years of age (Shiri et al., 2006).

Medial epicondylitis or "golfer's elbow" is a less common pathology resulting from excessive use of the flexor/pronator muscle group. Chronic and repetitive contractile stress exerted on muscular and tendinous structures of the medial epicondyle leads to underlying degenerative changes (M. C. Ciccotti et al., 2004). Medial epicondylitis is mostly seen in the fourth and fifth decades with a similar male-to-female prevalence rate (Bennett, 1994).

# LATERAL EPICONDYLITIS

## Pathophysiology

Lateral epicondylitis is considered to be an incorrect technical term by some researchers, because the underlying pathology is shown to be degenerative as opposed to inflammatory. Therefore, "lateral epicondylopathy" might be a more descriptive and correct way to identify the pathology (De Smedt et al., 2007) (Regan et al., 1992). Ischemic stress may be an important etiological factor considering the relatively avascular structures of both the tendon and the tenoperiosteal junction. Histologic examinations show angiofibroblastic hyperplasia, i.e., vascular granulation tissue and fibroblast invasion of collagen structures (Nirschl & Pettrone, 1979).

Initial degenerative changes occur predominantly in the origin of the extensor carpi radialis brevis (ECRB) and less commonly involve the common extensor origin. Playing tennis especially during a backhand move exerts greater stress on the ECRB tendon than on any other extensor tendon (Lenoir et al., 2019). Moreover, anatomical studies demonstrated that the ECRB is in direct contact with the humero-radial joint capsule making it prone to injury due to the transmission of joint loads. Friction between the lower aspect of the ECRB and the capitellum during flexion-extension movements of the elbow is another possible mechanism leading to lateral epicondylitis (Nimura et al., 2014) (Bunata et al., 2007).

In addition to the aforementioned processes, repetitive mechanical stress and the subsequent microtrauma are crucial factors leading to lateral epicondylitis.

## Diagnosis

Lateral epicondylitis usually presents with pain and tenderness localized to the lateral aspect of the elbow, i.e., slightly anterior and distal to the lateral epicondyle. Pain may occasionally radiate to the distal arm and proximal forearm. It has an insidious onset and patients rarely mention acute traumatic injuries. Common complaints include difficulty shaking hands and lifting weights when the elbow is extended, and decreased handgrip strength which impedes athletic and everyday activities. Physical examination reveals tenderness above the lateral epicondyle. Pain and disturbance can be reproduced when the patient is asked to extend and radially rotate their wrist against resistance while the elbow is extended and the forearm is pronated, during a positive Cozen's test. Gardner introduced the chair test as a highly sensitive tool in which the patient is asked to lift a chair while the elbow is extended and the forearm is pronated to provoke pain in the lateral aspect of the elbow (Gardner, 1970).

Imaging modalities are not generally indicated in lateral epicondylitis but rather used in recalcitrant cases and as tools to navigate the physician through differential diagnosis. Standard anteroposterior and lateral radiographs are mostly normal, although occasional calcifications around the origin of the common extensor tendon may be detected. Magnetic resonance imaging (MRI) may demonstrate increased signal intensity on T2-weighted images especially around the tendon origin. Peripheral edema can be seen as increased signal intensity in neighboring soft tissues. MRI is useful in distinguishing the presence and severity of tendon fissures, and important for the selection of surgical cases (Jeon et al., 2018). Ultrasonography (US) is a favorable first-line imaging modality. US enables the visualization of the common extensor tendon beginning from the musculotendinous junction to the lateral epicondyle. Bone irregularity, tendon thickening, tendinosis and calcification may be detected via US making it a practical, cost-effective and safe imaging method (Walz et al., 2010).

It is also important to exclude other factors that can cause lateral elbow pain. Differential diagnosis includes pain radiating from the neck and shoulder pathologies, humeroradial arthritis, osteochondritis dissecans, inflammatory diseases and nerve entrapment syndromes. Posterior interosseous nerve entrapment and radial tunnel syndrome can mimic lateral epicondylitis. However, tenderness is observed to be 3-4 cm distal to the lateral epicondyle rather than directly above it. Electromyographic studies should be employed to exclude nerve entrapment syndromes. Absence of pain/discomfort during stress tests and absence of pathology on MRI and US examinations should suggest causes other than lateral epicondylitis. In this case, the upper extremity including the neck region should be thoroughly evaluated to determine the underlying pathology (Brummel et al., 2014).

### Treatment

Treatment methods include the discontinuation of exacerbating activities, the application of cold packs, rest, oral analgesics such as non-steroidal anti-inflammatory drugs (NSAID), corticosteroid injections, bracing and physical therapy. Lateral epicondylitis is generally seen among amateur tennis players, therefore it is crucial to inform the patients regarding the correct forehand/backhand techniques, racquet grip size and tension recommendations (Tosti et al., 2013) (Nirschl & Pettrone, 1979). Eccentric extensor muscle strengthening is a promising new exercise approach which significantly improves pain and weakness-related complaints (Cullinane et al., 2014). Corticosteroid injections around the peritendinous area are widely used, and quite effective in relieving the pain in the acute period. However, adverse effects have been reported and long-term consequences are questionable (Altay et al., 2002). Other treatment options are platelet rich plasma (PRP) injection, extra-corporeal shock wave therapy (ESWT), high voltage galvanic stimulation and acupuncture. Recalcitrant cases may qualify as surgical candidates. Surgical treatment ensures the debridement of degenerative tissue which has high patient satisfaction rates (Dunn et al., 2008).

## Medial Epicondylitis

### Pathophysiology

Medial epicondylitis or "golfer's elbow" is a medially located elbow pathology resulting from common flexor tendon degeneration and repetitive microtrauma. Medial epicondylitis comprises 9.8% to 20% of all epicondylitis cases (M. C. Ciccotti et al., 2004). The overall prevalence is reported to be below 1% with the peak incidence occurring in the fourth through to sixth decades of life. Men and women are equally affected (Amin et al., 2015).

Repetitive valgus overload and eccentric loading of the muscles especially in golfers and throwing athletes may eventually exceed the strength of the flexor-pronator muscle group and can lead to medial epicondylitis (Walz et al., 2010). The flexor-pronator muscle group includes the flexor carpi radialis, pronator teres, palmaris longus, flexor digitorum superficialis and flexor carpi ulnaris. Medial epicondylitis primarily originates from injury of the flexor carpi radialis, pronator teres and/or palmaris longus. Involvement of the flexor carpi ulnaris and the inferior aspect of the flexor sublimis can also be seen, although occasionally.

The medial collateral ligament (MCL) or the "ulnar collateral ligament" is a crucial stabilizing structure which resists valgus stress. MCL injury can be detected as an accompanying or facilitating injury in medial epicondylitis cases. The ulnar nerve which runs through the cubital tunnel should also be evaluated as a nerve injury due to epicondylitis, or contractile forces transmitted on the nerve is possible. Therefore a medial epicondylitis diagnosis should be assessed along with possible MCL tears, ulnar nerve compression or subluxation (Saliman et al., 2006)

Pathogenesis of medial epicondylitis is similar to that of lateral epicondylitis for the most part: Repetitive stress causing degeneration, angiofibroblastic hyperplasia, and granulation tissue formation paving the way for tendinosis and tendon fissures (Jobe & Ciccotti, 1994).

## Diagnosis

A typical presentation for medial epicondylitis would include pain and discomfort on the medial aspect of the elbow, tenderness that is usually localized to the medial epicondyle and gradual onset of the symptoms. Patients can be throwing athletes who play golf or tennis, or manual workers with jobs demanding a forceful grip, weight lifting or vibratory tool use (Descatha et al., 2003) (Vangsness & Jobe, 1991). Elbow pain worsens with physical activity and especially in the chronic phase it is not alleviated by rest. Physical examination demonstrates tenderness 5 to 10 mm distal and anterior to the medial epicondyle, i.e., the insertion point of the pronator-flexor musculature. Soft tissue inflammation and swelling may occasionally accompany it (M. G. Ciccotti & Ramani, 2003). Moreover, when the patient is asked to flex their wrist and to pronate their forearm against resistance, medial elbow pain is provoked (Pienimäki et al., 2011).

Imaging studies are normal for the majority of cases. However, plain radiography might show punctuate calcifications of the common flexor tendon and MCL. MRI is quite beneficial in diagnosing common flexor tendon pathologies such as tendinosis and ruptures. High signal intensity in the common flexor tendon and the peritendinous soft tissue on T2-weighted sequences suggests medial epicondylitis (Walz et al., 2010). US is a practical modality for primary evaluation of the patient. Common flexor tendon continuity, echogenicity, a fibrillar pattern and cortex irregularity are important variables to observe. Dynamic examination is another advantage of US, although sensitivity and specificity may vary according to the user's expertise (Gündüz et al., 2012).

Ulnar neuritis and ulnar collateral ligament instability should be considered when a medial epicondylitis patient is being examined. These pathologies may coexist especially in athletes due to increased valgus stress (M. C. Ciccotti et al., 2004). Ulnar neuritis presents with medial elbow pain and numbness/tingling complaints in the $4^{th}$ and $5^{th}$ digits. Compressing the ulnar nerve at the elbow level will exacerbate and radiate the pain and numbness towards the fingers (Plancher et al., 1996). In order to assess ulnar collateral ligament instability, the clinician must perform the valgus stress test or the "milking test" (pulling the thumb while the elbow is flexed and the forearm is supinated). Presence of pain directly above the ulnar collateral ligament can be considered as a positive result for both tests (M. C. Ciccotti et al., 2004).

## Treatment

Similar to lateral epicondylitis, primary treatment of medial epicondylitis is the cessation of aggravating athletic and occupational activities. Methods to improve throwing techniques and diminish valgus stress can be employed on an individual basis after careful review of the daily activities. Ice application 3 to 5 times a day and NSAID use for 10 to 14 days are primarily recommended (Jobe & Ciccotti, 1994). If the pain persists despite these measures, night splinting might be considered. Local corticosteroid injection in the close vicinity of the affected tendon insertion can also be performed. Results of the corticosteroid injections are similar to those of lateral epicondylitis. Studies have shown significant pain relief following the injection; however, long-term efficacy is still controversial (Stahl & Kaufman, 1997). A one-year follow-up showed the recurrence of symptoms in up to 54% of patients who initially expressed pain relief (Price et al., 1991). High-voltage galvanic stimulation, ultrasound and ESWT are other physical therapy modalities that can be used in medial epicondylitis treatment. After a patient's symptoms have subsided, a tailored rehabilitation program should be started. Wrist and elbow range of motion exercises, followed by eccentric strengthening exercises can be performed. If conservative treatment for 3 to 6 months proves to be ineffective, surgery should be considered. For professional athletes, an earlier surgical intervention is indicated. Surgical techniques include the excision of the degenerated peritendinous tissue, debridement, and reattachment of the pronator-flexor tendon complex to its insertion on the medial epicondyle (M. C. Ciccotti et al., 2004).

## Conclusion

Both lateral and medial epicondylitis are widely encountered pathologies causing elbow pain, while the former is more common and more extensively studied. Professional athletes and manual workers comprise a substantial group of the patient population. Epicondylitis can be summarized as a degenerative process due to repetitive microtrauma and increased joint loads. It is defined by tendinosis, fissures or partial tears and an incomplete reparative process. A meticulous physical examination should guide the clinician towards the epicondylitis diagnosis, but imaging modalities like MRI and US are helpful in excluding other sources of elbow pain and in determining the extent of the injury. After establishing the diagnosis, the patient should be recommended to cease provocative activities. A tailored rehabilitation program is important to regain strength and stability. Surgery is indicated in complex and recalcitrant cases, although the majority of cases tend to resolve following conservative therapy.

## References

Altay, T., Günay, I., & Oztürk, H. (2002). Local injection treatment for lateral epicondylitis. *Clin Orthop Relat Res*, 398(May), 127-130.

Amin, N. H., Kumar, N. S., & Schickendantz, M. S. (2015). Medial epicondylitis: Evaluation and management. In *Journal of the American Academy of Orthopaedic Surgeons* (Vol. 23, Issue 6, pp. 348-355). Lippincott Williams and Wilkins. https://doi.org/10.5435/JAAOS-D-14-00145.

Bennett, J. B. (1994). Lateral and medial epicondylitis. In *Hand Clinics* (Vol. 10, Issue 1, pp. 157-163). https://doi.org/10.1016/s0749-0712(21)01042-8.

Brummel, J., Baker, C. L., & Hopkins, R. (2014). Epicondylitis: Lateral. In *Sports Medicine and Arthroscopy Review* (Vol. 22, Issue 3). Lippincott Williams and Wilkins. https://doi.org/10.1097/JSA.0000000000000024.

Bunata, R. E., Brown, D. S., & Capelo, R. (2007). Anatomic factors related to the cause of tennis elbow. *Journal of Bone and Joint Surgery - Series A*, 89(9), 1955-1963. https://doi.org/10.2106/JBJS.F.00727.

Calfee, R. P., Patel, A., DaSilva, M. F., & Akelman, E. (2008). Management of lateral epicondylitis: Current concepts. *Journal of the American Academy of Orthopaedic Surgeons*, 16(1), 19-29. https://doi.org/10.5435/00124635-200801000-00004.

Ciccotti, M. C., Schwartz, M. A., & Ciccotti, M. G. (2004). Diagnosis and treatment of medial epicondylitis of the elbow. In *Clinics in Sports Medicine* (Vol. 23, Issue 4, pp. 693-705). W. B. Saunders. https://doi.org/10.1016/j.csm.2004.04.011.

Ciccotti, M. G., & Ramani, M. N. (2003). Medial Epicondylitis. *Techniques in Hand and Upper Extremity Surgery*, 7(4), 190-196. https://doi.org/10.1097/00130911-200312000-00010.

Cullinane, F. L., Boocock, M. G., & Trevelyan, F. C. (2014). Is eccentric exercise an effective treatment for lateral epicondylitis? A systematic review. *Clinical Rehabilitation*, 28(1), 3-19. https://doi.org/10.1177/0269215513491974.

De Smedt, T., De Jong, A., Van Leemput, W., Lieven, D., & Van Glabbeek, F. (2007). Lateral epicondylitis in tennis: Update on aetiology, biomechanics and treatment. In *British Journal of Sports Medicine* (Vol. 41, Issue 11, pp. 816-819). Br J Sports Med. https://doi.org/10.1136/bjsm.2007.036723.

Descatha, A., Leclerc, A., Chastang, J. F., & Roquelaure, Y. (2003). Medial epicondylitis in occupational settings: Prevalence, incidence and associated risk factors. In *Journal of Occupational and Environmental Medicine* (Vol. 45, Issue 9, pp. 993-1001). J Occup Environ Med. https://doi.org/10.1097/01.jom.0000085888.37273.d9.

Dunn, J. H., Kim, J. J., Davis, L., & Nirschl, R. P. (2008). Ten- to 14-year follow-up of the Nirschl surgical technique for lateral epicondylitis. *American Journal of Sports Medicine*, 36(2), 261-266. https://doi.org/10.1177/0363546507308932.

Gardner, R. C. (1970). Tennis elbow: diagnosis, pathology and treatment. Nine severe cases treated by a new reconstructive operation. *Clinical Orthopaedics and Related Research*, 72, 248-253.

Gündüz, R., Malas, F. Ü., Borman, P., Kocaoğlu, S., & Özçakar, L. (2012). Physical therapy, corticosteroid injection, and extracorporeal shock wave treatment in lateral epicondylitis: Clinical and ultrasonographical comparison. *Clinical Rheumatology*, 31(5), 807-812. https://doi.org/10.1007/s10067-012-1939-y.

Jeon, J. Y., Lee, M. H., Jeon, I. H., Chung, H. W., Lee, S. H., & Shin, M. J. (2018). Lateral epicondylitis: Associations of MR imaging and clinical assessments with treatment options in patients receiving conservative and arthroscopic managements. *European Radiology*, 28(3), 972-981. https://doi.org/10.1007/s00330-017-5084-5.

Jobe, F. W., & Ciccotti, M. G. (1994). Lateral and Medial Epicondylitis of the Elbow. *The Journal of the American Academy of Orthopaedic Surgeons*, 2(1), 1-8.

Lenoir, H., Mares, O., & Carlier, Y. (2019). Management of lateral epicondylitis. In *Orthopaedics and Traumatology: Surgery and Research* (Vol. 105, Issue 8, pp. S241-S246). Elsevier Masson SAS. https://doi.org/10.1016/j.otsr.2019.09.004.

Morris, H. (1883). Lawn-tennis elbow. *British Medical Journal*, 2, 557.

Nimura, A., Fujishiro, H., Wakabayashi, Y., Imatani, J., Sugaya, H., & Akita, K. (2014). Joint capsule attachment to the extensor carpi radialis brevis origin: An anatomical study with possible implications regarding the etiology of lateral epicondylitis. *Journal of Hand Surgery*, 39(2), 219-225. https://doi.org/10.1016/j.jhsa.2013.11.036.

Nirschl, R., & Pettrone, F. (1979). Tennis elbow. The surgical treatment of lateral epicondylitis. *J Bone Joint Surg Am*, 61(6A), 832-839.

Pienimäki, T., Siira, P., & Vanharanta, H. (2011). Widespread pain in chronic epicondylitis. *European Journal of Pain*, 15(9), 921-927. https://doi.org/10.1016/j.ejpain.2011.04.002.

Plancher, K. D., Halbrecht, J., & Lourie, G. M. (1996). Medial and lateral epicondylitis in the athlete. *Clin Sports Med*, 15(2), 283-305.

Price, R., Sinclair, H., Heinrich, I., & Gibson, T. (1991). Local injection treatment of tennis elbow-hydrocortisone, triamcinolone and lignocaine compared. *Rheumatology*, 30(1), 39-44. https://doi.org/10.1093/rheumatology/30.1.39.

Priest, J. D., Braden, V., & Goodwin Gerberich, S. (1980). The elbow and tennis, Part 1: An analysis of players with and without pain. *Physician and Sportsmedicine*, 8(4), 80-91. https://doi.org/10.1080/00913847.1980.11710917.

Regan, W., Wold, L. E., Coonrad, R., & Morrey, B. F. (1992). Microscopic histopathology of chronic refractory lateral epicondylitis. *The American Journal of Sports Medicine*, 20(6), 746-749. https://doi.org/10.1177/036354659202000618.

Saliman, J. D., Beaulieu, C. F., & McAdams, T. R. (2006). Ligament and tendon injury to the elbow: Clinical, surgical, and imaging features. In *Topics in Magnetic Resonance Imaging* (Vol. 17, Issue 5, pp. 327-336). Top Magn Reson Imaging. https://doi.org/10.1097/RMR.0b013e3180421c9e.

Shiri, R., & Viikari-Juntura, E. (2011). Lateral and medial epicondylitis: Role of occupational factors. In *Best Practice and Research: Clinical Rheumatology* (Vol. 25, Issue 1, pp. 43-57). Bailliere Tindall Ltd. https://doi.org/10.1016/j.berh.2011.01.013.

Shiri, R., Viikari-Juntura, E., Varonen, H., & Heliövaara, M. (2006). Prevalence and determinants of lateral and medial epicondylitis: A population study. *American Journal of Epidemiology*, 164(11), 1065-1074. https://doi.org/10.1093/aje/kwj325.

Stahl, S., & Kaufman, T. (1997). The efficacy of an injection of steroids for medial epicondylitis: A prospective study of sixty elbows. *Journal of Bone and Joint Surgery - Series A*, 79(11), 1648-1652. https://doi.org/10.2106/00004623-199711000-00006.

Tosti, R., Jennings, J., & Sewards, J. M. (2013). Lateral epicondylitis of the elbow. In *American Journal of Medicine* (Vol. 126, Issue 4). *Am J Med*. https://doi.org/10.1016/j.amjmed.2012.09.018.

Vangsness, C. T., & Jobe, F. W. (1991). Surgical treatment of medial epicondylitis. Results in 35 elbows. *Journal of Bone and Joint Surgery - Series B*, 73(3), 409-411. https://doi.org/10.1302/0301-620x.73b3.1670439.

Walz, D. M., Newman, J. S., Konin, G. P., & Ross, G. (2010). Epicondylitis: Pathogenesis, imaging, and treatment. *Radiographics*, 30(1), 167-184. https://doi.org/10.1148/rg.301095078.

In: Musculoskeletal Pain (Common Clinical Presentations) ISBN: 978-1-68507-410-4
Editors: Mehmet Cenk Turgut and Serdar Toy 

*Chapter 20*

# ACHILLES TENDINOPATHY

***Mehmed Nuri Tütüncü****
Department of Orthopedics and Traumatology,
Kars Harakani State Hospital, Kars, Turkey

## ABSTRACT

Achilles tendinopathy is one of the most common overuse pathologies of the foot and ankle, usually presenting with pain and edema around the tendon. Although the etiology is not fully deciphered, it is reported to be multifactorial. Achilles tendinopathy has been shown to be more common in athletes and overweight individuals. Increased involvement in sportive activities worldwide has also led to an increase in the frequency of Achilles tendinopathy. Anatomical classification is used to define two groups: insertional and non-insertional tendinopathy. Histopathological studies of Achilles tendinopathy reported that degenerative signs were encountered as opposed to inflammatory ones.

The Achilles tendinopathy diagnosis can be readily made with a detailed anamnesis, a thorough physical examination and imaging aids. Pain is the prominent symptom. Several special tests can also be used during the physical examination. An initial evaluation is usually carried out with plain radiography. However, MRI is the most sensitive modality, and it is thus considered to be the gold standard in imaging.

Conservative treatment modalities are considered to be the first-line treatment methods in Achilles tendinopathy. Conservative methods include cryotherapy, NSAID use, activity modification and physical therapy. Cases that do not benefit from conservative methods can be treated surgically. Although surgical results are generally satisfactory, complications such as surgical site infections may be encountered.

* Corresponding Author's E-mail: mnuritutuncu@hotmail.com.

## INTRODUCTION

The name "Achilles tendon" is derived from the great warrior Achilles in Greek mythology. According to mythology, he was killed during the Trojan War by being shot in the heel, which was the only vulnerable part of his body. In addition, the word "Achilles" is etymologically associated with the concepts of pain, grief and weakness (Nagy, 1994).

Stress-induced trauma and rupture are most frequently seen in the Achilles tendon when compared to other tendinous structures of the foot and ankle. Achilles tendinopathy is a clinical condition characterized by pain and localized edema around the tendon (Wren et al., 2001). The term Achilles tendinopathy has been used to describe clinical entities such as Achilles tendinitis (acute inflammation of the tendon), Achilles tendinosis (a chronic process due to repetitive microtrauma to the tendon) and Achilles paratenonitis (acute inflammation of the paratenon). In recent studies, it has been reported that the main pathology is not inflammation, but a pathological condition characterized by degeneration and associated incomplete recovery periods. Accordingly, tendinopathy can be a more appropriate term in describing this pathology (Abate et al., 2009, Longo et al., 2009).

## ETIOLOGY AND EPIDEMIOLOGY

Achilles tendinopathy is one of the most widely encountered overuse injuries in the foot and ankle. The annual incidence of Achilles tendon pathologies in the USA is reported to be between 6% and 18% (Kujala et al., 2005). It is more common in athletes and the middle-aged, overweight population (Kalebo et al., 1990). Due to increased participation in sports activities in recent years, the frequency of Achilles tendinopathy has escalated (Aicale et al., 2018). In a study conducted with runners and age- and sex-matched controls, the frequency of Achilles tendinopathy was found to be 10 times higher in the runner group (Rolf and Movin, 1997). Other competitive sports also tend to increase the frequency of Achilles tendinopathy.

The etiology of Achilles tendinopathy has not been fully deciphered, possibly due to its multifactorial nature. Etiological factors can be divided into extrinsic and intrinsic groups. Extrinsic factors include poor technique, improper equipment or surface, a recent change in exercise intensity in professional athletes, the middle-aged sedentary group engaging in sportive activities and increased mechanical overload in general. Extrinsic factors play a more substantial role in acute tendon pathologies (Murtaugh and Ihm, 2013). Intrinsic causes on the other hand, can be listed as tendon hypoxia, age, gender, hyperlipidemia, steroid use, lower extremity malalignment, pes cavus and lateral ankle instability. Intrinsic factors are more prominent in chronic tendon pathologies (Irwin,

2010; Maganaris et al., 2008). Repetitive traumas that exceed the physiological capacity cause micro-tears, creating the pattern for tendinopathy.

## Classification and Pathophysiology

Achilles tendinopathy can be classified according to symptom duration or anatomical location. It can be categorized as acute (<2 weeks), subacute (2-6 weeks), or chronic (>6 weeks) according to the duration of symptoms. It can be divided into insertional (the area where the Achilles tendon attaches to the calcaneus) or non-insertional according to the anatomical position (Van Dijk et al., 2011).

In Achilles tendinopathy, degeneration is observed instead of inflammation which is more commonly seen in tendinitis. In a study conducted with patients who were operated for Achilles tendinopathy, pathological examinations of the specimens did not show inflammatory cells or mediators, instead 97% demonstrated signs of degenerative processes (Kannus and Jozsa, 1991). Histological studies have detected increased tenocyte and glycosaminoglycan concentration, abnormal fiber structure and neovascularization (Irwin, 2010; Alfredson, 2002). Mucoid and lipoid degeneration may be frequently encountered in the Achilles tendon. In mucoid degeneration, mucoid patches and vacuoles that usually contain glycosaminoglycans are seen between the fibers of the tendon. In lipoid degeneration however, fat deposition in the tendon is observed. Macroscopically, the tendon becomes gray or brown in mucoid degeneration and yellow in lipoid degeneration (Maffulli et al., 2000; Jozsa, 1997).

The pathophysiology of pain – the most common finding of Achilles tendinopathy – has not been elucidated yet. Although inflammation is not included in the pathogenesis of tendinopathy, pain is prominent, which could be elicited by neovascularization (Maffulli et al., 2004).

## Clinical Presentation and Physical Examination

Patients with Achilles tendinopathy often express pain and discomfort at the beginning or end of activities. In the acute period, there may be swelling and redness around the tendon. As the injury becomes chronic complaints may generally decrease, but pain can sometimes persist. Symptoms are not severe in the early phase and progress over time; therefore, an initial medical examination can be delayed (Paavola et al., 2002).

Achilles tendinopathy can be diagnosed by a thorough patient history and meticulous physical examination. Patients should be examined without lower body clothing, in standing and supine positions. Any signs of possible deformity and malalignment should be noted. Comparison with the contralateral side in terms of atrophy and leg length should be performed (Leppilahti et al., 1991).

Pain may occur at the attachment site of the tendon to the calcaneus in insertional tendinopathy and 2 to 6 cm above the insertion site in non-insertional tendinopathy. Tendon thickening, palpable nodules, warmth, crepitation, and redness can usually be detected by palpation (Wilson et al., 2018; Cook et al., 2002).

There are some special tests that are used in the examination of Achilles tendinopathy, the first one being the arc sign. Observing the movement of a palpable nodule during flexion and dorsiflexion of the ankle is considered to be a positive result. For the Royal London Hospital test, the painful area is determined by palpation during plantar flexion and the neutral position. Pain relief following dorsiflexion in the designated area indicates a positive result (Longo et al., 2018). In insertional tendinopathy, because patients experience severe pain while pointing their toes to the floor, they fail to stand for long periods. In chronic tendinopathies, the Thompson test can be performed especially if a tear is suspected (Maffulli et al., 2003).

## IMAGING

Imaging modalities are quite useful in reaching a definitive diagnosis of Achilles tendinopathy following a comprehensive patient history and physical examination. Conventional radiography, magnetic resonance imaging (MRI) and ultrasonography (US) are frequently used imaging methods. Radiological evaluation should start with an ankle (lateral view) radiography in the standing position. Enthesopathies, calcifications within the tendon and Haglund deformities can be detected via radiography (Cheng et al., 2007). US, being a practical, affordable, radiation-free and real-time examination tool can also be used for Achilles tendinopathy assessment. User dependency and low sensitivity are disadvantages of the US examination. Acute and chronic pathologies can easily be distinguished via US imaging. In acute pathologies, the tendon seems to be thick and edematous, and fluid accumulation in the peritendinous area can be observed, while in chronic pathologies, peritendinous adhesions, calcifications and nodules can be detected (Martin et al., 2018). In addition, patients with suspected partial or complete tears can benefit from a detailed US examination performed during dorsiflexion and the neutral position in order to determine the type and extent of the tear. In a study conducted with Doppler US, it was shown that the Doppler flow did not correlate with pain, but correlated with an increased tendon anteroposterior diameter which was associated with the presence of tendinopathy (Malliaras et al., 2008).

MRI is the most commonly used imaging modality in the diagnosis of Achilles tendinopathy. It has numerous advantages such as being non-invasive, radiation-free and a high-resolution imaging tool. MRI has a higher sensitivity (96%) in Achilles tendinopathy detection when compared to other imaging modalities (Garras et al., 2012). MRI findings that suggest tendinopathy are loss of the anterior concavity as a result of tendon thickening, remodeling into a convex shape, inflammation at the tendon insertion site, and changes in the retrocalcaneal bursa. Signs of degeneration are usually more evident on gradient echo T2 sequences. Mucinous and myxoid degeneration findings can be detected as hyperintense lesions. Different stages of the chronic degeneration process can be observed simultaneously with MRI. When planning surgery, the thickness, percentage and length of the affected tendon area can be calculated (Chandnani and Bradley, 1994).

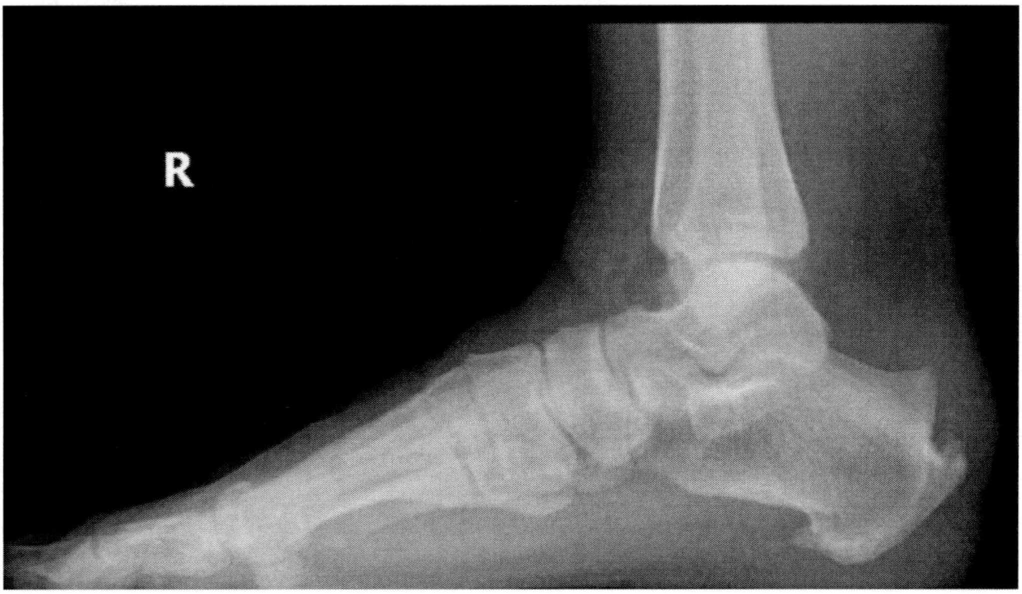


Figure 1. Haglund deformity seen on lateral ankle radiography.

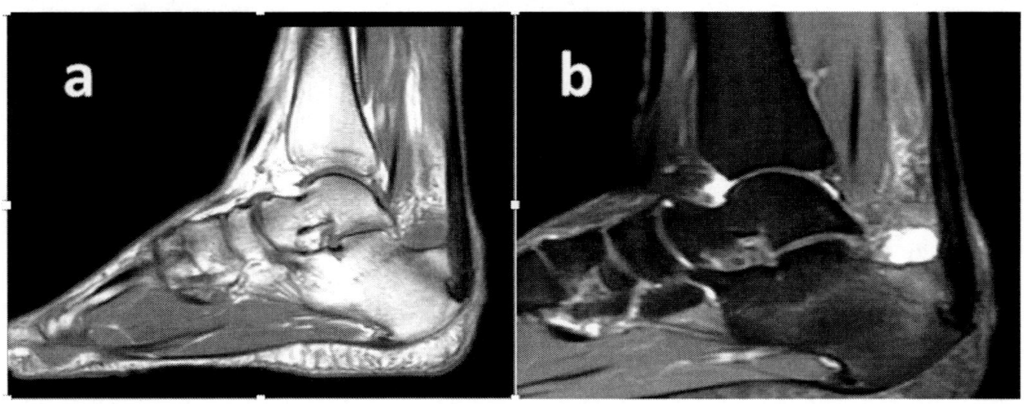


Figure 2. Sagittal T1-weighted (a) and T2-weighted (b) MRI images of an insertional Achilles tendinopathy showing tendon thickening, increased signal in the interstitial area, edema of the Kager fat pad and Haglund deformity.

## TREATMENT

Conservative methods are usually preferred as the initial treatment in Achilles tendinopathy. Detection at an early stage leads to a better prognosis, while the percentage of successfully treated patients decreases in neglected cases (Sorosky et al., 2004). The primary goal of conservative treatment should be pain relief and the restoration of function. Conservative methods should be employed for at least 3 to 6 months, and surgical treatment options can be assessed in recalcitrant and complex cases (Kader et al., 2002).

At first, patients should be recommended to rest, apply ice, use non-steroidal anti-inflammatory drugs (NSAID), and cease exacerbating activities. Possible underlying factors should be investigated. The restriction of athletic activities, a review of recent changes in the training program, and a detailed lower extremity examination regarding possible malalignment or deformity should be performed (Scott et al., 2013). Immobilization options may be considered depending on the severity of the symptoms. Night splinting, walking boots and orthoses can be offered to patients with severe symptoms. However, immobilization should not be prolonged, and a rehabilitation program should be implemented without delay (Irwin, 2010). Shoe modifications and heel pads are also used during the treatment. Glyceryl trinitrate patches can also be applied for the acceleration of the healing process and palliation of pain (Murrell et al., 1997).

Physical therapy is a crucial component of the conservative management of Achilles tendinopathy – restoring function and preventing a recurrence of pathology. After pain palliation is provided, an exercise program should be initiated to ensure tendon healing (Silbernagel et al., 2001). Exercises can be prescribed either as a home program or under the supervision of a physiotherapist. Eccentric strengthening exercises are shown to be highly effective in Achilles tendinopathy. Strengthening programs performed with gradually increasing loads have been reported to accelerate tendon remodeling (Sussmilch-Leitch et al., 2012).

Although no consensus has been reached regarding the dose, frequency and efficacy of extracorporeal shock-wave therapy (ESWT), it is a widely used treatment modality in Achilles tendinopathy. It is suggested that ESWT contributes to soft tissue reorganization and inhibits pain generation through pain receptors (Gerdesmeyer et al., 2015). Since high-energy ESWT can be quite painful for the patient, local anesthesia may be required. Therefore, low-energy ESWT is more often preferred. ESWT has been reported to be more effective when an eccentric strengthening exercise program is added to the treatment plan (Rompe et al., 2007). Low level laser therapy, deep friction massage, and therapeutic US are among the other methods used (Ramirez et al., 1997; Gehlsen et al., 1999; Tsai et al., 2014).

Injections are frequently administered for Achilles tendinopathy. There are numerous studies reporting the efficacy of platelet rich plasma (PRP) treatment during the tendon repair process (de Mos et al., 2008). PRP injections performed under US are reported to reduce pain in the short term, however long-term results are questionable considering the recurrence of symptoms after the initial period (Kaux et al., 2015). In addition, there are studies suggesting that PRP contributes to tendon repair in Achilles tendon rupture, but is not beneficial in the treatment of Achilles tendinopathy (Sadoghi et al., 2013). Corticosteroid injections may cause tendon rupture, therefore intratendinous application is controversial (Coombes et al., 2010). However, retrocalcaneal bursitis frequently coexists with insertional tendinopathy, and injection into the bursa is recommended in such cases (Checa et al., 201). Prolotherapy, sclerotherapy and hyaluronic acid injections can also be considered (Kaplan et al., 2019).

Patients who fail to respond to conservative treatment for at least 3 to 6 months can be considered for surgery. Surgical interventions should aim to remove adhesions and degenerative tissues and obtain a healthy/intact tendon structure (Kannus and Jozsa, 1991). Areas to be excised or debrided should be determined during preoperative planning (Filardo et al. 2010). For insertional tendinopathy, the degenerative area in the insertion site should be debrided, the associated calcaneal prominence and/or Haglund deformity should be treated, and a retrocalcaneal bursectomy should be performed, if necessary (Wiegerinck et al., 2013). For non-insertional tendinopathy, the degenerative tendon section should be debrided and nodules should be excised. There are studies showing that multiple longitudinal tenotomies induce recovery by increasing the blood flow to the region (Friedrich et al., 2001). If more than 50% of the tendon is to be resected, reconstruction with augmentation or grafting should be considered (Irwin, 2010). Surgical results are generally considered as good or excellent, but it should be kept in mind that complications such as superficial wound problems and infections are not rare (Paavola et al., 2000).

## CONCLUSION

Achilles tendinopathy is a very common pathology that presents with pain, swelling and loss of function. Multiple factors are influential in the etiology. Degeneration – as opposed to inflammation – plays an important role in the pathophysiology. A radiograph should be the first imaging test to be requested, but MRI is the most sensitive imaging modality. Conservative methods should be preferred in the initial period. Prognosis is favorable in early diagnosis and conservative treatment methods, which are RICE (rest, ice, compression elevation), NSAIDs, exercise, physical therapy and injections, usually suffice in this period. Surgical interventions are indicated in patients with recalcitrant symptoms despite conservative treatment for at least 3 to 6 months. Surgical results are generally considered to be successful.

## REFERENCES

Abate, M., Silbernagel, K. G., Siljeholm, C., Di Iorio, A., De Amicis, D., Salini, V., Werner, S. & Paganelli, R. (2009). Pathogenesis of tendinopathies: inflammation or degeneration?. *Arthritis research & therapy*, *11*(3), 235. https://doi.org/10.1186/ar2723.

Aicale, R., Tarantino, D. & Maffulli, N. (2018). Overuse injuries in sport: a comprehensive overview. *Journal of orthopaedic surgery and research*, *13*(1), 309. https://doi.org/10.1186/s13018-018-1017-5.

Alfredson, H., Bjur, D., Thorsen, K., Lorentzon, R. & Sandström, P. (2002). High intratendinous lactate levels in painful chronic Achilles tendinosis. An investigation using microdialysis technique. *Journal of orthopaedic research: official publication of the Orthopaedic Research Society*, *20*(5), 934–938. https://doi.org/10.1016/S0736-0266(02)00021-9.

Chandnani, V. P. & Bradley, Y. C. (1994). Achilles tendon and miscellaneous tendon lesions. *Magnetic resonance imaging clinics of North America*, *2*(1), 89–96.

Checa, A., Chun, W. & Pappu, R. (2011). Ultrasound-guided diagnostic and therapeutic approach to Retrocalcaneal Bursitis. *The Journal of rheumatology*, *38*(2), 391–392. https://doi.org/10.3899/ jrheum.100920.

Cook, J. L., Khan, K. M. & Purdam, C. (2002). Achilles tendinopathy. *Manual therapy*, *7*(3), 121–130. https://doi.org/ 10.1054/math.2002.0458.

Coombes, B. K., Bisset, L. & Vicenzino, B. (2010). Efficacy and safety of corticosteroid injections and other injections for management of tendinopathy: a systematic review of randomised controlled trials. *Lancet (London, England)*, *376*(9754), 1751–1767. https://doi.org/10.1016/S0140-6736(10)61160-9.

de Mos, M., van der Windt, A. E., Jahr, H., van Schie, H. T., Weinans, H., Verhaar, J. A. & van Osch, G. J. (2008). Can platelet-rich plasma enhance tendon repair? A cell culture study. *The American journal of sports medicine*, *36*(6), 1171–1178.

Filardo, G., Presti, M. L., Kon, E. & Marcacci, M. (2010). Nonoperative biological treatment approach for partial Achilles tendon lesion. *Orthopedics*, *33*(2), 120–123. https://doi.org/10.3928/ 01477447-20100104-31.

Friedrich, T., Schmidt, W., Jungmichel, D., Horn, L. C. & Josten, C. (2001). Histopathology in rabbit Achilles tendon after operative tenolysis (longitudinal fiber incisions). *Scandinavian journal of medicine & science in sports*, *11*(1), 4–8. https://doi.org/10.1034/j.1600-0838.2001.011001004.x.

Garras, D. N., Raikin, S. M., Bhat, S. B., Taweel, N. & Karanjia, H. (2012). MRI is unnecessary for diagnosing acute Achilles tendon ruptures: clinical diagnostic criteria. *Clinical orthopaedics and related research*, *470*(8), 2268–2273. https://doi.org/10.1007/s11999-012-2355-y.

Gehlsen, G. M., Ganion, L. R. & Helfst, R. (1999). Fibroblast responses to variation in soft tissue mobilization pressure. *Medicine and science in sports and exercise*, *31*(4), 531–535. https://doi.org/10.1097/ 00005768-199904000-00006.

Gerdesmeyer, L., Mittermayr, R., Fuerst, M., Al Muderis, M., Thiele, R., Saxena, A. & Gollwitzer, H. (2015). Current evidence of extracorporeal shock wave therapy in chronic Achilles tendinopathy. *International journal of surgery (London, England)*, *24*(Pt B), 154–159. https://doi.org/10.1016/ j.ijsu.2015.07.718.

Irwin, T. A. (2010). Current concepts review: insertional Achilles tendinopathy. *Foot & ankle international*, *31*(10), 933–939. https://doi.org/10.3113/FAI.2010.0933.

Jozsa, L. K. P. (1997). *Human Tendon: Anatomy, Physiology and Pathology*. Champaign: Human Kinetics.

Kader, D., Saxena, A., Movin, T. & Maffulli, N. (2002). Achilles tendinopathy: some aspects of basic science and clinical management. *British journal of sports medicine*, *36*(4), 239–249. https://doi.org/10.1136/bjsm.36.4.239.

Kannus, P. & Józsa, L. (1991). Histopathological changes preceding spontaneous rupture of a tendon. A controlled study of 891 patients. *The Journal of bone and joint surgery. American volume*, *73*(10), 1507–1525.

Kaplan, K., Olivencia, O., Dreger, M., Hanney, W. J. & Kolber, M. (2019). *Achilles Tendinopathy: An Evidence-Based Overview for the Sports Medicine Professional, Strength and Conditioning Journal*, *41*(5), 24-40. doi: 10.1519/SSC.0000 000000000485.

Kaux, J. F., Drion, P., Croisier, J. L. & Crielaard, J. M. (2015). Tendinopathies and platelet-rich plasma (PRP): from pre-clinical experiments to therapeutic use. *Journal of stem cells & regenerative medicine*, *11*(1), 7–17. https://doi.org/10. 46582/jsrm.1101003.

Kälebo, P., Goksör, L. A., Swärd, L. & Peterson, L. (1990). Soft-tissue radiography, computed tomography, and ultrasonography of partial Achilles tendon ruptures. *Acta radiologica (Stockholm, Sweden: 1987)*, *31*(6), 565–570.

Kujala, U. M., Sarna, S. & Kaprio, J. (2005). Cumulative incidence of Achilles tendon rupture and tendinopathy in male former elite athletes. *Clinical journal of sport medicine: official journal of the Canadian Academy of Sport Medicine*, *15*(3), 133–135. https://doi.org/10.1097/01.jsm.0000165347.55638.23.

Leppilahti, J., Orava, S., Karpakka, J. & Takala, T. (1991). Overuse injuries of the Achilles tendon. *Annales chirurgiae et gynaecologiae*, *80*(2), 202–207.

Longo, U. G., Ronga, M. & Maffulli, N. (2018). Achilles Tendinopathy. *Sports medicine and arthroscopy review*, *26*(1), 16–30. https://doi.org/10.1097/JSA.000 0000000000185.

Longo, U. G., Ronga, M. & Maffulli, N. (2009). Achilles tendinopathy. *Sports medicine and arthroscopy review*, *17*(2), 112–126. https://doi.org/10.1097/JSA.0b01 3e3181a3d625.

Lu, C. C., Cheng, Y. M., Fu, Y. C., Tien, Y. C., Chen, S. K. & Huang, P. J. (2007). Angle analysis of Haglund syndrome and its relationship with osseous variations and Achilles tendon calcification. *Foot & ankle international*, *28*(2), 181–185. https://doi.org/10.3113/ FAI.2007.0181.

Maffulli, N., Khan, K. M. & Puddu, G. (1998). Overuse tendon conditions: time to change a confusing terminology. *Arthroscopy: the journal of arthroscopic & related surgery: official publication of the Arthroscopy Association of North America and the International Arthroscopy Association*, *14*(8), 840–843. https://doi.org/10.1016/ s0749-8063(98)70021-0.

Maffulli, N., Barrass, V. & Ewen, S. W. (2000). Light microscopic histology of Achilles tendon ruptures. A comparison with unruptured tendons. *The American journal of sports medicine*, *28*(6), 857–863. https://doi.org/10.1177/03635465000280061401.

Maffulli, N., Kenward, M. G., Testa, V., Capasso, G., Regine, R. & King, J. B. (2003). Clinical diagnosis of Achilles tendinopathy with tendinosis. *Clinical journal of sport medicine: official journal of the Canadian Academy of Sport Medicine*, *13*(1), 11–15. https://doi.org/10.1097/00042752-200301000-00003.

Maffulli, N., Sharma, P. & Luscombe, K. L. (2004). Achilles tendinopathy: aetiology and management. *Journal of the Royal Society of Medicine*, *97*(10), 472–476. https://doi.org/10.1258/ jrsm.97.10.472.

Maganaris, C. N., Narici, M. V. & Maffulli, N. (2008). Biomechanics of the Achilles tendon. *Disability and rehabilitation*, *30*(20-22), 1542–1547. https://doi.org/10.1080/ 09638280701785494.

Malliaras, P., Richards, P. J., Garau, G. & Maffulli, N. (2008). Achilles tendon Doppler flow may be associated with mechanical loading among active athletes. *The American journal of sports medicine*, *36*(11), 2210–2215. https://doi.org/10.1177/ 0363546508319052.

Martin, R. L., Chimenti, R., Cuddeford, T., Houck, J., Matheson, J. W., McDonough, C. M., Paulseth, S., Wukich, D. K. & Carcia, C. R. (2018). Achilles Pain, Stiffness, and Muscle Power Deficits: Midportion Achilles Tendinopathy Revision 2018. *The Journal of orthopaedic and sports physical therapy*, *48*(5), A1–A38. https://doi.org/10.2519/jospt.2018.0302.

Murrell, G. A., Szabo, C., Hannafin, J. A., Jang, D., Dolan, M. M., Deng, X. H., Murrell, D. F. & Warren, R. F. (1997). Modulation of tendon healing by nitric oxide.

*Inflammation research: official journal of the European Histamine Research Society ...* [et al.], *46*(1), 19–27. https://doi.org/10.1007/s000110050027.

Murtaugh, B. & Ihm, J. M. (2013). Eccentric training for the treatment of tendinopathies. *Current sports medicine reports*, *12*(3), 175–182. https://doi.org/10.1249/JSR.0b013e3182933761.

Nagy, G. (1994). The Name of Achilles: Questions of Etymology and "Folk-Etymology". *Illinois Classical Studies*, *19*, 3-9. Retrieved May 9, 2021, from http://www.jstor.org/stable/23065415.

Paavola, M., Orava, S., Leppilahti, J., Kannus, P. & Järvinen, M. (2000). Chronic Achilles tendon overuse injury: complications after surgical treatment. An analysis of 432 consecutive patients. *The American journal of sports medicine*, *28*(1), 77–82. https://doi.org/10.1177/ 03635465000280012501.

Paavola, M., Kannus, P., Orava, S., Pasanen, M. & Järvinen, M. (2002). Surgical treatment for chronic Achilles tendinopathy: a prospective seven month follow up study. *British journal of sports medicine*, *36*(3), 178–182. https://doi.org/10.1136/bjsm.36.3.178.

Ramirez, A., Schwane, J. A., McFarland, C. & Starcher, B. (1997). The effect of ultrasound on collagen synthesis and fibroblast proliferation *in vitro*. *Medicine and science in sports and exercise*, *29*(3), 326–332. https://doi.org/10.1097/00005768-199703000-00007.

Rolf, C., & Movin, T. (1997). Etiology, histopathology, and outcome of surgery in achillodynia. *Foot & ankle international*, *18*(9), 565–569. https://doi.org/10.1177/107110079701800906.

Rompe, J. D., Nafe, B., Furia, J. P. & Maffulli, N. (2007). Eccentric loading, shock-wave treatment, or a wait-and-see policy for tendinopathy of the main body of tendo Achillis: a randomized controlled trial. *The American journal of sports medicine*, *35*(3), 374–383. https://doi.org/10.1177/0363546506295940.

Sadoghi, P., Rosso, C., Valderrabano, V., Leithner, A. & Vavken, P. (2013). The role of platelets in the treatment of Achilles tendon injuries. *Journal of orthopaedic research: official publication of the Orthopaedic Research Society*, *31*(1), 111–118. https://doi.org/ 10.1002/jor.22199.

Scott, A., Huisman, E. & Khan, K. (2011). Conservative treatment of chronic Achilles tendinopathy. *CMAJ: Canadian Medical Association journal = journal de l'Association medicale canadienne*, *183*(10), 1159–1165. https://doi.org/10.1503/cmaj.101680.

Silbernagel, K. G., Thomeé, R., Thomeé, P. & Karlsson, J. (2001). Eccentric overload training for patients with chronic Achilles tendon pain--a randomised controlled study with reliability testing of the evaluation methods. *Scandinavian journal of medicine & science in sports*, *11*(4), 197–206. https://doi.org/10.1034/j.1600-0838.2001.110402.x.

Sorosky, B., Press, J., Plastaras, C. & Rittenberg, J. (2004). The practical management of Achilles tendinopathy. *Clinical journal of sport medicine: official journal of the Canadian Academy of Sport Medicine*, *14*(1), 40–44. https://doi.org/10.1097/00042752-200401000-00007.

Sussmilch-Leitch, S. P., Collins, N. J., Bialocerkowski, A. E., Warden, S. J. & Crossley, K. M. (2012). Physical therapies for Achilles tendinopathy: systematic review and meta-analysis. *Journal of foot and ankle research*, *5*(1), 15. https://doi.org/10.1186/1757-1146-5-15.

Tsai, W. C., Cheng, J. W., Chen, J. L., Chen, C. Y., Chang, H. N., Liao, Y. H., Lin, M. S. & Pang, J. H. (2014). Low-level laser irradiation stimulates tenocyte proliferation in association with increased NO synthesis and upregulation of PCNA and cyclins. *Lasers in medical science*, *29*(4), 1377–1384. https://doi.org/10.1007/s10103-014-1528-1.

van Dijk, C. N., van Sterkenburg, M. N., Wiegerinck, J. I., Karlsson, J. & Maffulli, N. (2011). Terminology for Achilles tendon related disorders. *Knee surgery, sports traumatology, arthroscopy: official journal of the ESSKA*, *19*(5), 835–841. https://doi.org/10.1007/s00167-010-1374-z.

Wiegerinck, J. I., Kerkhoffs, G. M., van Sterkenburg, M. N., Sierevelt, I. N. & van Dijk, C. N. (2013). Treatment for insertional Achilles tendinopathy: a systematic review. *Knee surgery, sports traumatology, arthroscopy: official journal of the ESSKA*, *21*(6), 1345–1355. https://doi.org/10.1007/s00167-012-2219-8.

Wilson, F., Walshe, M., O'Dwyer, T., Bennett, K., Mockler, D. & Bleakley, C. (2018). Exercise, orthoses and splinting for treating Achilles tendinopathy: a systematic review with meta-analysis. *British journal of sports medicine*, *52*(24), 1564–1574. https://doi.org/10.1136/bjsports-2017-098913.

Wren, T. A., Yerby, S. A., Beaupré, G. S. & Carter, D. R. (2001). Mechanical properties of the human Achilles tendon. *Clinical biomechanics (Bristol, Avon)*, *16*(3), 245–251. https://doi.org/ 10.1016/s0268-0033(00)00089-9.

In: Musculoskeletal Pain (Common Clinical Presentations) ISBN: 978-1-68507-410-4
Editors: Mehmet Cenk Turgut and Serdar Toy 

*Chapter 21*

# PLANTAR HEEL PAIN

***Hakan Özbay*[*], MD***
Department of Orthopedics and Traumatology,
Ağrı Training and Research Hospital, Ağrı, Turkey

## ABSTRACT

Plantar heel pain which sometimes seriously disrupts the activities of daily living is one of the main reasons for admission to orthopedic outpatient clinics. Although pain may originate due to rheumatological, inflammatory, neurological, or oncological reasons, the most common cause is plantar fasciitis. History and physical examination are the mainstays of the diagnosis, and imaging tools or electromyography can be used to exclude several reasons for plantar heel pain. The localization or distribution of the pain, the age of the patient, unilateral or bilateral involvement, accompanying symptoms like burning or paresthesia, and some physical examination tests are generally enough to make a prompt diagnosis. Conservative treatment options like oral nonsteroidal anti-inflammatory drugs, shoe modifications, and physical therapy modalities are generally satisfactory to relieve symptoms, and surgery is rarely needed in recalcitrant cases.

**Keywords:** foot, heel, plantar fasciitis, physical therapy, surgery

## INTRODUCTION

Plantar heel pain is one of the most common complaints that orthopedic surgeons are likely to encounter in outpatient clinics. It is generally caused by plantar fasciitis which is the diagnosis of exclusion. Plantar fasciitis is an overuse injury characterized by

[*] Corresponding Author's E-mail: ozbayhakan@yahoo.com.

inflammation at the origin of the plantar fascia and pain in the inferomedial aspect of the calcaneal tuberosity. The annual cost of plantar heel pain in the US is estimated at approximately $284 million (Tong and Furia, 2010). Musculoskeletal, inflammatory, and neurological diseases may present with plantar heel pain and these diseases should be investigated especially in atypical clinical presentation. A thorough history and physical examination are usually enough to make a proper diagnosis in almost all cases, but diagnostic modalities exist as a helpful adjunct (Cullen and Singh, 2006).

Conservative interventions are the mainstay of the treatment regardless of diagnosis. Oral or local anti-inflammatory medications, shoe inserts or orthosis, physical therapy exercises, and extracorporeal shock-wave therapy are included. Surgery is an option for patients who are not responsive to conservative treatment for at least six months (Young et al., 2001).

## Etiology

Plantar heel pain, with or without the calcaneal heel spur, is described as soreness or tenderness under the heel, and may be experienced by 10% of the population at any time in their life. The pain often radiates from the central part or medial of the heel pad to the medial longitudinal arch of the foot. The term "plantar fasciitis" is a common cause of heel pain in adults, described as a self-limited inflammatory condition that extends along the plantar fascia. Some causes of plantar heel pain such as tendinitis or retrocalcaneal bursitis are well understood but the precise cause of the pain is still uncertain. Some occupations, such as police or military personnel are more susceptible to plantar heel pain, because of prolonged standing or repetitive stress. Factors that have been proposed for the etiology of plantar heel pain are aging, obesity, anatomical and biomechanical factors, occupational factors and acute injuries (Landorf and Menz, 2008).

The precise etiology and the exact cause of the painful heel are uncertain. Obesity is one of the etiological factors for increased risk of developing plantar heel pain in 40% of men and 90% of women. Individuals whose body mass index is >30 kilograms/square meter are also at increased risk for the development of plantar fasciitis (van Leeuwen et al., 2016).

The heel pad is a shock absorber structure on the soles of the feet. It distributes body weight and absorbs shock while walking, running, and jumping. Heel pad displacement occurs during walking or running to dissipate the impact of energy and elastic recoil recovers part of the impacted energy. Loss of the elasticity of the plantar heel pad is yet another factor in plantar heel pain. The collagen and water content, as well as the elastic fibrous tissue of the plantar heel pad decrease with aging. These degenerative changes with increasing age, also named as plantar fat pad atrophy, can account in part for plantar heel pain (Yi et al., 2011).

**Table 1. Etiological factors for plantar heel pain**

| |
|---|
| Aging |
| Obesity |
| Anatomical factors |
| Biomechanical causes |
| Occupational factors |
| Acute injury |

## ANATOMY

The plantar fascia is a strong connective tissue that extends from its origin at the os calcis to its insertion at the heads of the metatarsals. So, it crosses all the plantar aspect of the foot longitudinally. This longitudinal arch is the strongest ligamentous band of all the other ligaments. The plantar fascia comprises three bundles: medial, central, and lateral bundles with the central bundle being most commonly affected. It arises from the medial tubercle of the os calcis and divides into five limbs to the heads of the metatarsals. The other ligaments are short and long plantar ligaments (Kirkpatrick et al., 2017).

The origin of the long plantar ligament is the os calcis and the insertion is the bases of the second to fifth metatarsals. The short plantar ligament runs from the os calcis to the navicula. The long plantar ligament is separated from the plantar fascia by the quadratus plantae, flexor digitorum brevis, abductor hallucis, and abductor digiti minimi. Chronic overuse or repetitive microtrauma leads to microtears and recurrent inflammation at the origin of the plantar fascia and inferomedial muscularity containing the abductor hallucis, flexor digitorum brevis, and quadratus plantae (Kirkpatrick et al., 2017).

The plantar fascia is innervated by the posterior tibial nerve. It provides branches to the medial calcaneal and the first branch of the lateral plantar nerve which is more important. Baxter's neuritis is the entrapment of the first branch of the lateral plantar nerve which is a possible cause of plantar heel pain. Although the patients with plantar fasciitis describe tenderness only at the medial tubercle, Baxter's neuritis causes tenderness all along the nerve (Stecco et al., 2013).

## BIOMECHANICS

The plantar fascia is one of the most important static supports of the longitudinal arch of the foot. The plantar fascia is under constant strain as it is pulled distally around the drum of the metatarsal heads, as the toes are dorsiflexed. So, the elevation of the longitudinal arch occurs by tightening after traction on the origin of the plantar fascia.

This mechanism is described as the "windlass mechanism" by Hicks et al., (Hicks et al., 1954).

Some diseases such as pes cavus, pes planus, shortening of the Achilles tendon, or varus deformity of the hindfoot can increase the repetitive stress on the plantar fascia and disrupt the windlass mechanism (Van Wyngarden, 1997). So, disruption of the windlass mechanism and increased stress put the patient at increased risk for plantar heel pain. Limitation in ankle dorsiflexion is believed to be one of the risk factors for painful heels (Riddle et al., 2003).

The principal stress on the plantar fascia occurs during walking. The plantar fascia is also responsible for assisting in the push-off power during ambulation. It is relaxed in the "heel strike" period of the stance phase and tightens maximally at the end of the push-off phase. Athletes participating in gymnastics or racquet sports complain of painful heel because of the contribution of the plantar fascia to push-off power during walking, running, or jumping (Tsai et al., 1999).

## Clinical Examination

The diagnosis of plantar heel pain is based on history and physical examination. A detailed history and particularly physical examination are generally enough to detect the underlying pathology for the painful heel. Physical examination of the foot also has great importance and ease of practice because of the subcutaneous location of underlying structures (Thompson et al., 2014).

People with painful heels are usually between 40 and 70 years old, male and active, with unilateral symptoms. Individuals <40 years old with bilateral plantar heel pain should be investigated to rule out rheumatoid arthritis, ankylosing spondylitis, and Reiter syndrome. Differential diagnosis of plantar heel pain is summarized in Table 2.

People with plantar fasciitis usually complain about pain under the heel pad, especially at the inferomedial aspect of the calcaneal tuberosity, worsening in the morning while getting out of bed. The reason for this symptom is believed to be due to the contracted or stiff plantar fascia in the morning. The pain diminishes after the patient ambulates for a few steps after rising from bed. Patients don't complain about the pain during the day, but mention that pain increases toward the end of the day and is relieved by rest. The duration of symptoms can vary from weeks to years. The pain is usually unilateral, but bilateral feet are affected in 15-30% of patients (Thompson et al., 2014). The typical location of the pain on the medial aspect of the foot in different clinical scenarios is shown in Figure 1.

On physical examination of the foot with plantar fasciitis, localized pain and tenderness at the inferomedial aspect of the calcaneal tuberosity are typical (Figure 1). Patients can report pain radiating to the calf or toes. Some patients can refuse to bear weight on their calcaneal region, and they can represent with toe-walking on the affected side in unilateral involvement.

**Table 2. Differential diagnosis of painful heel**

| |
|---|
| Musculoskeletal |
| Plantar fasciitis |
| Fat pad syndrome |
| Calcaneal stress fracture or contusion |
| Flexor hallucis longus/posterior tibial tendinitis |
| Achilles' tendinopathy |
| Neurological |
| Tarsal tunnel syndrome |
| Diabetic/alcoholic neuropathy |
| Entrapment neuropathies (Baxter's neuritis, medial calcaneal, and abductor digiti quinti nerve entrapment) |
| Lumbosacral radiculopathy |
| Inflammatory |
| Rheumatoid arthritis |
| Reiter syndrome |
| Ankylosing spondylitis |
| Others |
| Retrocalcaneal bursitis |
| Haglund's disease |
| Tumors |
| Infections |
| Plantar fascia rupture |
| Calcaneal apophysitis (Sever disease) |

Heel pain is reproduced with passive dorsiflexion of the metatarsophalangeal (MTP) joints (Windlass test) while the patient's knee is flexed to 90 degrees in a non-weight bearing position (Figure 2). The ankle is stabilized by the examiner, and the MTP joint is extended. If the pain is produced at the end range of the passive extension due to excessive tightening of the plantar fascia, the Windlass test is positive. Other causes of painful heel should be investigated if history and physical examination are not typical for plantar fasciitis (De Garceau et al., 2003).

Calcaneal stress fractures are usually seen in military recruits and result from repetitive compressive loads after weight-bearing activities. Patients usually mention a sudden increase in their running activities. On physical examination, there will be pain on palpation at both the medial and lateral sides of the calcaneus (Welck et al., 2017).

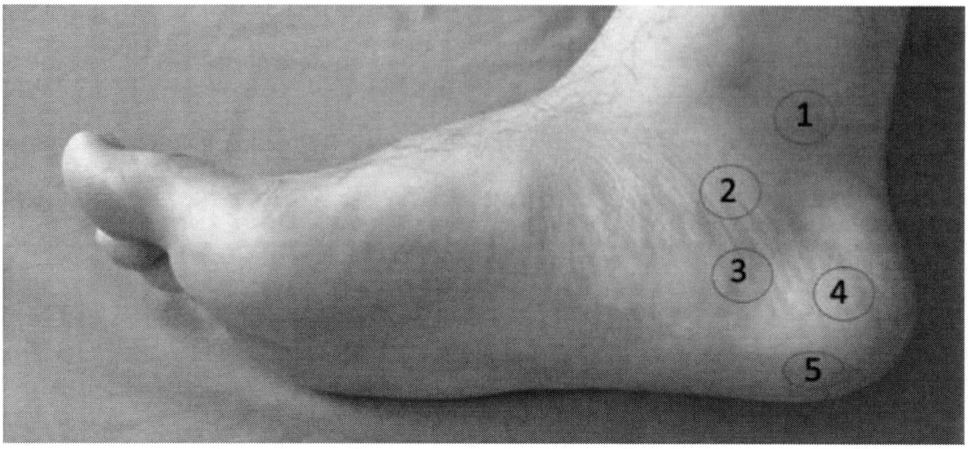


Source: from the author's individual archives.

Figure 1. Typical locations of heel pain in different diseases on the medial aspect of the calcaneus. 1: Tarsal tunnel syndrome 2: Baxter nerve entrapment 3: Plantar fasciitis 4: Calcaneus stress fracture 5: Heel fat pad atrophy.

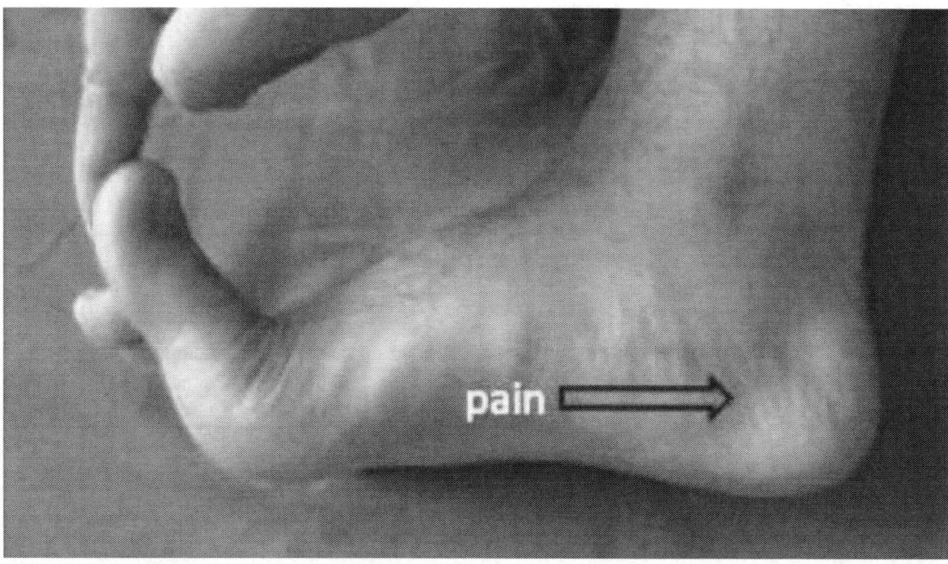


Source: from the author's individual archives.

Figure 2. Windlass test for the physical examination of plantar fasciitis.

Heel fat pad syndrome is typically due to atrophy of the heel fat pad. The typical location of the pain is the center of the heel (Figure 1). Patients will typically complain of pain increasing with walking on hard surfaces. Palpation or applying pressure on the plantar side of the center of the heel may elicit sharp or stabbing pain.

Tarsal tunnel syndrome is a compressive neuropathy of the tibial nerve generally caused by space-occupying lesions such as ganglion cysts. Patients report sharp, burning pain in the medial aspect of the foot, numbness, or intermittent paresthesias in the plantar side of the foot. Tinel's sign is a positive percussion test of the tibial nerve reproducing symptoms on the medial aspect of the heel. Baxter's nerve entrapment is another clinical entity that can be confused with plantar fasciitis because of its close proximity to the typical location in the medial aspect of the calcaneus (Ahmad et al., 2012).

The first branch of the lateral plantar nerve (the branch to the abductor digiti quinti) is compressed between the fascia of the abductor hallucis longus and the quadratus plantae. This nerve can also be affected by the inflammation of the plantar fascia. So, plantar fasciitis and Baxter's nerve entrapment can overlap in the same patient and discrimination is not always possible (Cullen and Singh, 2006).

Patients with diabetic or alcoholic neuropathies usually represent a history of burning pain and numbness. A thorough neurological examination is essential in the detection of the neuropathic source of heel pain (Sidon et al., 2019). A history of fever or malaise, unilateral swelling, and erythema of the foot is an indicator of infections of the foot (Aiyer et al., 2019). Foot tumors are rare. Soft tissue tumors are easily palpable because of the subcutaneous location of masses on the foot. Bone tumors of the calcaneus are also rare and can be detected by radiological examination (Murai et al., 2018).

## Radiographic Findings

Radiographic studies such as radiographs, ultrasound, computed tomography (CT), magnetic resonance imaging (MRI), or bone scans are useful to rule out mechanical causes of the painful heel. Otherwise, these modalities are not usually helpful in the diagnosis or treatment of plantar fasciitis. In 50% of the patients who are diagnosed with plantar fasciitis, lateral calcaneal radiographs indicate a heel spur. But calcaneal spurs on these radiographs have no clinical significance (Figure 3).

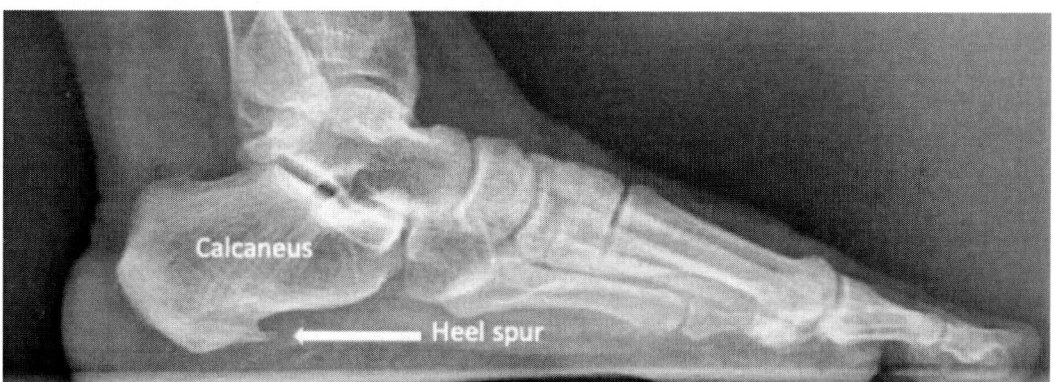


Source: from the author's individual archives.

Figure 3. Lateral calcaneal radiography of a patient with calcaneal heel spur.

Weight-bearing calcaneal radiographs are used to detect or rule out calcaneus stress fractures. But, it should be kept in mind that radiographs may not become positive for the first 4 weeks. Bone scans can be used to rule out calcaneus stress fractures in the acute setting.

Ultrasonography is a helpful diagnostic modality for the diagnosis of plantar fasciitis. It is not an optimal diagnostic tool to rule out other pathological conditions of the foot. MRI can be used to evaluate the bony structures and soft tissues of the foot, and also to rule out diseases other than plantar fasciitis. It is preferred to use this for the atypical symptomatic presentation of heel pain to rule out malignities, osteomyelitis, flexor hallucis longus or posterior tibial tendinitis, calcaneal stress fracture or contusion, and plantar fascia rupture (McNally and Shetty, 2010).

Electrodiagnostic studies can be performed to rule out radiculopathies or peripheral neuropathies in patients with a neurological etiology of plantar heel pain. Electromyography of the abductor digiti minimi or abductor hallucis muscle is more likely to be abnormal in patients with entrapment of the lateral or medial plantar nerve, respectively (Schon et al., 1993).

## TREATMENT

Conservative measures are generally sufficient for the resolution of the symptoms within 12 months in almost 90% of the patients despite the lack of understanding of the exact cause of plantar heel pain. Only 10% of the patients do not benefit from conservative interventions and symptoms persist longer than 12 months. Conservative interventions include oral nonsteroidal anti-inflammatory drugs (NSAIDs), shoe inserts or modifications, local corticosteroid injections, specific physical therapy exercises for plantar fascia stretching and strengthening, casting, botulinum toxin type A injection, extracorporeal shock wave therapy, and, rigid or semi-rigid orthosis (Ahmad et al., 2017; Donley et al., 2007).

The patient should be advised to be patient, that symptoms may persist for over twelve months and conservative treatment should be continued for at least six months. Some of the patients (approximately 10% of all patients) who do not respond to conservative treatment and whose symptoms persist over 12 months, require surgery to relieve symptoms. The American Orthopedic Foot and Ankle Society (AOFAS) also recommends a minimum of 6 to 12 months of conservative treatment before surgery. Although a painful heel is one of the most common complaints in orthopedic outpatient clinics, surgery is required in extremely rare conditions for recalcitrant cases.

Conservative treatment aims to achieve three main principles: to diminish pain and inflammation, reduce the stress of tissue, and restore strength and flexibility. There is not a universally accepted protocol for the treatment of plantar heel pain. Generally, combinations of different nonsurgical interventions are used to treat this challenging clinical entity. The University of Pittsburgh Medical Center Foot and Ankle Clinic has suggested a standardized protocol for the conservative management of insertional heel pain that includes: taking NSAIDs for four weeks, using an orthosis or heel cup at all times when wearing shoes, wearing a night splint, and taking part in a plantar fascia and Achilles stretching program. However, the success rate was not satisfactory, with 51% being asymptomatic after four months (Lareau et al., 2014).

Fat pad atrophy of the heel is a different clinical entity that needs a unique treatment modality. Advanced age, trauma, inflammatory diseases, and corticosteroid injections are the main causes of heel fat pad atrophy; and treatment principles should focus on the etiology. Heel cups, pads, or orthotics are the mainstay of the treatment. An augmenting plantar subdermal region injection of liquid silicone is an alternative treatment method. Also, rheumatological and neurological causes of plantar heel pain should be addressed in atypical cases, and treatment should be constructed accordingly (Lim et al., 2016).

In cases that are unresponsive to conservative treatment for at least nine to twelve months, surgical treatment is the choice. Patients should be informed about the complications and the possibility of no improvement in symptoms after surgery. Endoscopic and open surgical options include the release of the structures at the anterior aspect of the calcaneal tuberosity, gastrocnemius recession, elevation of the heel pad, neurolysis (nerve to the abductor digiti minimi or calcaneal nerve), osteotomy of the calcaneus, excision of the medial inferior tuberosity of the calcaneus, drilling decompression of the calcaneus, and calcaneal neurectomy (Barrett et al., 1995).

## CONCLUSION

Plantar heel pain is defined as soreness or tenderness of the central heel which often radiates to the medial tubercle of the calcaneus, or along the plantar fascia into the medial longitudinal arch of the foot. Plantar fasciitis is the most common cause of the painful heel with typical characteristics of clinical features. But other causes should be investigated with a thorough history and examination or additional radiographic studies. Plantar heel pain requires a differential diagnosis with consideration for appropriate management. Nonoperative interventions are the first line of treatment to relieve the symptoms in most patients. But surgical options should be kept in mind for recalcitrant cases.

## References

Ahmad, J., Ahmad, S. H., & Jones, K. (2017). Treatment of Plantar Fasciitis with Botulinum Toxin. *Foot & ankle international*, 38(1), 1-7.

Ahmad, M., Tsang, K., Mackenney, P. J., & Adedapo, A. O. (2012). Tarsal tunnel syndrome: A literature review. *Foot and ankle surgery: official journal of the European Society of Foot and Ankle Surgeons*, 18(3), 149-152.

Aiyer, A., Raikin, S., & Parvizi, J. (2019). 2018 International Consensus Meeting on Musculoskeletal Infection: Findings of the Foot and Ankle Work Group. *Foot & ankle international*, 40(1_suppl), 1S.

Barrett, S. L., Day, S. V., Pignetti, T. T., & Egly, B. R. (1995). Endoscopic heel anatomy: analysis of 200 fresh frozen specimens. *The Journal of foot and ankle surgery: official publication of the American College of Foot and Ankle Surgeons*, 34(1), 51-56.

Cullen, N. P., & Singh, D. (2006). Plantar fasciitis: a review. *British journal of hospital medicine (London, England: 2005)*, 67(2), 72-76.

De Garceau, D., Dean, D., Requejo, S. M., & Thordarson, D. B. (2003). The association between diagnosis of plantar fasciitis and Windlass test results. *Foot & ankle international*, 24(3), 251-255.

Donley, B. G., Moore, T., Sferra, J., Gozdanovic, J., & Smith, R. (2007). The efficacy of oral nonsteroidal anti-inflammatory medication (NSAID) in the treatment of plantar fasciitis: a randomized, prospective, placebo-controlled study. *Foot & ankle international*, 28(1), 20-23.

Hicks, J. H. (1954). The mechanics of the foot. II. The plantar aponeurosis and the arch. *Journal of anatomy*, 88(1), 25-30.

Kirkpatrick, J., Yassaie, O., & Mirjalili, S. A. (2017). The plantar calcaneal spur: a review of anatomy, histology, etiology and key associations. *Journal of anatomy*, 230(6), 743-751.

Landorf, K. B., & Menz, H. B. (2008). Plantar heel pain and fasciitis. *BMJ clinical evidence*, 2008, 1111.

Lareau, C. R., Sawyer, G. A., Wang, J. H., & DiGiovanni, C. W. (2014). Plantar and medial heel pain: diagnosis and management. *The Journal of the American Academy of Orthopaedic Surgeons*, 22(6), 372-380.

Lim, A. T., How, C. H., & Tan, B. (2016). Management of plantar fasciitis in the outpatient setting. *Singapore medical journal*, 57(4), 168-171.

McNally, E. G., & Shetty, S. (2010). Plantar fascia: imaging diagnosis and guided treatment. *Seminars in musculoskeletal radiology*, 14(3), 334-343.

Murai, N. O., Teniola, O., Wang, W. L., & Amini, B. (2018). Bone and Soft Tissue Tumors about the Foot and Ankle. *Radiologic clinics of North America*, 56(6), 917-934.

Riddle, D. L., Pulisic, M., Pidcoe, P., & Johnson, R. E. (2003). Risk factors for Plantar fasciitis: a matched case-control study. *The Journal of bone and joint surgery. American volume*, 85(5), 872-877.

Schon, L. C., Glennon, T. P., & Baxter, D. E. (1993). Heel pain syndrome: electrodiagnostic support for nerve entrapment. *Foot & ankle*, 14(3), 129-135.

Sidon, E., Rogero, R., McDonald, E., Daecher, A., Shakked, R., Pedowitz, D. I., Fuchs, D., Daniel, J. N., & Raikin, S. M. Prevalence of Neuropathic Pain Symptoms in Foot and Ankle Patients, *Foot Ankle Int*. 2019 Jun;40(6):629-633.

Stecco, C., Corradin, M., Macchi, V., Morra, A., Porzionato, A., Biz, C., & De Caro, R. (2013). Plantar fascia anatomy and its relationship with Achilles tendon and paratenon. *Journal of anatomy*, 223(6), 665-676.

Thompson, J. V., Saini, S. S., Reb, C. W., & Daniel, J. N. (2014). Diagnosis and management of plantar fasciitis. *The Journal of the American Osteopathic Association*, 114(12), 900-906.

Tong, K. B., & Furia, J. (2010). Economic burden of plantar fasciitis treatment in the United States. *American journal of orthopedics (Belle Mead, N. J.)*, 39(5), 227-231.

Tsai, W. C., Wang, C. L., Hsu, T. C., Hsieh, F. J., & Tang, F. T. (1999). The mechanical properties of the heel pad in unilateral plantar heel pain syndrome. *Foot & ankle international*, 20(10), 663-668.

van Leeuwen, K. D., Rogers, J., Winzenberg, T., & van Middelkoop, M. (2016). Higher body mass index is associated with plantar fasciopathy/'plantar fasciitis': systematic review and meta-analysis of various clinical and imaging risk factors. *British journal of sports medicine*, 50(16), 972-981.

van Wyngarden, T. M. (1997). The painful foot, Part II: Common rearfoot deformities. *American family physician*, 55(6), 2207-2212.

Welck, M. J., Hayes, T., Pastides, P., Khan, W., & Rudge, B. (2017). Stress fractures of the foot and ankle. *Injury*, 48(8), 1722-1726.

Yi, T. I., Lee, G. E., Seo, I. S., Huh, W. S., Yoon, T. H., & Kim, B. R. (2011). Clinical characteristics of the causes of plantar heel pain. *Annals of rehabilitation medicine*, 35(4), 507-513.

Young, C. C., Rutherford, D. S., & Niedfeldt, M. W. (2001). Treatment of plantar fasciitis. *American family physician*, 63(3), 467-478.

In: Musculoskeletal Pain (Common Clinical Presentations) ISBN: 978-1-68507-410-4
Editors: Mehmet Cenk Turgut and Serdar Toy 

*Chapter 22*

# SINUS TARSI SYNDROME

***Serdar Toy**, MD***
Department of Orthopedics and Traumatology,
Ağrı Training and Research Hospital, Ağrı, Turkey

## ABSTRACT

Sinus tarsi syndrome is a clinical disease characterized by chronic anterolateral ankle soreness, that occurs following severe ankle injuries. As a result of traumatic injuries, the ligaments in the sinus tarsi cavity are damaged. The sinus tarsi cavity is filled with fibrotic tissue remnants and synovitis following ligament injuries. Synovitis and fibrotic tissue deposits accumulate in this space and stimulate the chronic inflammatory process.

Patients with sinus tarsi syndrome have ankle sprain caused by the supination/inversion mechanism. Acute ankle sprain typically presents with pain associated with anterolateral ankle swelling, ecchymosis, and tenderness. Conservative treatment is the first treatment method to be applied in sinus tarsi syndrome. If conservative treatments fail, surgical treatment becomes necessary. The aim is to excise the sinus tarsi contents and to clean the fibrotic tissues and synovial hypertrophy.

## INTRODUCTION

Sinus tarsi syndrome is a symptomatic disease that causes persistent discomfort on the anterolateral side of the ankle. Sinus tarsi syndrome develops after traumatic injuries of the ankle (Helgeson, 2009). Especially walking on rough ground, crouching, and bending the ankle cause pain. Patients with sinus tarsi syndrome experience more pain as pressure is applied to the anterolateral side of the foot. The average age of patients

* Corresponding Author's E-mail: serdartoy737@gmail.com.

suffering from sinus tarsi syndrome is 20-30 years. At least 70% of these patients have only one or more trauma histories, such as ankle rotation or sprain that have not been treated correctly. After exercise, patients often complain of swelling in front of the lateral malleolus and ankle instability (Schwarzenbach, Dora, Lang, & Kissling, 1997).

The sinus tarsi is located lateral to the ankle, distal to the lateral malleolus and slightly anterior to it. It is a space outlined by the talus' neck and the calcaneus' anterosuperior aspect. As a funnel-shaped tarsal canal, the sinus tarsi opens medially, posterior to the sustentaculum tali of the calcaneus. The sinus tarsi divides the subtalar joint into anterior and posterior parts (Lektrakul et al., 2001; Rosenberg, Beltran, & Bencardino, 2000; Shear, Baitch, & Shear, 1993). This space runs obliquely from posteromedially to anterolaterally. The extensor retinaculum covers the lateral surface of the sinus tarsi. The cervical and talocalcaneal ligaments are located within the sinus tarsi (Bilstrom, O'Rourke, & Deodhar, 2008). Injuries to these ligaments in the sinus tarsi cause fibrotic tissue debris and hypertrophic synovium deposits. Fibrotic tissue remnants and hypertrophic synovium deposits cause sinus tarsi syndrome (Shear et al., 1993). Sinus tarsi syndrome accompanies subtalar instability that develops with inversion injuries of the ankle (Bilstrom et al., 2008).

## Etiology

In 1958, O'Connor (O'Connor, 1958) presented that tension and injury caused by the healing of the ligament could cause pain in sinus tarsi syndrome. In 1960, Brown (Brown, 1960) suggested that a herniation in this area was responsible. In an article published by Claustre et al., (Claustre, Simon, & Allieu, 1979) in 1979, clinical and radiological studies reported that no findings indicated neither bone lesions nor ligament injuries. The authors also stated that the talocalcaneal and talocalcaneonavicular joints had no restriction of mobility. There are several theories as to the causes of persistent pain in sinus tarsi syndrome. These theories include damage to the sinus tarsi ligaments (Borrelli & Arenson, 1987; Claustre et al., 1979), bleeding into the sinus tarsi (Arias, 1986; Taillard, Meyer, Garcia, & Blanc, 1981), arthritis or synovitis of the subtalar joint (Arias, 1986; Taillard et al., 1981), and chronic fibro-adipose tissue inflammation within the sinus tarsi (Claustre et al., 1979; Taillard et al., 1981). In 1997, Schwarzenbach et al., (Schwarzenbach et al., 1997) suggested that fibrotic modifications in the wall and surrounding tissues occurring as a result of trauma, which caused increased intra-sinus tension and decreased venous drainage, might be a contributing component to the development of sinus tarsi syndrome. Recent studies explained the etiological cause of sinus tarsi syndrome as subtalar joint instability because of synovitis and fibrous tissue infiltration following ligament injuries in the sinus tarsi space (Frey, Feder, & DiGiovanni, 1999; Pisani, Pisani, & Parino, 2005).

Sinus tarsi syndrome was thought to occur following damage to the talocrural interosseous and cervical ligaments following a single traumatic event or recurrent ankle sprains (primarily because of a weak anterior talofibular ligament) (Budny, 2004; Pisani et al., 2005). These injuries induce subtalar joint instability, resulting in an increased pronation and supination motions. These extreme movements in the subtalar joint create excessive forces on the subtalar joint synovial and sinus tarsi tissues (Helgeson, 2009). These intense forces cause persistent inflammation and fibrous tissue invasion within the sinus tarsi, resulting in anterolateral ankle pain characteristic of sinus tarsi syndrome (Pisani et al., 2005). These traumatic injuries damage the tibiotalar and talocalcaneal ligaments due to excessive movement and instability in the hindfoot and midfoot.

Sinus tarsi syndrome might be associated with ankle sprains leading to talocrural joint instability. Keefe and Haddad (Keefe & Haddad, 2002) reported that subtalar joint instability was seen in 10% to 25% of individuals with persistent talocrural joint instability. Hertel et al., (Hertel, Denegar, Monroe, & Stokes, 1999) reported that 75 per cent of patients with repeated ankle sprain exhibited increased talocrural and subtalar joint motions. Hubbard and Hertel (Hubbard & Hertel, 2006) stated that most patients had injuries of the subtalar joint ligaments after ankle sprains.

## DIAGNOSIS

Patients with sinus tarsi syndrome have ankle sprain caused by the supination/inversion mechanism. Injury to the subtalar joint may occur in patients who are particularly interested in jumping sports in the case of sudden stops following a leap or fall. This process is considered to be the source of a "whiplash injury" to the hindfoot as the talus moves forward on the calcaneus (Keefe & Haddad, 2002). This mechanism can also result in damage to the talocrural joint ligaments.

Acute ankle sprain typically presents with pain associated with anterolateral ankle swelling, ecchymosis, and tenderness. Since the development of synovitis and fibrotic tissues associated with sinus tarsi syndrome takes time, patients with subtalar joint injuries may not exhibit symptoms that may initially be localized on the sinus tarsi. Patients experience instability in their ankles while walking on uneven roads, stepping on the curb, and running (Budny, 2004; Keefe & Haddad, 2002; Shear et al., 1993). Athletes with subtalar instability experience serious difficulties during the activities they do, especially on hard floors, because these activities cause excessive supination and pronation in the subtalar joint (Keefe & Haddad, 2002; Thermann, Zwipp, & Tscherne, 1997).

Medial and lateral subtalar joint displacement and subtalar joint distraction, performed by moving the calcaneus in the transverse plane over a stabilized talus, are used to test the stability of the subtalar joint (Hertel et al., 1999; Hubbard & Hertel,

2006). Thermann et al., (Thermann et al., 1997) described a stability test that reproduced the instability of the subtalar joint. This test is performed by keeping the talocrural joint in a fixed position and bringing the ankle to 10-degree dorsiflexion. The patient is placed on the examination table in the supine position. The examiner stabilizes the forefoot and applies calcaneal tilt and rotation stress. The examiner then applies an inversion force to the forefoot. The inspector evaluates whether there is extreme calcaneal medial shift and the instability and symptoms associated with the patient's complaint (Figure 1).

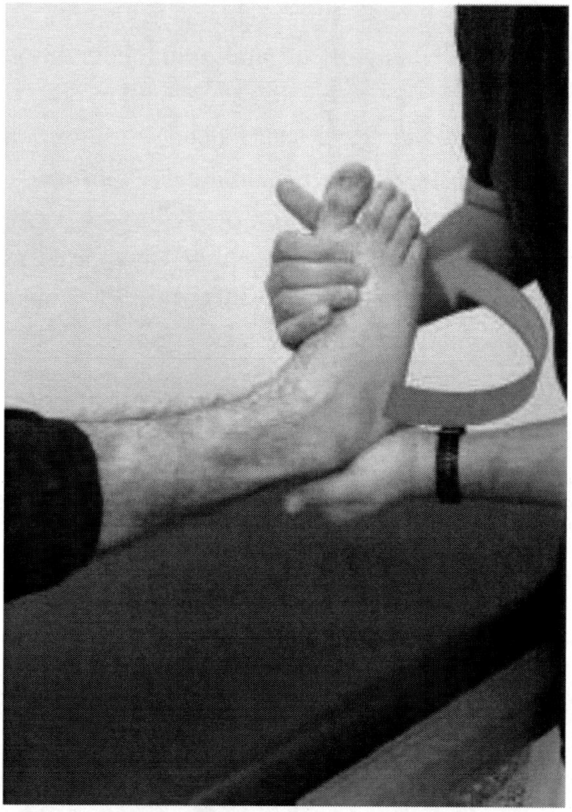

Source: from the author's individual archives.

Figure 1. A clinical test is to confirm subtalar instability.

## Imaging Techniques

Imaging is required in patients with suspected subtalar joint instability or sinus tarsi syndrome. Whilst imaging tests are proposed to measure the subtalar joint stability, the majority of these approaches have low specificity and inconsistency for subtalar joint instability (Hertel et al., 1999; Keefe & Haddad, 2002). Subtalar joint radiography is usually evaluated with Broden stress radiography. This is an oblique tangent radiograph that comes from the vertical line with angles such as 10, 20, 30, and 40 degrees, with the patient in the supine position, the knee joint in slight flexion, the leg in 45 degrees of internal rotation, and the beam targeting the lateral malleolus. Stress fluoroscopy is a method developed to view subtalar joint movements utilizing low levels of radiation in real time. The benefits of fluoroscopy over radiography are that fluoroscopy allows the investigator to simulate movements that cause the patient to feel instability or discomfort.

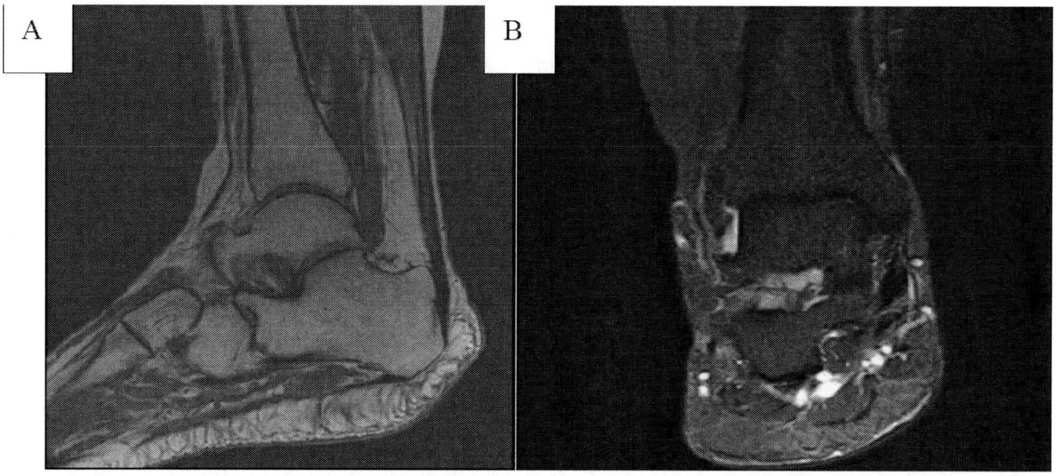


Source: from the author's individual archiveso.

Figure 2. MR images of a 45-year-old female patient with sinus tarsi syndrome (A. T1-weighted sagittal MR image, sinus tarsi ligaments (interosseous talocalcaneal and cervical ligaments), and inferior extensor retinaculum were observed. In addition, chronic inflammation and edema were seen. B. T2-weighted coronal MR image was observed).

Magnetic resonance imaging (MRI) seems to be the most effective tool for seeing components inside the sinus tarsi, particularly the cervical and interosseous ligaments. One of the most striking findings for patients suffering from sinus tarsi syndrome is a bright signal on the T2-weighted view of the area containing fatty tissue within the sinus tarsi. This tissue shows infiltration or replacement by inflammatory cells of fibrotic tissue (Klein & Spreitzer, 1993; Lektrakul et al., 2001). MRI findings may show structural abnormalities of the cervical and interosseous ligaments, as well as degenerative changes in the subtalar joint (Lektrakul et al., 2001; Pisani et al., 2005) (Figure 2).

## TREATMENT

Conservative treatment is the first treatment method to be applied in sinus tarsi syndrome. Conservative treatment includes bandages to restrict excessive movements of the ankle (Figure 3), heel supports, proprioception exercises, and standard physical therapy modalities such as ice, elevation, and ultrasound for swelling. Oral NSAIDs could be given as an adjunct to these, or an intra-articular injection of a single dose steroid + a local anesthetic mixture (Figure 4) could be applied (Ferkel, Karzel, Del Pizzo, Friedman, & Fischer, 1991; Scranton, 1994).

Exercises to increase the subtalar joint stability and the function of the lower extremities should form the basis of medical interventions for sinus tarsi syndrome (Helgeson, 2009). Joint stability is based on passive range of motion of the joints, dynamic muscle reactions, and neurological responses. The hindfoot dynamic muscular and neurological responses should be adjusted to compensate for losing passive stabilization in treating sinus tarsi syndrome.

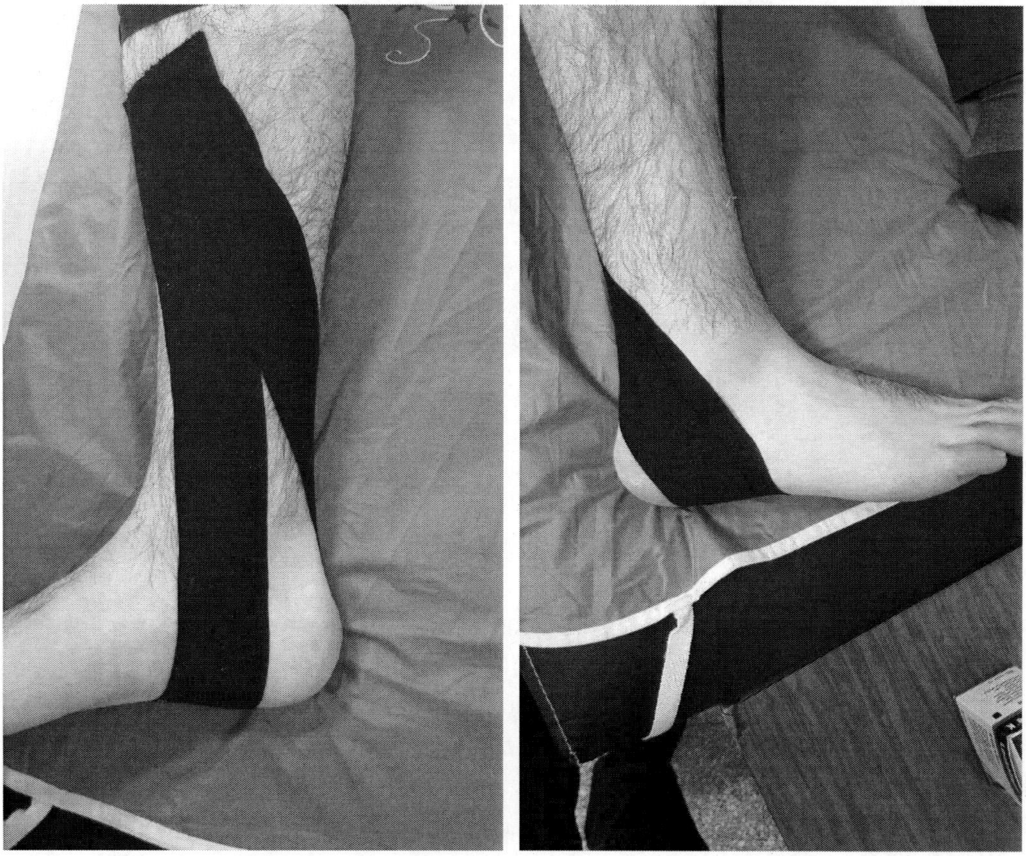

Source: from the author's individual archives.

Figure 3. Stabilizing bandage for the hindfoot. A) A calcaneal sling with a long strip to control hindfoot pronation. B) Heel lock strips to control hindfoot supination.

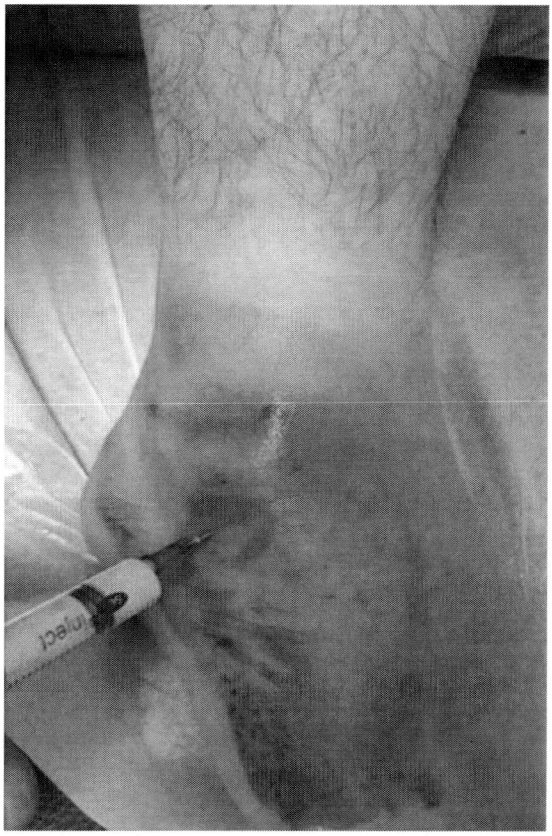

Source: from the author's individual archives.

Figure 4. Intra-articular injection of corticosteroid + local anesthetic.

If conservative treatments fail, surgical treatment becomes necessary. Surgical intervention historically consisted of draining the sinus tarsi contents. Meanwhile, subtalar joint decompression can also be performed by subtalar joint arthroscopy (Fried & Dobbs, 1985; Klein & Spreitzer, 1993; O'Connor, 1958; Taillard et al., 1981). The aim is to excise the sinus tarsi contents and to clean the fibrotic tissues and synovial hypertrophy. An incision is performed on the sinus tarsi parallel to skin tension that has been relaxed. The middle dorsal cutaneous nerve emerges slightly anterior to the incision. The sural and one branch of the middle dorsal cutaneous nerve may be transverse from the sinus tarsi. Sometimes these nerves can be sacrificed. A sharp dissection is used to deepen the incision to the level of the inferior extensor retinaculum. When the deep fascia covering the sinus tarsi is opened, the contents of the sinus come out. Although it is known that damaged ligaments will contribute to the inflammation process, there is some debate over whether the interosseous talocalcaneal ligament should be excised. It should be kept in mind that the vascular supply of the talus will be seriously impaired when the sinus tarsi is completely cleared. After the damaged tissues in the sinus tarsi are removed, the posterior facet of the talus is examined. Arthrodesis is considered if there are severe degenerative changes in the articular surface of the talus posterior facet. After the surgical area is closed, a sterile and pressed dressing is made. A weight bearing walking cast is applied to the patient for 2-4 weeks postoperatively. A rarely performed major hindfoot fusion may be required in cases of recurrent, persistent sinus tarsi syndrome. Subtalar or triple arthrodesis can be applied to patients with chronic pain to relieve symptoms.

## CONCLUSION

It is crucial to be able to diagnose sinus tarsi syndrome. Many patients are undertreated because of misdiagnosis. It is necessary to evaluate the patient presenting with ankle pain in terms of sinus tarsi syndrome.

## REFERENCES

Arias, C., S. A. Abdulle and J. Wagner. (1986). Conception actuelle du sinus du tarse. *Rev. Med. Brux.*, 7:323-326.

Bilstrom, E., O'Rourke, K. S., & Deodhar, A. (2008). Injection of the subtalar joint and sinus tarsi. *J Musculoskeletal Med.,* 25(1), 29.

Borrelli, A., & Arenson, D. (1987). Sinus tarsi syndrome and its relationship to hallux abducto valgus. *J Am Podiatr Med Assoc.,* 77(9), 495-499.

Brown, J. E. (1960). The sinus tarsi syndrome. *Clin Orthop Relat Res.,* 18, 231-233.

Budny, A. (2004). Subtalar joint instability: current clinical concepts. *Clin Podiatr Med Surg.,* 21(3), 449-460.

Claustre, J., Simon, L., & Allieu, Y. (1979). Le syndrome du sinus du tarse existe-t-il. *Rheumatologie,* 31, 19-23. [Does tarsal sinus syndrome exist.]

Ferkel, R. D., Karzel, R. P., Del Pizzo, W., Friedman, M. J., & Fischer, S. P. (1991). Arthroscopic treatment of anterolateral impingement of the ankle. *Am J Sports Med.,* 19(5), 440-446.

Frey, C., Feder, K. S., & DiGiovanni, C. (1999). Arthroscopic evaluation of the subtalar joint: does sinus tarsi syndrome exist? *Foot Ankle Int.,* 20(3), 185-191.

Fried, A., & Dobbs, B. (1985). Sinus tarsi synovectomy. A possible alternative to a subtalar joint fusion. *J Am Podiatr Med Assoc.,* 75(9), 494.

Helgeson, K. (2009). Examination and intervention for sinus tarsi syndrome. *N Am J Sports Phys Ther.,* 4(1), 29.

Hertel, J., Denegar, C. R., Monroe, M. M., & Stokes, W. L. (1999). Talocrural and subtalar joint instability after lateral ankle sprain. *Med Sci Sports Exerc.,* 31(11), 1501-1508.

Hubbard, T. J., & Hertel, J. (2006). Mechanical contributions to chronic lateral ankle instability. *Sports Med.,* 36(3), 263-277.

Keefe, D. T., & Haddad, S. L. (2002). Subtalar instability. Etiology, diagnosis, and management. *Foot Ankle Clin.,* 7(3), 577-609.

Klein, M., & Spreitzer, A. (1993). MR imaging of the tarsal sinus and canal: normal anatomy, pathologic findings, and features of the sinus tarsi syndrome. *Radiology,* 186(1), 233-240.

Lektrakul, N., Chung, C. B., Lai, Y. M., Theodorou, D. J., Yu, J., Haghighi, P., . . . Resnick, D. (2001). Tarsal sinus: arthrographic, MR imaging, MR arthrographic, and pathologic findings in cadavers and retrospective study data in patients with sinus tarsi syndrome. *Radiology,* 219(3), 802-810.

O'Connor, D. (1958). Sinus tarsi syndrome. Clinical entity. *J. Bone Joint Surg.,* 40, 720.

Pisani, G., Pisani, P. C., & Parino, E. (2005). Sinus tarsi syndrome and subtalar joint instability. *Clin Podiatr Med Surg.,* 22(1), 63-77.

Rosenberg, Z. S., Beltran, J., & Bencardino, J. T. (2000). MR imaging of the ankle and foot. *Radiographics,* 20(suppl_1), S153-S179.

Schwarzenbach, B., Dora, C., Lang, A., & Kissling, R. (1997). Blood vessels of the sinus tarsi and the sinus tarsi syndrome. *Clin Anat.,* 10(3), 173-182.

Scranton, P. (1994). Arthroscopic treatment of symptomatic anterior ankle impingement lesions in the athlete. *Sports Med Arthrosc Rev.,* 2(4), 289-292.

Shear, M. S., Baitch, S. P., & Shear, D. B. (1993). Sinus tarsi syndrome: the importance of biomechanically-based evaluation and treatment. *Arch Phys Med Rehabil.,* 74(7), 777-781.

Taillard, W., Meyer, J. M., Garcia, J., & Blanc, Y. (1981). The sinus tarsi syndrome. *Int Orthop.,* 5(2), 117-130.

Thermann, H., Zwipp, H., & Tscherne, H. (1997). Treatment algorithm of chronic ankle and subtalar instability. *Foot Ankle Int.,* 18(3), 163-169.

In: Musculoskeletal Pain (Common Clinical Presentations) ISBN: 978-1-68507-410-4
Editors: Mehmet Cenk Turgut and Serdar Toy 

*Chapter 23*

# TARSAL TUNNEL SYNDROME

***Mehmet Çetin**, MD***
Department of Orthopedics and Traumatology,
Ağrı Training and Research Hospital, Ağrı, Turkey

## ABSTRACT

Tarsal tunnel syndrome represents an entrapment neuropathy, which is rare, insufficiently diagnosed and often confused with other clinical conditions. There are contradictions in diagnosing and treating the most frequently observed entrapment neuropathy of the foot. Treatment includes conservative methods such as analgesics and physical therapy and rehabilitation or surgical procedures. In this chapter, the etiology, pathophysiology, diagnostic methods, and treatments of tarsal tunnel syndrome are reviewed by employing a systematic approach.

## INTRODUCTION

Tarsal tunnel syndrome (TTS) constitutes the most frequent compressive neuropathy of the foot. It represents an entrapment neuropathy that emerges due to the compressed posterior tibial nerve or its branches (lateral plantar, medial plantar, and calcaneal nerves) in the fibro-osseous tunnel under the flexor retinaculum in the ankle's medial part. However, unlike carpal tunnel syndrome, which is a similar counterpart on the hand, TTS is a clinical entity that is misunderstood to a considerable extent. There are still contradictions and differences regarding diagnosing and treating tarsal tunnel syndrome. Proximal tarsal tunnel syndrome mostly comes to mind when tarsal tunnel syndrome is

* Corresponding Author's E-mail: cetotemm@gmail.com.

mentioned. However, forgetting the presence of distal tarsal tunnel syndrome may result in treatment failure. It is possible to divide tarsal tunnel entrapment into proximal and distal syndromes. Here, proximal syndrome describes the entire tibial nerve being compressed, while distal syndrome describes one or more of the terminal branches being compressed.

## Anatomy

The tibial nerve, one of the terminal branches of the two sciatic nerves, descends the leg's posterior aspect with the posterior tibial vessels. The mentioned vessel-nerve, which progresses between the muscles in the proximal leg, becomes superficial in the distal. This tunnel is an area with a width of 2.5-3.0 cm in which various structures are closely in contact with each other.

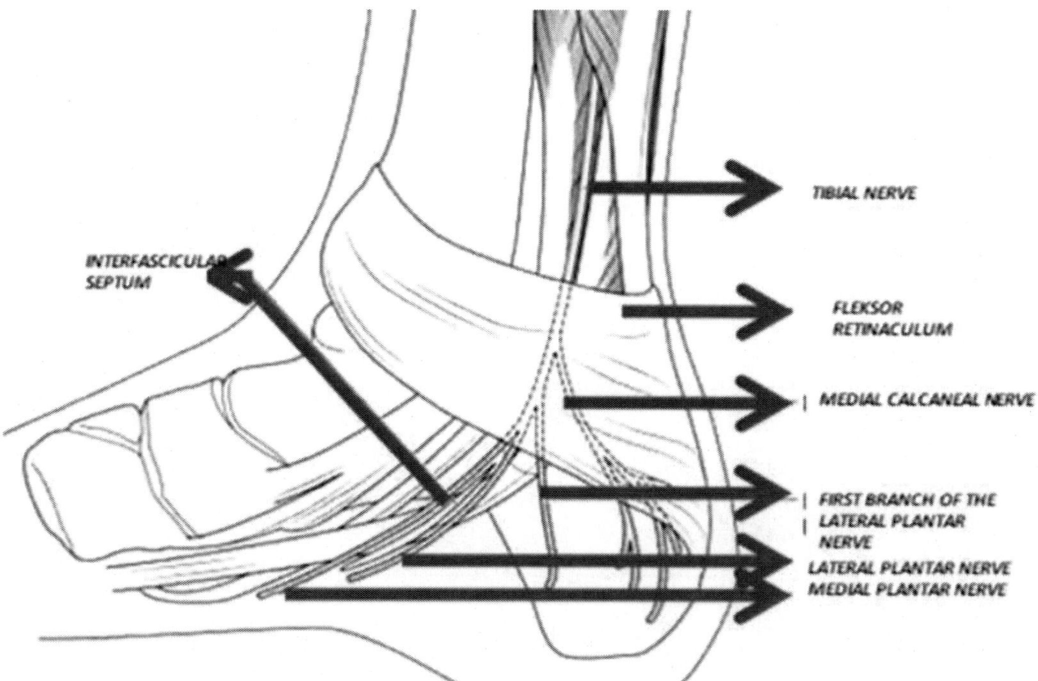


Source: from https://www.phxfootankle.com/blog/tarsal-tunnel-syndrome-treatment-and-management.

Figure 1. Anatomy of the Tarsal Tunnel.

The tarsal tunnel involves many significant structures. It involves the tendons of the flexor digitorum longus, posterior tibialis and flexor hallucis longus muscles. Moreover, the posterior tibial artery and vein and the posterior tibial nerve pass through it. They are the tibialis posterior tendon, FDL tendon, posterior tibial artery and vein, posterior tibial nerve and FHL tendon from medial to lateral.

Various tendons represent three separate fibro-osseous compartments, and the tibial artery and nerve are usually attached to this septum through the surrounding dense areolar tissue layer. The tibial nerve may be compressed behind the medial malleolus below the flexor retinaculum, and there are also other points at which compression may occur. The tibial nerve extension includes the compression of the plantar nerves at the abductor hallucis level as it enters the foot. On the sole, there are three firm fascial septa that represent possible nerve entrapment sites attached to the tibial nerve, and their branches are closely associated with these septa. The compartments are the deep fascia of the medial septum abductor hallucis, the dorsal extension of the lateral border of the middle septum plantar aponeurosis, and the dorsal extension of the lateral border of the lateral septum lateral band, the plantar aponeurosis. The posterior tibial nerve is often divided into the medial and lateral plantar and calcaneal branches at the medial malleolus-calcaneal level within the tarsal tunnel. The calcaneal branch originates from the tibial nerve by 69-90% in the proximal zone, and the rest originates from the lateral plantar nerve. The lateral and medial plantar branches ensure the motor innervation of the intrinsic foot muscles and the sensory innervation of the sole. The calcaneal branch is sensory only and ensures the sensory innervation of the heel.

## ETIOLOGY

The actual incidence of tarsal tunnel syndrome is not clear. It was found to be observed by 0.4%-0.5% of subjects in electrophysiological studies. The association of the syndrome with traumatic and inflammatory etiologies was established. Nevertheless, other causative factors were also investigated, and a specific cause of TTS was detected in approximately 80% of subjects.

Trauma is the most frequent cause of TTS. Displaced fractures of the tarsal bones, calcaneus or distal tibia, ankle strain injuries, flexor hallucis longus, flexor digitorum longus and posterior tibial tenosynovitis, epineural scarring of the tibial nerve due to bleeding in the tarsal tunnel, and sudden overload in runners may be due to chronic anterior exercise-induced compartment syndrome in athletes, especially in those involved in athleticism. Some hypotheses regarding the pathophysiology of tarsal tunnel syndrome have been suggested. McComas and Upton defined the "double-crush" phenomenon in 1973. Local damage to any part of the nerve may lead to the disruption of other axons along the nerve tract, and these neurons become more prone to compression trauma than under normal conditions. McComas and Upton indicated that the majority (75%) of subjects having a peripheral lesion also had a second lesion elsewhere. These lesions were first identified with an increase in the incidence of carpal tunnel syndrome in cases with brachial plexus injury. Another example of the "double crush" phenomenon is S1 root compression, which results in an increase in the possibility of compression neuropathy in the tarsal tunnel.

**Table 1. Etiology of Tarsal Tunnel**

| Extrinsic Causes | Intrinsic Causes |
|---|---|
| Trauma | Ganglion, lipoma, neoplasm, neuroma |
| Anatomical-biomechanical anomalies (valgus or varus hindfoot, tarsal coalition) | Varicose veins |
| Shoes that do not fit well | Arterial insufficiency |
| Scar after surgery | Hypertrophic flexor retinaculum |
| Generalized lower extremity edema | Accessory muscles (soleus, etc.) |
| Systemic inflammatory arthropathies | Tendinopathy |
| Scar tissue after surgery | Tenosynovitis |

## Clinical Features and Diagnosis

It is more common after the age of 40 and proportionately more frequent in females than males. The symptoms are usually insidious, exacerbated with activity, and often resolve with rest and elevation of the lower limb. Tarsal tunnel syndrome may cause pain, numbness, electrical sensations in the feet, burning, and tingling in the big toe and soles of the feet and heels. However, the most frequently observed symptoms are burning and tingling in the soles or both of them and night-time exacerbation of symptoms. The earliest finding is a decreased sense of two-point discrimination in the foot plantar part. As the disease progresses, hypoesthesia emerges in the dermatome of the involved nerve. Patients' pain is usually triggered by percussion along the tibial nerve, which indicates Tinel's positive sign. When varicose veins are the cause of TTS, Turk's test, which is performed with the placement of a tourniquet over the malleolus at a pressure between systolic and diastolic, may be performed. The impaired sensory distribution of the plantar nerve terminal branches represents another common objective finding. Furthermore, the compressed digital nerve and the continuous inversion of the hindfoot can cause the reproduction of symptoms distally or even spread proximally. Examining the tibial nerve, and medial and lateral plantar nerves separately is important to determine whether one or both will be influenced.

## Electrodiagnostic Studies

Electrophysiological studies are usually the gold standard for TTS conducted to determine sensory and motor latencies.

Conduction is found to be slow in sensory nerves, and motor evoked potentials have increased latency and reduced amplitude in motor nerves. It is necessary to know that the TN and its branches represent mixed nerves to understand nerve conduction studies in TTS. Today, nerve conduction velocity and electromyography are the objective quantitative test with the highest reliability utilized in TTS, and conduction problems are generally observed in the lateral plantar nerve. Nevertheless, unlike electrophysiological studies conducted in the upper extremities, obtaining sensory and motor responses in studies in the lower extremities may be challenging due to reasons such as edema and foot deformity. The following algorithm can be applied in patients with TTS. TTS is diagnosed if foot pain and paresthesia, a positive Tinel's sign, and a positive electrodiagnostic study triad are present. In the presence of two findings, it is possible that the subject has TTS, and further evaluation is required. In the presence of one finding, the subject does not have TTS and must be evaluated for other differential diagnoses. Nevertheless, the postoperative clinical outcome is not correlated with the findings of preoperative electrodiagnostic studies.

## Imaging

Radiographs or computed tomography can help to assess bone deformities. Magnetic resonance imaging (MRI) is capable of detecting the soft tissue mass in the tunnel, and the etiology that is responsible for the compression and its relationship with the tibial nerve can be detected in MRI. If surgery is planned, it can provide valuable preoperative findings. Ultrasound can provide information about compression status and nerve variations by describing the complex tarsal tunnel anatomy and its components. Ganglion, varicose veins, lipomas, tenosynovitis and talocalcaneal coalition can be determined with diagnostic ultrasound. Doppler high-resolution US can be helpful in measuring a peripheral nerve's cross-sectional area.

## Differential Diagnosis

Diabetic and peripheral neuropathy, plantar fasciitis, rheumatoid arthritis, metatarsalgia and Morton's neuroma are pathologies that must be primarily evaluated in the differential diagnosis of tarsal tunnel syndrome. Morton's neuroma, which is one of the most frequently observed pathologies, is a fibrous degenerative condition induced by the compressed plantar digital nerve. Although it is most common between the heads of the 3rd and 4th metatarsals, it can be found between all successive metatarsals. Like TTS, the early symptom of Morton's neuroma is pain. However, pain localization is more common in the metatarsal heads.

## TREATMENT

We can classify the treatment of tarsal tunnel syndrome as conservative and surgical.

### Conservative Treatment

In conservative treatment, physiotherapy, injections, non-steroidal anti-inflammatory drugs, and orthosis can be utilized, and weight loss and immobilization are recommended. Foot-ankle orthosis is used for immobilization. If there is a flexible foot deformity, an orthosis that will keep the foot in a neutral position is recommended. In the heel with valgus deformity, medial heel wedges and medial longitudinal arch supports provide positive results. It is necessary to consider non-steroidal anti-inflammatory drugs for a short period of time, especially in patients with tenosynovitis. It is possible to try pregabalin, gabapentin and tricyclic antidepressants in patients with neuropathic pain. Injections into the third canal of the tarsal tunnel can have some benefits. Administering lidocaine or bupivacaine to the tibial nerve for anesthetic purposes will cause significant relief and also help to identify and localize the nerve branches for the further isolation of the problem. In persistent cases of TTS, corticosteroid injection can be administered which significantly reduces the symptoms. However, attention should be paid to avoiding administering the injection into the adjacent tibialis posterior tendon. Iontophoresis, ultrasound, phonophoresis, and E-stimulation are physical therapy soft tissue modalities with some benefits. Moreover, calf stretching and nerve mobility or nerve gliding can be helpful with symptoms. It may be helpful to strengthen the tibialis posterior. Activity modification also takes part in symptom management. It is possible to utilize kinesiology tapes for arc support and the reduction of biomechanical stress. Although different outcomes are obtained in treating TTS, to our mind, it is necessary to apply physical therapy prior to considering surgical treatment in the majority of patients. However, space-occupying lesions or traumatic ones in TTS etiologies must be evaluated surgically.

## Surgical Treatment

There is an indication for surgery if the symptoms of the patient cannot be resolved with conservative treatment or in the case of the identification of a definitive cause of the entrapment. There is usually a good response to surgical treatment in subjects having symptoms induced by a space-occupying lesion. Abnormally slow nerve conduction along the posterior tibial nerve represents a precursor of unsuccessful conservative treatment.

A surgical indication is indisputable in the presence of a space-occupying formation pressing on the nerve in the tarsal tunnel. It is possible to consider surgical treatment in subjects not responding to conservative treatment applied for 3 months. Surgical treatment includes releasing the flexor retinaculum to the proximal sustentaculum tali close to the medial malleolus.

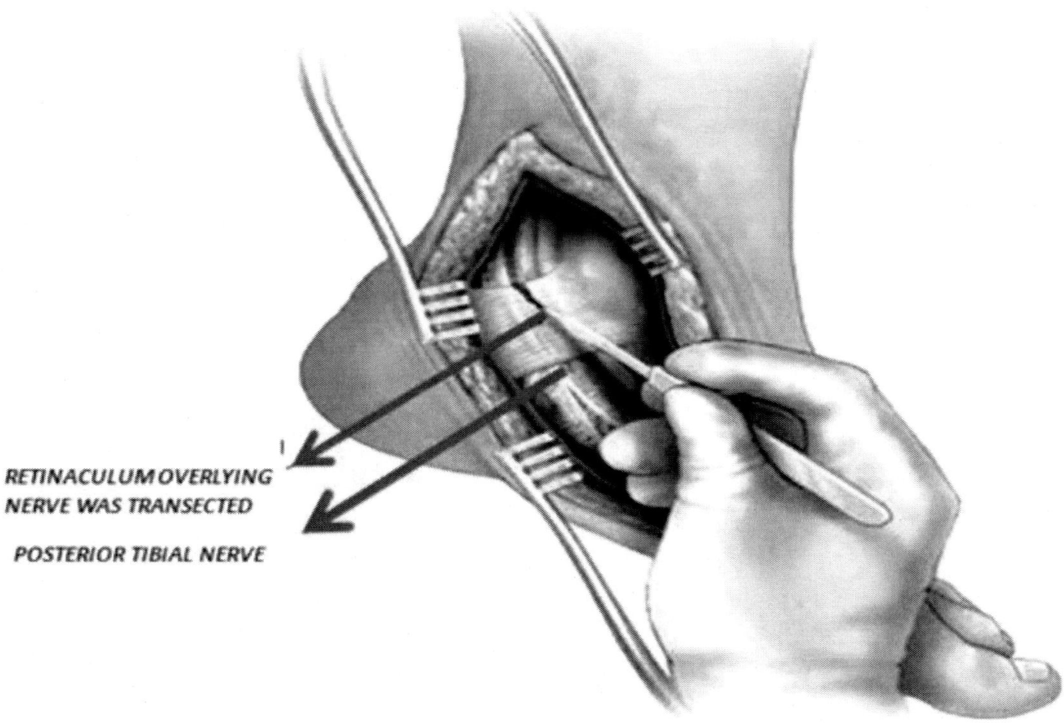


Source: from http://www.southfloridasportsmedicine.com/tarsal-tunnel.html.

Figure 2. Flexor Retinaculum Incision.

The objective of surgery is to release the tarsal tunnel to include both the proximal and distal zones. In the distal zone, the canals that the lateral and plantar branches enter under the abductor hallucis should be released about 3 cm toward the sole, and the fibrous bands, if any, should be cut. There is a tendency for a better response to surgical decompression in patients with a positive preoperative Tinel's sign. There is a tendency for a better response to surgery in patients at a younger age and subjects having a short history of symptoms, a clear etiology, an early diagnosis, and no previous ankle pathology.

The use of endoscopic and minimally invasive surgical methods has increased in recent years.

## Conclusion

Tarsal tunnel syndrome represents an entrapment neuropathy, which often accompanies other foot pathologies and can therefore be overlooked. The diagnosis is established as a result of clinical and physical examination. A complementary test, electromyography and MRI assist us in confirming the diagnosis and offering patients the best treatment. Electrophysiological studies are regarded as the gold standard diagnostic test, and normal findings usually show abnormalities, despite not eliminating the possibility of compression. The correct identification of the pathology causing tarsal tunnel syndrome and other accompanying pathologies affects the surgical success. It is recommended that patients should be assessed in detail prior to surgery and that they should be adequately enlightened about the post-surgical expectations.

## References

Almeida, D. F., Scremin, L., Zúniga, S. F., & Oh, S. J. (2010). Focal conduction block in a case of tarsal tunnel syndrome. *Muscle & nerve*, *42*(3), 452–455.

Cimino W. R. (1990). Tarsal tunnel syndrome: review of the literature. *Foot & ankle*, *11*(1), 47–52.

DiStefano, V., Sack, J. T., Whittaker, R., & Nixon, J. E. (1972). Tarsal-tunnel syndrome. Review of the literature and two case reports. *Clinical orthopaedics and related research*, *88*, 76–79.

Erickson, S. et al., (1990). MR imaging of the tarsal tunnel and related spaces: normal and abnormal findings with anatomic correlation. *AJR. American journal of roentgenology*, *155*(2), 323–328.

Galardi, G. et al., (1994). Electrophysiologic studies in tarsal tunnel syndrome. Diagnostic reliability of motor distal latency, mixed nerve and sensory nerve conduction studies. *American journal of physical medicine & rehabilitation*, *73*(3), 193–198.

Hudes K. (2010). Conservative management of a case of tarsal tunnel syndrome. *The Journal of the Canadian Chiropractic Association*, *54*(2), 100–106.

Kaplan, P. E., & Kernahan, W. T., Jr (1981). Tarsal tunnel syndrome: an electrodiagnostic and surgical correlation. *The Journal of bone and joint surgery. American volume*, *63*(1), 96–99.

Lopez-Ben R. (2011). Imaging of nerve entrapment in the foot and ankle. *Foot and ankle clinics*, *16*(2), 213–224.

Oh, S. J., Sarala, P. K., Kuba, T., & Elmore, R. S. (1979). Tarsal tunnel syndrome: electrophysiological study. *Annals of neurology*, *5*(4), 327–330.

Patel A. T., et al.; American Association of Neuromuscular and Electrodiagnostic Medicine. Usefulness of electrodiagnostic techniques in the evaluation of suspected tarsal tunnel syndrome: an evidence-based review. *Muscle Nerve*. 2005 Aug; 32(2):236-40.

Pfeiffer, W. H., & Cracchiolo, A., 3rd (1994). Clinical results after tarsal tunnel decompression. *The Journal of bone and joint surgery. American volume*, *76*(8), 1222–1230.

Pickard, J. D., Robinson, A. H., & Bearcroft, P. W. (2006). Posterior tarsal tunnel syndrome: an unusual unrelated cause of late pain after lumbar spine surgery. *British journal of neurosurgery*, *20*(5), 331–332.

Rozmaryn, L. M., Dovelle, S., Rothman, E. R., Gorman, K., Olvey, K. M., & Bartko, J. J. (1998). Nerve and tendon gliding exercises and the conservative management of carpal tunnel syndrome. *Journal of hand therapy: official journal of the American Society of Hand Therapists*, *11*(3), 171–179.

Sammarco, G. J., & Chang, L. (2003). Outcome of surgical treatment of tarsal tunnel syndrome. *Foot & ankle international*, *24*(2), 125–131.

Singh, G., & Kumar, V. P. (2012). Neuroanatomical basis for the tarsal tunnel syndrome. *Foot & ankle international*, *33*(6), 513–518.

Upton, A. R., & McComas, A. J. (1973). The double crush in nerve entrapment syndromes. *Lancet (London, England)*, *2*(7825), 359–362.

Watson, B. V., Algahtani, H., Broome, R. J., & Brown, J. D. (2002). An unusual presentation of tarsal tunnel syndrome caused by an inflatable ice hockey skate. *The Canadian journal of neurological sciences.* [*Le journal canadien des sciences neurologiques*], *29*(4), 386–389.

In: Musculoskeletal Pain (Common Clinical Presentations) ISBN: 978-1-68507-410-4
Editors: Mehmet Cenk Turgut and Serdar Toy 

*Chapter 24*

# HALLUX VALGUS AND HALLUX RIGIDUS

***Khalid Bunyatov**, MD**
Department of Orthopedics and Traumatology,
Sultanbeyli Ersoy Hospital, Istanbul, Turkey

## ABSTRACT

Hallux valgus is a combination of deformities involving complex abnormalities of the first metatarsophalangeal joint. Hallux valgus is defined as an increase in the outward axis of the big toe relative to the axis of the first metatarsal. The main complaint of patients is the formation of a painful lump in the medial of the first metatarsophalangeal joint. Sometimes a lump without pain causes cosmetic complains. Though the deformity generally occurs because of idiopathic reasons, choice of narrow-toed, high-heeled shoes is also among the etiological reasons that contribute to the emergence of the clinic. It has treatment methods from shoe modification to surgical treatment. Hallux rigidus is degenerative arthritis of the first metatarsophalangeal joint. It occurs idiopathically as well as secondary to some ligament tissue diseases. The main complaint of patients is pain. Conservative and surgical treatment methods are available in its treatment.

**Keywords:** hallux valgus, hallux rigidus

## INTRODUCTION

Hallux valgus is a clinical diagnosis involving the first metatarsophalangeal joint, which defines an increase in the outward axis of the big toe relative to the axis of the first metatarsal. The hallux valgus term was first described as "Hallux Abducto

* Corresponding Author's E-mail: khalid_bunyatov@yahoo.com.

Valgus"(Burns &Mecham, 2014) by Carl Hueter in 1877. The center of the deformation occurs in the first metatarsophalangeal joint. This joint and the first metatarsocuneiform joint stability become weak because muscle tendons do not adhere to them. The first metatarsophalangeal joint is supported by two collateral ligaments in the medial and lateral. The plantar part of the joint is supported by the plantar plate. Other than that, the plantar part of the joint is supported by two tendons of the flexor hallucis brevis muscle, tendons of the abductor and adductor hallucis muscles, the plantar aponeurosis and sesamoid bones. On the contrary, the dorsal part of the joint is only supported by the joint capsule and the extensor hallucis longus and extensor hallucis brevis muscles. The dorsolateral and dorsomedial parts of the joint become weak and are prone to deformity(Coughlin & Jones, 2007). Tendon shortening and thickening result in the later stages of the deformity to the active pulling of the abductor hallucis muscle. This results in an indication for routine release of this tendon during surgical procedures(Jastifer et al., 2014).

Hallux rigidus is the clinical table that refers to arthrosis of the first metatarsophalangeal joint. The foot is seen in the second most common pathology after hallux valgus in first row pathologies. It is more common in adults (Coughlin &Shurnas, 2003).

## ETIOLOGY

The etiological causes are divided into extrinsic and intrinsic in the development of hallux valgus. The choice of narrow-toed, high-heeled shoes and overloading are extrinsic factors. On the other hand, the presence of hallux valgus, especially juvenile hallux valgus, in societies that do not wear shoes suggests that shoe wear is not very important in the etiology (Coughlin, 1995). Intrinsic causes such as genetic factors, gender (it is more common in women), ligament laxity (Marfan syndrome, Ehlers-Danlos syndrome, rheumatoid arthritis), age, the morphology of the tarsometatarsal joint, the morphology of the metatarsophalangeal joint, pes planus, strained Achilles tendon, and cerebral palsy play a role in the development of hallux valgus (Hecht & Lin, 2014).

The degenerative process that increases with age in adults is held responsible for the development of hallux rigidus. As the degenerative process may develop idiopathically, it may also develop as a result of reasons such as trauma, systemic joint and ligament tissue diseases, and infection.

## Radiological Evaluation

Properly taken graphs are always important in the evaluation of foot pathologies. Foot graphs should be taken with weight-bearing. The graphs are taken with the x-ray tube focused on the midtarsal joint at a distance of 100 cm from the foot and tilted towards the ankle at 15 degrees (Takakura, Tanaka, Kumai, & Tamai, 1995). In addition to the anterior-posterior, oblique, and lateral graphs, which are standard foot graphs, a sesamoid tangential graph can also be taken to evaluate the position of the sesamoid bones. The tarsometatarsal joint, other foot pathologies and hallux valgus specific angles are evaluated in direct graphs.

### Hallux Valgus Angle

This is the angle between the axis of the first metatarsal and the axis of the proximal phalanx in the anterior-posterior foot graphs with weight-bearing (Figure 1). A normal angle is 15° and under.

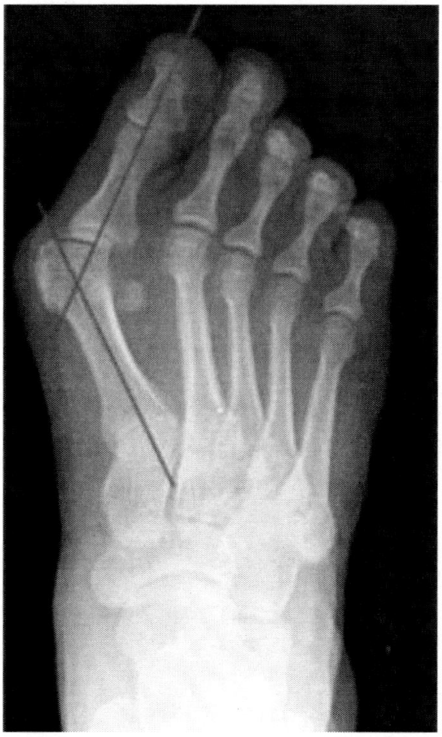

Figure 1. The source is from the author's archive.

## Intermetatarsal Angle

This is the angle between the axis of the first and second metatarsals in the anterior-posterior foot graphs with weight-bearing (Figure 2). A normal angle is 10° and under.

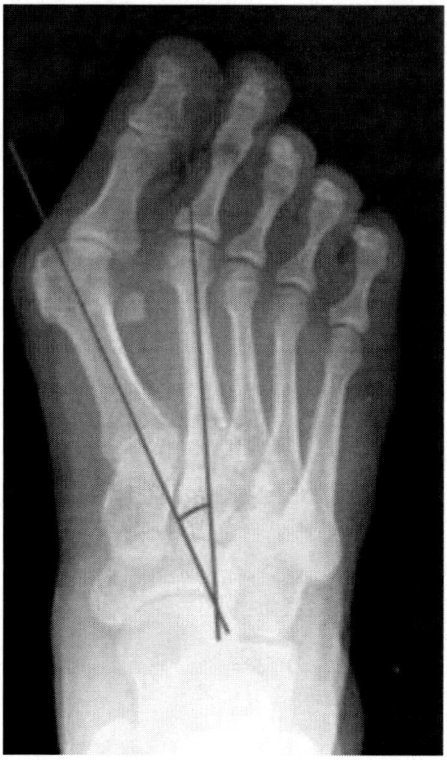

Figure 2. The source is from the author's archive.

## Hallux Valgus Interphalangeal Angle

This is the angle between the axis of the proximal and distal phalanges in the anterior-posterior foot graphs with weight-bearing (Figure 3). The normal angle is between 0 and 10°.

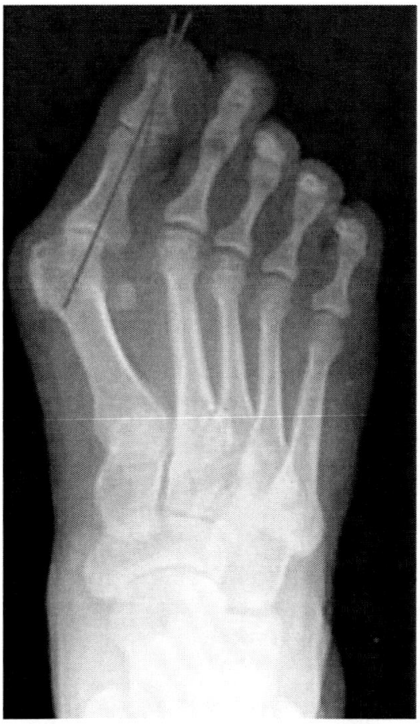

Figure 3. The source is from the author's archive.

## Distal Metatarsal Articular Angle

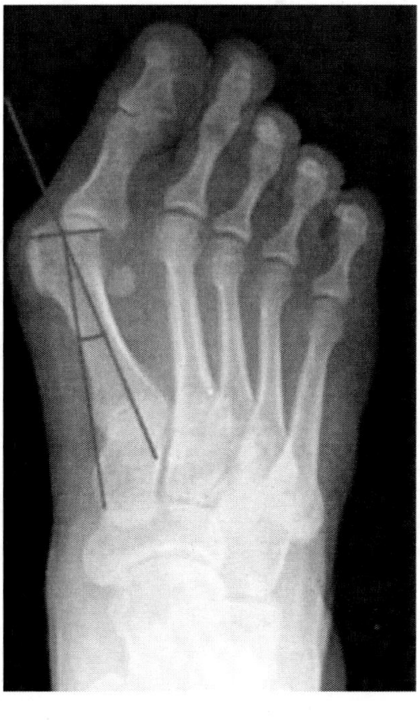

Figure 4. The source is from the author's archive.

This is the angle between the axis of the first metatarsal axis and the axis drawn longitudinal to the line connecting the first metatarsal distal joint endpoints in anterior-posterior foot graphs with weight-bearing (Figure 4). The normal angle is 6° and under.

## Distal Metatarsophalangeal Joint Adjustment

This is the adjustment of the line connecting the distal joint endpoints of the first metatarsal and the line connecting the proximal joint endpoints of the proximal phalanx (Figure 5). Normally these two lines are parallel to each other, and a divergence up to 3° is considered to be normal.

As with all foot pathologies, hallux rigidus should be evaluated with foot graphs taken with weight-bearing (Shereff & Baumhauer, 1998). Degenerative joint radiological findings such as narrowing of the joint space, osteophyte formation, subchondral sclerosis and cysts are seen on the graphs (Figure 6).

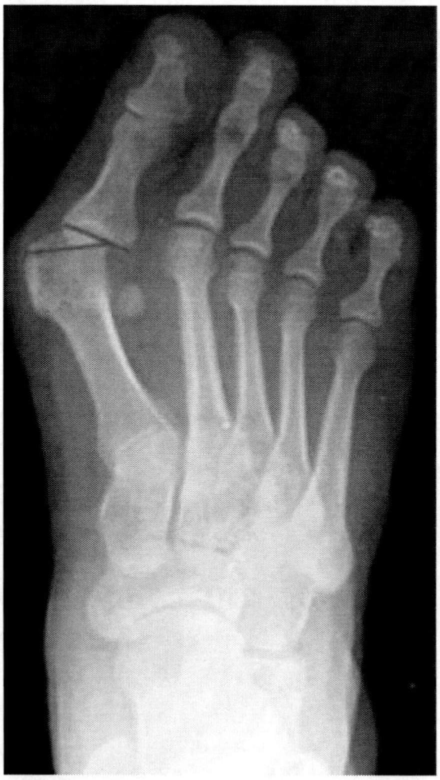

Figure 5. The source is from the author's archive.

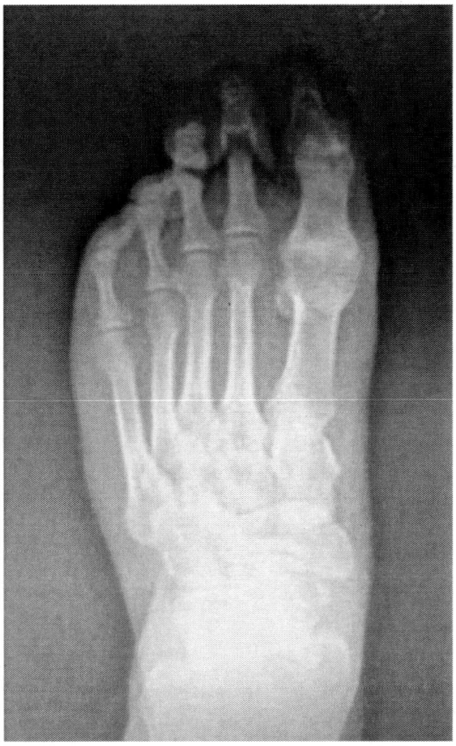

Figure 6. The source is from the author's archive.

## Clinical Evaluation

Deformity is not always the reason for patients being admitted to the hospital. Generally, the reason for patients being admitted to the hospital is a bunion in the 1st metatarsophalangeal joint medial and secondary pain for it. Other than that, patients in the young population rarely consult a doctor with aesthetic concerns. Erythema on the bunion, ulcer, other toe problems, a painful bunionette on the distal lateral of the 5th metatarsal, and metatarsalgia are reasons for presenting to the clinic in severe deformity cases (Pinney, Song, & Chou, 2006).

Pain, swelling, redness, and especially dorsiflexion restriction in the first metatarsophalangeal joint are priority clinical findings. In hallux rigidus, decreased dorsiflexion and plantar flexion in the 1st metatarsophalangeal joint due to arthrosis may cause secondary metatarsalgia as a result of transferring the load to the lateral foot during the pushing phase of walking (Hamid & Parekh, 2015).

# TREATMENT

Hallux valgus treatment is not performed primarily for cosmetic reasons; on the contrary, it aims to relieve pain and ensure that patients may walk comfortably (Tai et al., 2008). Sometimes, young patient groups in particular seek treatment for aesthetic concerns, with the idea of solving the problem so they can wear high heels and narrow-toed box shoes. There is a combination of conservative and surgical treatment. Conservative treatment includes non-steroidal anti-inflammatory drugs, protective orthoses, and shoe modifications. It should be noted that orthoses do not straighten the deformity in the hallux valgus (Tai et al., 2008). The main purpose of surgical treatment is to treat the complaints of patients. It is not appropriate to recommend surgical treatment because of the deformity or because of the thought that the deformity may increase. While planning the surgical treatment, a clinical and radiological evaluation of the additional pathologies that may cause the development of hallux valgus, systemic diseases (rheumatoid arthritis), cerebral palsy, other structural problems of the foot, and the first metatarsal-medial cuneiform joint should be made and the treatment decision should be made accordingly. Today, biplanar osteotomies are widely used in surgical treatment, the best known being osteotomy defined by Chevron. The choice of the surgical treatment of hallux valgus is made by considering the clinical and radiological evaluation of the deformity, as well as the presence of additional pathologies causing the deformity (Table 1).

After surgery, patients are provided with a hard-soled hallux valgus slipper to bear as much weight as they can tolerate, weight-bearing walking is started according to the radiographs taken at the 6th week, and full weight-bearing is started at the 12th week. It is recommended to use a toe separator or gauze bandage for an average of 12 weeks (Trnka, 2005).

Hallux rigidus is treated conservatively and surgically. NSAIDs (nonsteroid anti-inflammatory drugs), activity modification, choosing wide-toed, hard-soled, and non-high-heeled shoes, and intra-articular steroid injection are recommended in conservative treatment. Surgical treatment is indicated in patients who do not respond to conservative treatment. In surgical treatment, the purpose is to relieve pain and ensure that the patient can walk comfortably. In stage 1, hallux rigidus, debridement, and orientation osteotomies of the first metatarsal head; cheilectomy in stage 2; and fusion of the first metatarsopharyngeal joint in stages 3 and 4 are the preferred surgical approaches (Keiserman, Sammarco, & Sammarco, 2005).

**Table 1. Hallux valgus surgical treatment algorithm**

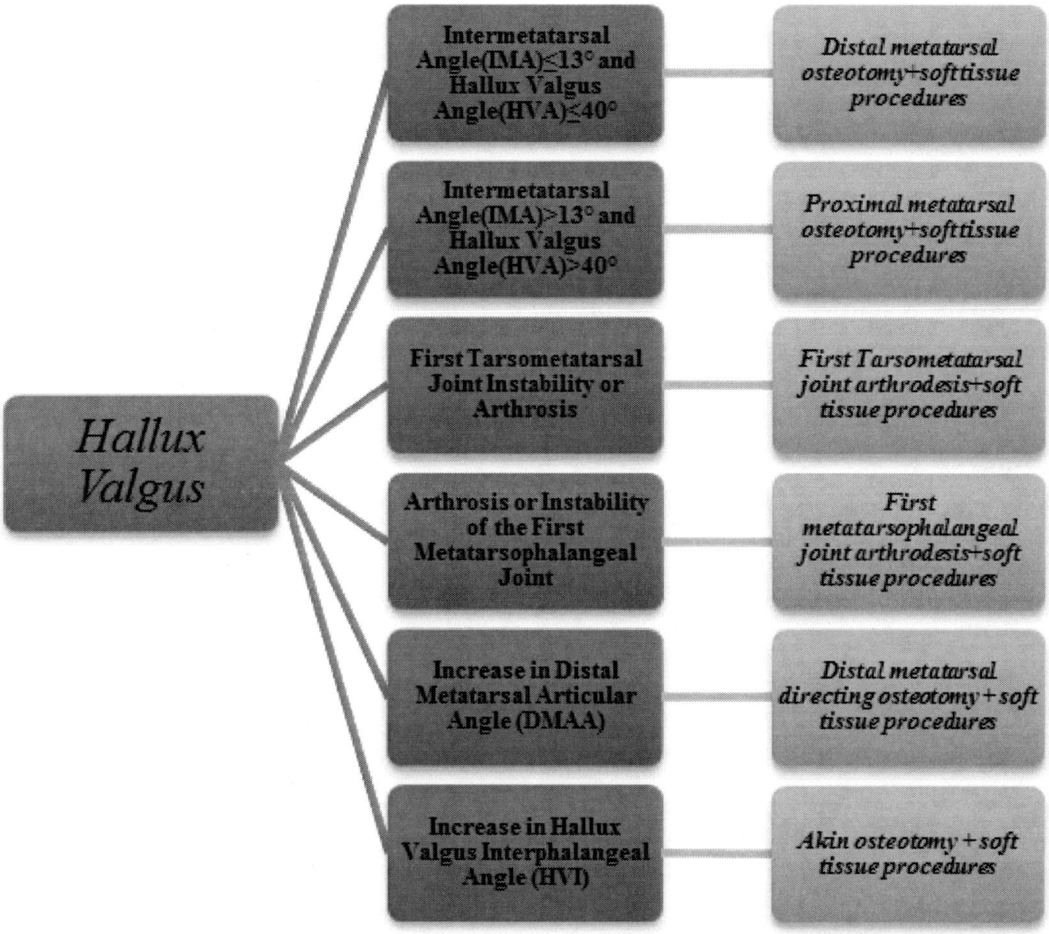


## Conclusion

Nowadays, hallux valgus and hallux rigidus appear as deformities that mostly affect the female gender. They are clinical conditions that affect the daily comfort of patients causing both pain and cosmetic problems. Though conservative treatment results in successful clinical results, sometimes surgical treatment is applied due to unresponsive pain in conservative treatment, cosmetic reasons, and reasons involving choosing modern shoes. Both clinical conditions are among the reasons for patients to consult a doctor complaining of pain and cosmetic problems caused by the deformity. Above all, relief of pain and comfortable living should be the main aims in treatment, and cosmetic reasons should always be a dual treatment option for both diseases.

## REFERENCES


Burns, P. R., & Mecham, B. (2014). Biodynamics of hallux abductovalgus etiology and preoperative evaluation. *Clinics in podiatric medicine and surgery, 31*(2), 197-212.

Coughlin, M. J. (1995). Juvenile hallux valgus: etiology and treatment. *Foot & ankle international, 16*(11), 682-697.

Coughlin, M. J., & Jones, C. P. (2007). Hallux valgus: demographics, etiology, and radiographic assessment. *Foot & ankle international, 28*(7), 759-777.

Coughlin, M. J., & Shurnas, P. S. (2003). Hallux rigidus: demographics, etiology, and radiographic assessment. *Foot & ankle international, 24*(10), 731-743.

Hamid, K. S., & Parekh, S. G. (2015). Clinical presentation and management of hallux rigidus. *Foot and ankle clinics, 20*(3), 391-399.

Hecht, P. J., & Lin, T. J. (2014). Hallux valgus. *Medical Clinics, 98*(2), 227-232.

Jastifer, J. R., Coughlin, M. J., Doty, J. F., Stevens, F. R., Hirose, C., & Kemp, T. J. (2014). Sensory nerve dysfunction and hallux valgus correction: a prospective study. *Foot & ankle international, 35*(8), 757-763.

Keiserman, L. S., Sammarco, V. J., & Sammarco, G. J. (2005). Surgical treatment of the hallux rigidus. *Foot and ankle clinics, 10*(1), 75-96.

Pinney, S. J., Song, K. R., & Chou, L. B. (2006). Surgical treatment of severe hallux valgus: the state of practice among academic foot and ankle surgeons. *Foot & ankle international, 27*(12), 1024-1029.

Shereff, M. J., & Baumhauer, J. F. (1998). Current Concepts Review-Hallux Rigidus and Osteoarthrosis of the First Metatarsophalangeal Joint. *JBJS, 80*(6), 898-908.

Tai, C., Ridgeway, S., Ramachandran, M., Ng, V., Devic, N., & Singh, D. (2008). Patient expectations for hallux valgus surgery. *Journal of orthopaedic surgery, 16*(1), 91-95.

Takakura, Y., Tanaka, Y., Kumai, T., & Tamai, S. (1995). Low tibial osteotomy for osteoarthritis of the ankle. Results of a new operation in 18 patients. *The Journal of bone and joint surgery. British volume, 77*(1), 50-54.

Trnka, H.-J. (2005). Osteotomies for hallux valgus correction. *Foot and ankle clinics, 10*(1), 15-33.

In: Musculoskeletal Pain (Common Clinical Presentations) ISBN: 978-1-68507-410-4
Editors: Mehmet Cenk Turgut and Serdar Toy 

*Chapter 25*

# MORTON'S NEUROMA

***Fatih Durgut**, MD***
Department of Orthopedics and Traumatology,
Dicle University Medicine Faculty, Diyarbakır, Turkey

## ABSTRACT

Morton's neuroma is a degenerative neuropathy featuring fibrosis of the common interdigital nerve. Patients typically present with symptoms of forefoot pain that can be associated with burning, tingling or numbness between the toes. Morton's neuroma is primarily a clinical diagnosis; however, radiological assessment is frequently requested to aid or confirm the diagnosis. Surgery is considered if symptoms persist after 3 months of non-operative treatment.

## INTRODUCTION

Despite being mentioned for the first time by Civinini in 1835, it was first described as Morton's neuroma by Thomas George Morton in 1876 (Civinini, 1835; Morton, 1876). The etiology and pathology of Morton's neuroma, which is the most frequent cause of metatarsalgia, are not exactly known. It is not actually a neuroma and manifests itself with fibrosis in the digital nerve (Morscher, Ulrich, & Dick, 2000). It progresses with neural edema, axonal injury, and fibrosis in the digital nerve (Figure 1). It should be kept in mind that although it is most commonly observed in the third web space, it can also be observed in other web spaces (Kasparek & Schneider, 2013).

* Corresponding Author's E-mail: drdurgut84@hotmail.com.

Its prevalence in women is four times higher than in men, and it is thought that wearing high-heeled shoes causes pressure on the digital nerve in the metatarsal head region and repetitive irritation causes changes in the nerve.

## Presentation

Patients present to the clinician with burning pain. This pain may be accompanied by numbness in the affected digital nerve sensory areas. While the pain increases with walking and standing, it is relieved at rest. If this condition becomes chronic, the pain may become continuous (Mahadevan, Venkatesan, Bhatt, & Bhatia, 2015). Patients usually state that wearing shoes triggers pain, whereas wearing slippers reduces pain.

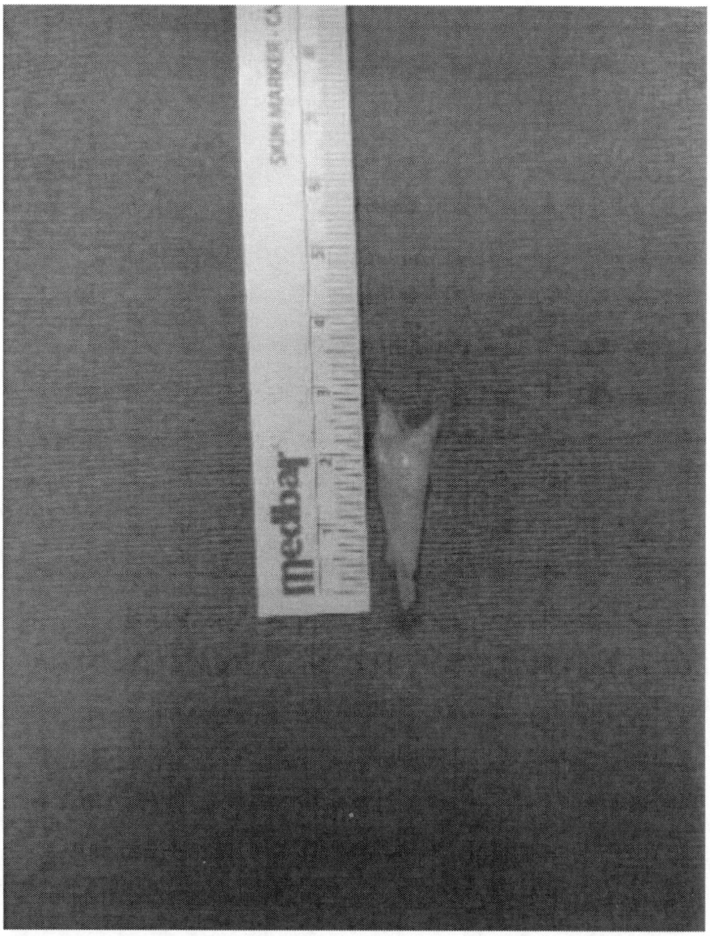


Figure 1. Abnormal nerve tissue.

The localization of the pain is usually in the web space, at the level of the metatarsal heads. Rarely, the pain may spread to the proximal (Di Caprio, Meringolo, Eddine, & Ponziani, 2018).

## Physical Examination

Patients should be in a sitting position and naked below the knees. The clinical examination starts with the observation of the patient's foot and lower leg. During the examination, the hind and midfoot should be evaluated. Patients should be evaluated for scars from previous surgery. The patient is asked to show the exact location of the pain. If the pain is in the dorsal region and above the metatarsal head, there may be synovitis, arthritis, or instability in the metatarsophalangeal joint. If the pain occurs in the intermetatarsal space and proximal to the MTP joint, a stress fracture should be considered. If the pain is on the plantar side of the metatarsal head, plantar plate degeneration and rupture should be considered.

Since the diagnosis of Morton's neuroma is based on the history and clinical examination, the patient's anamnesis should be carefully taken, and the physical examination should be carefully performed.

## Tests in Morton's Neuroma

### *Thumb and Index Finger Squeeze Test*

The web space where the patient has pain is squeezed between the thumb and index finger. In the presence of Morton's neuroma, squeezing the web space causes pain (Figure 2).

### *Mulder's Click Test*

The foot is placed in dorsiflexion. After placing the thumb and index finger in the painful web space, the metatarsal heads are squeezed by the other hand. If a jumping sensation occurs, the test is considered positive. If the neuroma is more than 1 cm, a click sound is heard (Figure 3).

### *Foot Squeeze Test*

Pain caused by squeezing the metatarsal heads indicates that the test is positive (Figure 4).

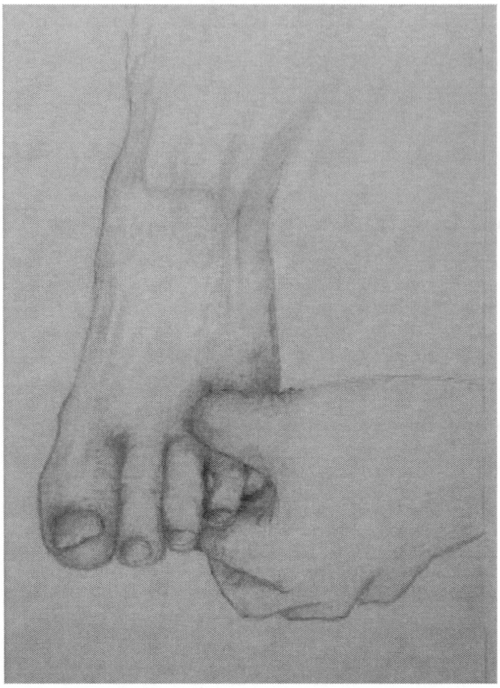

Figure 2. Thumb and index finger squeeze test.

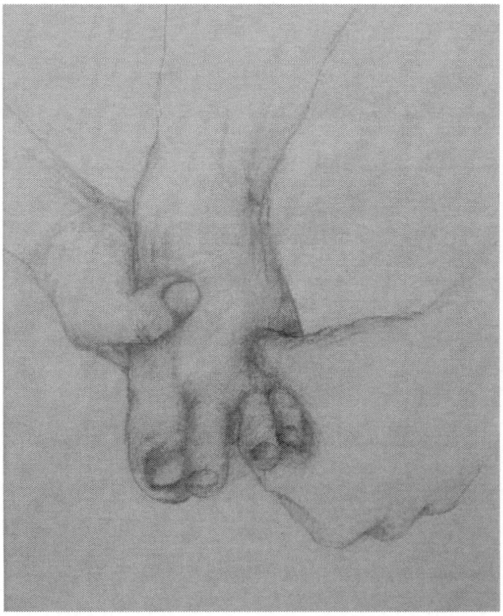

Figure 3. Mulder's click test.

### *Plantar Percussion Test*

The fingers are brought to dorsiflexion. Percussion is applied to the web space. Pain and numbness in the fingers indicate that the test is positive (Figure 5).

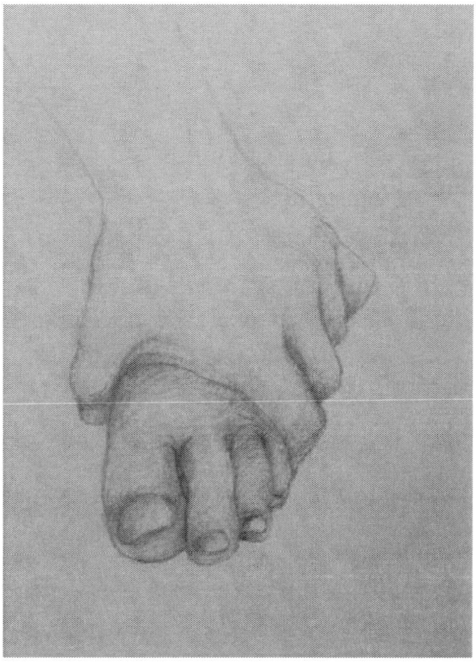

Figure 4. Foot squeeze test.

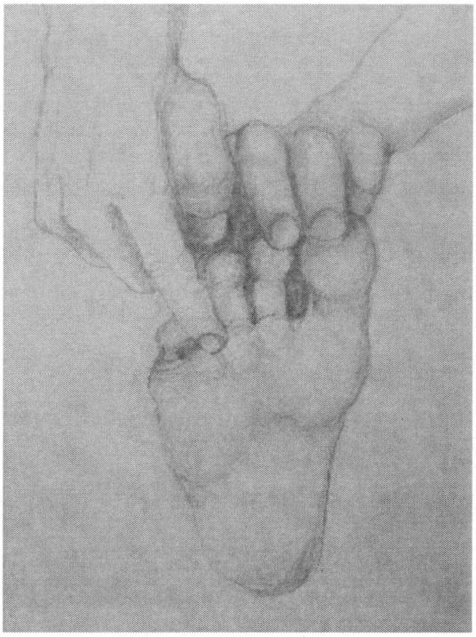

Figure 5. Plantar percussion test.

# IMAGING

The diagnosis of Morton's neuroma is established with clinical findings. Radiography is required to exclude metatarsalgia causes such as Freiberg, stress fracture, and joint subluxation.

Ultrasonography (USG) and magnetic resonance imaging (MRI) may be required to confirm the diagnosis of Morton's neuroma. Although the fact that USG is inexpensive is regarded as an advantage, it should be performed by specialists. MRI is the gold standard in confirming the diagnosis, and neuroma should be evaluated in T1 axial sections (Sharp, Wade, Hennessy, & Saxby, 2003; Torres-Claramunt, Ginés, Pidemunt, Puig, & De Zabala, 2012).

# TREATMENT

The treatment of Morton's neuroma can be divided into two: non-surgical and surgical. If patients do not benefit from conservative treatment of between 3 and 6 months, surgical treatment should be started. At first, nonsteroidal anti-inflammatory treatments should be administered in addition to shoe modification.

## Conservative Treatment

Among the conservative treatment options, patients should first be informed about the use of wide and comfortable shoes. The use of orthoses can reduce the burden on the neuroma and provide relief in patients' symptoms.

Corticosteroid injection is the most common conservative treatment method in Morton's neuroma (Gougoulias, Lampridis, & Sakellariou, 2019). Corticosteroid injection is thought to reduce inflammation around the neuroma, and as a result, local pressure and pain (Thomson et al., 2013). In addition to being repeatable, patients should be informed that steroid injection can cause thinning of the plantar fat pad, skin discoloration, and deviation in the fingers after joint capsule tears (van Vendeloo & Ettema, 2016). Symptoms can be relieved in 30% of patients after corticosteroid injection (Markovic, Crichton, Read, Lam, & Slater, 2008; Schon, 2014).

Alcohol is another injection method. Although successful results have been reported with this method, care should be taken before the application because one-third of patients go on to surgery and alcohol causes fibrosis in the surgical field, making surgery difficult (Bhatia & Thomson, 2020).

Radiofrequency application (15), extracorporeal shock wave therapy (16), laser therapy (17), botulinum toxin A treatment (18), and cryotherapy (19) are among other conservative treatment methods. These methods do not have long-term outcomes.

## Surgical Treatment

The neuroma can be excised with the dorsal or plantar approach. The dorsal approach is preferred in primary cases since it allows early weight-bearing during the postoperative period. On the other hand, the plantar approach is preferred in recurrence cases due to wound complications and scar problems (Thomson, Gibson, & Martin, 2004).

## Dorsal Approach

In the dorsal approach, the patient is in the supine position. The surgery is performed under a tourniquet. A 3-4 cm longitudinal incision is made from the web space, starting from the proximal part of the metatarsal head and extending to the distal (Figure 6). Subcutaneous tissues are passed through by blunt dissection. The distal transverse metatarsal ligament (DTML) is reached. After the DTML is cut, the distal branches of the digital nerve are found and explored. The nerve endings cut from the distal are dissected toward the metatarsal proximal and cut. The proximal part of the nerve is sutured into the muscle to prevent the development of a postoperative neuroma. The skin is closed.

## Plantar Approach

The plantar approach is usually preferred in recurrence cases. It is thought to be easier to reach and explore a nerve stump in the plantar approach (Johnson, Johnson, & Unni, 1988).

The plantar incision starts from the proximal part of the web space and requires a 4 cm incision proximally (Figure 7). The neuroma is reached after soft tissue dissection. After reaching the neuroma, exploration toward the proximal is performed until the healthy nerve tissue is reached. The neuroma part is excised, the remaining nerve tissue is embedded in the muscle, and the skin is closed.

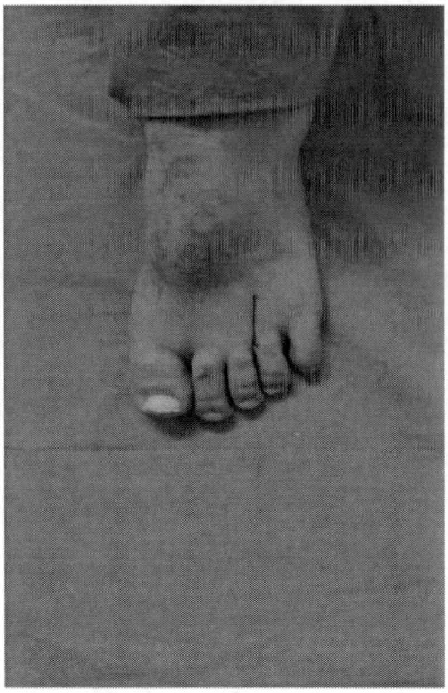

Figure 6. Dorsal approach.

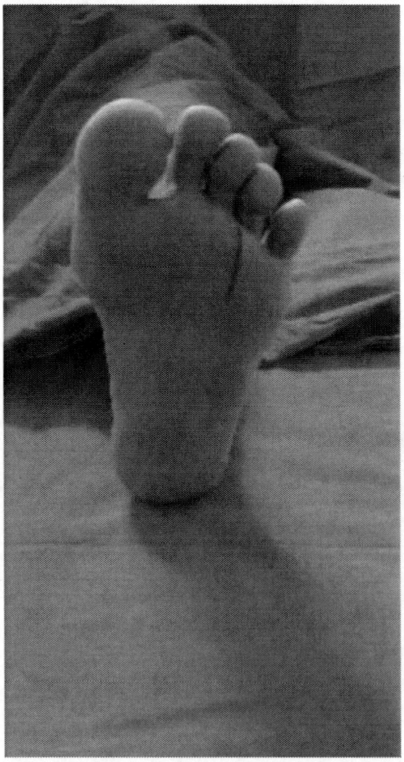

Figure 7. Plantar approach.

### Postoperative Care

During the postoperative period, bandages that protect the foot are applied. Early weight-bearing is allowed in patients undergoing surgery with the dorsal approach. Patients undergoing surgery with the plantar approach are allowed to bear weight after the wound is fully healed.

## Conclusion

Morton's neuroma is the most common cause of forefoot pain. The diagnosis of Morton's neuroma is established with the history and physical examination findings. Radiological procedures such as USG and MRI may be required to confirm the diagnosis. Direct radiography is necessary to exclude other problems that cause forefoot pain. Conservative methods are applied in the primary treatment of Morton's neuroma. Surgical treatment is applied in cases where conservative methods fail.

Pain complaints may persist in up to 30% of patients after surgery. Misdiagnosis, inadequate resection, the presence of adjacent neuromas, and the recurrence of a neuroma at the resected nerve end can be listed among the reasons for this. The correct diagnosis should be established, and an appropriate surgical method should be performed to increase the success rate after surgery.

## References

Bhatia, M., & Thomson, L. (2020). Morton's neuroma - Current concepts review. *Journal of clinical orthopaedics and trauma.*

Civinini, F. (1835). Su d'un nervoso gangliare rigonfiamento alla pianta del piede. *Lettera anatomica al Dr. Salomone Lampronti. Pistoia, Tip. Bracali.* [On a nervous ganglionic swelling on the sole of the foot. *Anatomical letter to Dr. Salomone Lampronti. Pistoia, Tip. Bracali*]

Di Caprio, F., Meringolo, R., Eddine, M. S., & Ponziani, L. (2018). Morton's interdigital neuroma of the foot: a literature review. *Foot and ankle surgery,* 24(2), 92-98.

Gougoulias, N., Lampridis, V., & Sakellariou, A. (2019). Morton's interdigital neuroma: instructional review. *EFORT open reviews,* 4(1), 14-24.

Johnson, J. E., Johnson, K., & Unni, K. K. (1988). Persistent pain after excision of an interdigital neuroma. Results of reoperation. *The Journal of bone and joint surgery. American volume,* 70(5), 651-657.

Kasparek, M., & Schneider, W. (2013). Surgical treatment of Morton's neuroma: clinical results after open excision. *International orthopaedics,* 37(9), 1857-1861.

Mahadevan, D., Venkatesan, M., Bhatt, R., & Bhatia, M. (2015). Diagnostic accuracy of clinical tests for Morton's neuroma compared with ultrasonography. *The Journal of Foot and Ankle Surgery,* 54(4), 549-553.

Markovic, M., Crichton, K., Read, J. W., Lam, P., & Slater, H. K. (2008). *Effectiveness of ultrasound-guided corticosteroid injection in the treatment of Morton's neuroma.*

Morscher, E., Ulrich, J., & Dick, W. (2000). Morton's intermetatarsal neuroma: morphology and histological substrate. *Foot & ankle international,* 21(7), 558-562.

Morton, T. G. (1876). A peculiar and painful affection of the fourth metatarsophalangeal articulation. *Am J Med Sci,* 71(35), 9.

Schon, L. (2014). An injection of corticosteroid plus anesthetic was more effective than anesthetic alone for Morton neuroma. *The Journal of bone and joint surgery. American volume,* 96(4), 334.

Sharp, R., Wade, C., Hennessy, M., & Saxby, T. (2003). The role of MRI and ultrasound imaging in Morton's neuroma and the effect of size of lesion on symptoms. *The Journal of bone and joint surgery. British volume,* 85(7), 999-1005.

Thomson, C. E., Beggs, I., Martin, D. J., McMillan, D., Edwards, R. T., Russell, D., . . . Gibson, J. A. (2013). Methylprednisolone injections for the treatment of Morton neuroma: a patient-blinded randomized trial. *JBJS,* 95(9), 790-798.

Thomson, C. E., Gibson, J. A., & Martin, D. (2004). Interventions for the treatment of Morton's neuroma. *Cochrane Database of Systematic Reviews* (3).

Torres-Claramunt, R., Ginés, A., Pidemunt, G., Puig, L., & De Zabala, S. (2012). MRI and ultrasonography in Morton's neuroma: diagnostic accuracy and correlation. *Indian journal of orthopaedics,* 46, 321-325.

van Vendeloo, S. N., & Ettema, H. B. (2016). Skin depigmentation along lymph vessels of the lower leg following local corticosteroid injection for interdigital neuroma. *Foot and ankle surgery,* 22(2), 139-141.

In: Musculoskeletal Pain (Common Clinical Presentations) ISBN: 978-1-68507-410-4
Editors: Mehmet Cenk Turgut and Serdar Toy 

*Chapter 26*

# RATIONAL USE OF DRUGS IN THE TREATMENT OF MUSCULOSKELETAL PAIN

***Hanzade Aybüke Ünal Artık*, MD and Fatma Ayşen Eren, MD***
[1]Department of Neurology,
Uşak Training and Research Hospital, Uşak, Turkey
[2]Department of Neurology,
Kanuni Training and Research Hospital, Istanbul, Turkey

## ABSTRACT

Musculoskeletal pain is frequently encountered in the community. In the treatment of musculoskeletal pain, the treatment scheme should be determined after the etiology of the pain has been carefully determined. Age, gender, comorbid diseases, medications used, and onset of pain should be considered in the selection of treatment. Pain management should be individualized on a patient basis. In this section, information about the non-steroidal anti-inflammatory drugs, opioids and adjuvant drugs which are frequently used in the treatment of musculoskeletal pain will be given.

## INTRODUCTION

Analgesics, which form the basis of pain treatment, are drugs used to control pain in acute and chronic pain syndromes. The history of the use of analgesic drugs, which are among the most frequently used drugs in society, dates back to ancient times. Advances in understanding the anatomical and physiological pathways of pain perception and

* Corresponding Author's E-mail: hanzadeunal@windowslive.com.

advances in drug pharmacology have led to new views and understanding. The important thing is which analgesics should be chosen to achieve the goal. After careful evaluation, the localization, duration, character, and temporal characteristics of pain should be determined. The age of the patient, the presence of liver-kidney problems that may affect the drug level, the severity and course of the disease, sociocultural characteristics, and the presence of analgesic or non-analgesic drugs should be taken into consideration (*NSAIDs: Therapeutic Use and Variability of Response in Adults – Up To Date*, n.d.). Non-steroidal anti-inflammatory drugs, opioids and adjuvant drugs are used in the treatment of musculoskeletal pain.

## Non-Steroidal Anti-Inflammatory Drugs

Non-steroidal anti-inflammatory drugs (NSAIDs) show analgesic, anti-inflammatory, and antipyretic effects by inhibiting the cyclooxygenase (COX) enzyme. The COX enzyme is involved in the conversion of prostaglandin, prostacyclin and thromboxane A2 from arachidonic acid (Ghosh et al., 2019). NSAIDs target two types of COX enzymes. COX-1 expression is present in all cells. COX-2 expression is induced by tissue damage (Atkinson & Fudin, 2020). The COX-1 enzyme is responsible for gastrointestinal mucosal integrity, platelet aggregation and renal flow regulation, and the balance of prostacyclin and thromboxane A2. COX-2 is mainly expressed in the kidney, brain, and blood vessels but induced by cytokine release after inflammation and/or injury. Therefore, COX-2 inhibition is targeted in pain management, and all NSAIDs show their analgesic effects through this pathway (Atkinson & Fudin, 2020). NSAIDs are divided into "nonselective," "COX-2 selective," and "COX-2 specific" according to their COX selectivity (Table 1).

**Table 1. NSAIDs by COX selectivity**

| Nonselective NSAIDs | COX-2 selective NSAIDs | COX-2 specific NSAIDs |
|---|---|---|
| Indomethacin | Meloxicam | Celecoxib |
| Piroxicam | Nimesulide | Rofecoxib |
| Sulindac | Etodolac | |
| Flurbiprofen | | |
| Ketoprofen | | |
| Ibuprofen | | |
| Naproxen | | |

NSAIDs differ in their side effect profiles depending on their COX selectivity. COX-1 inhibition causes an increase in the risk of gastrointestinal ulceration and bleeding through the inhibition of platelet aggregation. COX-2 selective NSAIDs can be used to reduce gastric side effects, and misoprostol or proton pump inhibitors can be added to the treatment. A history of ulcer, *Helicobacter pylori* infection, increasing age, and a high NSAID dose pose a risk for gastrointestinal bleeding (Atkinson & Fudin, 2020). With COX-1 and COX-2 inhibition, sodium and water retention, hypertension and renal damage may develop. Particular attention should be paid to sodium and water retention in patients with heart failure. COX-2 inhibition may cause myocardial infarction and stroke (Cooper et al., 2019). Selective COX-2 inhibitors are contraindicated in patients with ischemic heart disease, cerebrovascular disease, peripheral arterial disease, and moderate to severe heart failure (Shah & Mehta, 2012). In 2015, the FDA stated that cardiovascular events could occur with all NSAIDs. NSAIDs are contraindicated in patients with a history of coronary artery bypass graft surgery, and the benefit-risk ratio should be well evaluated in patients with a history of urticaria, angioedema, and bronchospasm (Brewer et al., 2010). NSAID use may worsen existing diseases in patients with asthma and renal and heart diseases. Anaphylaxis may develop in those with nasal polyps and a history of allergy (Eyichukwu, 2010). Acetaminophen has a weak anti-inflammatory effect compared to other NSAIDs. Adverse effects in the use of acetaminophen are rare, and it does not have a significant effect on the gastrointestinal and cardiovascular systems. Transient liver function test abnormalities were reported in the use of acetaminophen, and severe hepatic side effects may develop in long-term use at the maximum dose (Loveless & Fry, 2016). Oral NSAIDs are preferred in musculoskeletal pain that is unresponsive to acetaminophen (Cooper et al., 2019). NSAIDs are indicated for pain accompanying inflammation in acute trauma, chronic pain accompanied by inflammation (osteoarthritis and rheumatological diseases), bone metastasis, soft tissue rheumatism, neuritis, low back and neck pain, and myalgia (Eyichukwu, 2010) (Eyichukwu, 2010). NSAIDs and their doses commonly used in musculoskeletal pain are listed in Table 2 (*NSAIDs: Therapeutic Use and Variability of Response in Adults – Up To Date*, n.d.).

Although oral NSAIDs are effective in musculoskeletal pain, the use of topical NSAIDs in musculoskeletal pain has recently gained popularity due to their gastrointestinal, cardiovascular, renal, hepatic, and cerebrovascular side effects (Stanos, 2007). Topical NSAIDs are preferred, especially in the geriatric population over 75 years of age (Cooper et al., 2019). Topical NSAIDs should be applied to intact skin without lesions. They show their effect by inhibiting COX-2 in the tissue to which they are applied. Since the plasma concentration of the drug is very low due to its local application, its side effects are minimal compared to oral NSAIDs (Derry et al., 2016). The most common side effects are local skin reactions. However, as with their oral forms, topical agents have black box warnings for cardiovascular events, stroke, and gastrointestinal side effects (Brewer et al., 2010). Diclofenac, indomethacin, ketoprofen, ibuprofen, and piroxicam are NSAIDs with a topical form (Derry et al., 2016). There are three different topical diclofenac forms: the diclofenac hydroxyethylpyrrolidine (DHEP) patch, diclofenac sodium gel 1%, and diclofenac sodium 1.5% drop. Topical diclofenac was found to be superior to other topical NSAIDs in pain palliation, especially in soft tissue injuries (Stanos, 2007). There are various guidelines and expert recommendations for rational drug use according to musculoskeletal pain types. Acetaminophen or NSAID is the first-line drug of choice in addition to training and exercise in acute spinal pain (Loveless & Fry, 2016).

**Table 2. Commonly used oral NSAID dosing schedule**

| | Usual analgesic dosage | Maximum dosage |
|---|---|---|
| Acetaminophen | 325-650 mg every 4-6 h | 3000 mg |
| Naproxen | 250 mg every 6-8 h or 500 mg every 12 h (naproxen base)<br>275 mg every 6-8 h or 550 mg every 12 h (naproxen sodium) | 1000 mg (naproxen base)<br>1100 mg (naproxen sodium) |
| Ibuprofen | 200-400 mg every 4-6 h | 3200 mg |
| Ketoprofen | 50 mg every 6 h or 75 mg every 8 h<br>200 mg daily (ER form) | 300 mg |
| Flurbiprofen | 50 to 100 mg every 6-12 h | 300 mg |
| Diclofenac | 50 mg every 8-12 h (diclofenac potassium)<br>50 mg every 5 h or 75 mg every 12 h (diclofenac sodium)<br>100 mg daily (ER form) | 150 mg<br>The approved maximum daily dose in Canada is 100 mg |
| Etodolac | 200-400 mg every 6 to 8 h<br>400-1000 mg once daily (ER form) | 1000 mg<br>1200 mg (ER form) |
| Indomethacin | 25- 50 mg every 8-12 h<br>75-150 mg once daily (ER form) | 150 mg |
| Tolmetin | 400-600 mg every 8 h | 1800 mg |
| Sulindac | 150-200 mg every 12 h | 400 mg |
| Meloxicam | 7.5-15 mg once daily (tablet)<br>5-10 mg once daily (capsule) | 15 mg (tablet)<br>10 mg (capsule) |
| Piroxicam | 10-20 mg once daily | 20 mg |
| Mefenamic acid | 250 mg every 6 h | 1000 mg |
| Celecoxib | 200 mg daily or 100 mg every 12 h | 400 mg |

Abbreviations: hours (h); extended release (ER).
The recommended doses are adult patient doses.

In new-onset neck pain and cervical radiculopathy, experts recommend the use of NSAIDs after careful evaluation. Acupuncture, topical NSAID and exercise are recommended before NSAIDs in neck pain. In cervical radiculopathy, short-term NSAID use is recommended in cases in which pain control cannot be achieved with paracetamol (Kjaer et al., 2017). In low back pain, the use of acetaminophen alone is not recommended. Considering the individual comorbid conditions of patients, short-term NSAID use is recommended in appropriate patient populations (*NICE | The National Institute for Health and Care Excellence*, n.d.). Topical NSAID efficacy in low back pain has not been proven, but it can be used in neck pain because of the superficial anatomy of neck structures (Loveless & Fry, 2016). There is low-to-moderate evidence that nonselective COX inhibitors and selective COX-2 inhibitors are effective in short-term pain management in rotator cuff tendinopathy. Oral NSAIDs were found to be as effective as corticosteroid injections in short-term pain control (Boudreault et al., 2014). In the treatment of osteoarthritis, oral NSAID/selective COX-2 inhibitors are recommended if acetaminophen or topical NSAIDs are ineffective (Abdulla et al., 2013). In the geriatric population, in which musculoskeletal pain is common, guidelines recommend first-line acetaminophen for musculoskeletal pain, including osteoarthritis and low back pain (Abdulla et al., 2013). In the pediatric population, acetaminophen and ibuprofen can be used for musculoskeletal pain, but medication treatment should be discontinued as soon as possible (Banerjee & Butcher, 2020).

## Opioids

Opioids act by binding to peripheral and central mu, kappa and delta receptors. By binding to opioid receptors located at the presynaptic nerve endings, they provide analgesia with a decrease in the release of neurotransmitters such as glutamate and substance P, activation of GABA and an antagonistic effect on N-methyl-D-aspartate (NMDA) receptors (Trescot et al., 2008). Opioids are divided into weak (tramadol, codeine, hydrocodone) and strong (morphine, fentanyl, oxycodone, oxymorphone) according to their potency (Saba et al., 2017). The World Health Organization (WHO) recommends the use of opioids in pain unresponsive to NSAIDs and/or acetaminophen. Opioids should be used by titration. Before treatment, patients should be informed about the risk of addiction. Together, the patient and physician should decide on individualized treatment (*NICE | The National Institute for Health and Care Excellence*, n.d.). Care should be taken in terms of the development of misuse, abuse, and addiction. Opioid therapy should be discontinued as soon as possible (Busse et al., 2018). It should be carefully followed up for potential side effects such as sedation, nausea, vomiting, gastrointestinal spasm, pruritus, respiratory depression, constipation, immunosuppression, orthostatic hypotension, urinary retention, and opioid-induced hyperalgesia (Crofford, 2010). Sedation, nausea, vomiting, and pruritus are temporary side effects that usually last for 2-3 days, while constipation is persistent in most patients (Podichetty et al., 2003). With the use of opioids, falls and fractures may develop due to the drowsiness and dizziness effects of opioids in the geriatric population (Abdulla et al., 2013). In the pediatric population, the use of codeine and tramadol is contraindicated in children under 12 years of age (Banerjee & Butcher, 2020).

Although opioids are frequently used and effective analgesics in cancer pain, a systemic review and meta-analysis conducted in 2018 indicated that opioids provided minimal benefit in the treatment of non-cancer pain (Busse et al., 2018). It is stated that tramadol may be beneficial in the treatment of musculoskeletal pain in patients for whom NSAID and acetaminophen use is inappropriate or pain palliation cannot be achieved. Furthermore, using opioids in combination with NSAIDs or acetaminophen may provide additional benefits (Loveless & Fry, 2016). There are various guidelines and expert recommendations regarding the use of opioids in musculoskeletal pain types. In the knee osteoarthritis treatment algorithm published in 2019, weak opioids such as tramadol are recommended as the last trial in preoperative pharmacological treatment (Bruyère et al., 2019). In the NICE recommendations updated in 2016, weak opioids are recommended for patients with acute low back pain who do not respond to NSAID use and/or have NSAID contraindications. Moreover, the use of opioids in chronic low back pain and lumbar radicular pain is not recommended by NICE (*NICE | The National Institute for Health and Care Excellence*, n.d.). Although opioid analgesics cause short-term pain relief in chronic low back pain, this effect is minimal and not clinically significant (Shaheed et al., 2016).

## Adjuvant Analgesics

While adjuvant analgesics are used in the treatment of diseases other than pain, they are drugs belonging to different pharmacological groups, which are useful in some pain syndromes and show analgesic effects (Lussier et al., 2004). They are also called secondary analgesic, co-analgesic or adjuvant analgesic drugs (Lusser and Portenoy, 2003).

Adjuvant analgesics, which are present at every step of the analgesic treatment ladder recommended by the World Health Organization, take an important place in the treatment of chronic pain (Grond et al., 1999). One of the keys to success in pain treatment is the correct use of adjuvant drugs. According to the type of pain, its cause, accompanying symptoms, and the clinical characteristics of the patient, which adjuvant drug to choose for treatment should be decided. Adjuvant drugs not only increase analgesic effectiveness but also reduce drug side effects by reducing the doses of other analgesic drugs. The main adjuvant drugs are antiepileptics, antidepressants, local anesthetics, corticosteroids, and muscle relaxants (Moulin et al., 2007).

### Antidepressant Drugs

Antidepressants take an undeniable place in the treatment of chronic pain. The main mechanisms of action of antidepressant drugs include preventing peripheral sensitization by blocking sodium channels and preventing the reuptake of inhibitory neurotransmitters such as serotonin and noradrenaline between inhibitory neurons in the dorsal horn of the spinal cord and nociceptive neurons that provide transmission (Stahl et al., 2005). Antidepressant drugs can be mainly classified as TCA (tricyclic antidepressants), SNRI (selective noradrenaline reuptake inhibitors), and SSRI (selective serotonin reuptake inhibitors).

Among the tricyclic antidepressants, amitriptyline provides the best results in the treatment of neuropathic pain and is the most widely used. Attention should be paid to its anticholinergic and cardiac side effects (Magni, 1991).

Within the SNRI group, venlafaxine and duloxetine are used in the treatment of neuropathic pain. Since they do not have antihistaminergic and anticholinergic effects like TCAs, they have fewer side effects. During chronic use, a dose-dependent increase in blood pressure may develop (Stahl et al., 2005).

The same efficacy with TCAs was not demonstrated in the use of SSRIs in the treatment of neuropathic pain. Their use was recommended in patients with chronic neuropathic pain in the presence of comorbidities such as insomnia, depression, and anxiety (Max et al., 1992).

## Antiepileptic Drugs

This is a group of drugs that are frequently used in the treatment of neuropathic pain. The most important mechanisms of action of antiepileptics in neuropathic pain are blocking Na channels, affecting calcium transmission, decreasing the activity of glutamate, and activating the GABA system. Thus, synaptic transmission is suppressed, the repetitive firing threshold of nociceptive neurons is increased, and the discharges occurring in the dorsal root ganglia are reduced (Eisenberg et al., 2007).

Gabapentin is a GABA receptor agonist, and its analgesic and antiepileptic effect is achieved by the blockade of L-type calcium channels. It is excreted in the urine and a small amount in the feces without being metabolized to a large extent. Dose adjustment should be made in renal patients. The most common side effects are drowsiness, sedation, ataxia, and edema of the legs (Gottrup et al., 2004).

Pregabalin is a GABA analog and acts by binding to the alpha-2 delta subunit of the calcium channel on primary afferent neurons and preventing the release of pronociceptive neurotransmitters from the nerve terminal. Its elimination is similar to gabapentin, and dose adjustment should be made in renal patients. The most common side effects are dose-dependent and include dizziness, somnolence, dry mouth, and peripheral edema (Eisenberg et al., 2007).

## Corticosteroids

These are used in many diseases in medicine. Their use in the treatment of pain comes to the fore when inflammation and edema cause pain. The mechanism of action of corticosteroids prevents the formation of leukotrienes and prostaglandins by inhibiting the formation of cytokines (IL1, IL6, TNF), lymphokines and phospholipase A2 that cause inflammation. In this way, by preventing inflammation, they prevent the activation of the nociceptive neuron by means of chemical mediators and also prevent the mechanical stimulation of the nociceptive neuron with the anti-edema effect (Schwiebert et al., 1996).

They are mainly used as adjuvant analgesics in the treatment of chronic pain, in rheumatoid arthritis, radiculopathy, synovitis and entrapment neuropathies. Although there are studies showing that corticosteroids reduce short-term pain in the systemic treatment of acute radiculopathy, their efficacy in chronic low back and neck pain was not determined (Finckh et al., 2006). The efficacy of epidural corticosteroid injection was demonstrated in chronic low back and neck pain (Benyamin et al., 2009).

## Local Anesthetics

Local anesthetics are thought to provide analgesia in regional and systemic administration through sodium channel inactivation and inhibition of the action potential in the axon membrane. Interestingly, analgesic properties occur at subanesthetic doses (Knotkova & Pappagallo, 2007). Drugs in this group are not the first-choice drugs in chronic pain because they have severe side effects after systemic administration, but they can be used in cases of neuropathic pain resistant to other treatments (Glazer & Portenoy, 1991).

## Skeletal Muscle Relaxants

Skeletal muscle relaxants are used for spasticity associated with the upper motor neuron and peripheral musculoskeletal pain (Chou et al., 2004). Skeletal muscle relaxants are divided into two as antispastic and antispasmodic agents. Antispastic agents exert their effects through the spinal cord or directly through the skeletal muscle. They are often used in diseases that cause spasticity, such as cerebral palsy, multiple sclerosis, and spinal cord damage (See & Ginzburg, 2008). Baclofen, dantrolene, and tizanidine are drugs approved for the treatment of spasticity (Chou et al., 2004). Antispasmodic agents are used for musculoskeletal pain such as low back pain, radicular pain, and myofascial pain. Benzodiazepines, cyclobenzaprine, carisoprodol, metaxalone, chlorzoxazone, methocarbamol, tizanidine, and orphenadrine are antispasmodic agents (See & Ginzburg, 2008).

Cyclobenzaprine acts through 5 HT2 receptor antagonism (El-Tallawy et al., 2021). Cyclobenzaprine has a similar effect to tricyclic antidepressants in structure. It shows its antispasmodic effect mostly at the level of the brain stem (See & Ginzburg, 2008). Attention should be paid to the anticholinergic side effects (drowsiness, dry mouth, urinary retention, increased intraocular pressure), arrhythmia, seizure, and cardiac side effects of cyclobenzaprine (Toth & Urtis, 2004). Metaxalone's direct mechanism of action could not be defined, and it is thought to provide an antispasmodic effect by affecting signal modification from polysynaptic fibers involved in central nervous system depression and passive stretch control. Its side effects include drowsiness, leukopenia, hemolytic anemia, jaundice, nausea and vomiting (Toth & Urtis, 2004). Tizanidine is an alpha2 receptor agonist. It acts by motor neuron presynaptic inhibition. Although the mechanism of action of metaxalone is not known, it is thought to act by depressing the polysynaptic spinal reflex (Sullivan et al., 2007). Carisoprodol is a centrally acting skeletal muscle relaxant which is metabolized to meprobamate. Meprobamate is a risky molecule for drug addiction (See & Ginzburg, 2008). Caution should be exercised against sedation side effects in the use of carisoprodol (El-Tallawy et al., 2021).

Muscle relaxants can be used in the treatment of acute low back pain and soft tissue injury (Eyichukwu, 2010). There are studies showing that tizanidine may be effective in myofascial pain (Bair & Sanderson, 2011). The superiority of skeletal muscle relaxant agents to each other was not reported in the studies, and agents should be preferred according to adverse effects, comorbid diseases, and age (Sullivan et al., 2007). They should be used for a minimum time in musculoskeletal diseases, and skeletal muscle relaxants show a more central effect after 1-2 weeks of use. This situation also poses a risk for physical dependence. The moderate side effect of skeletal muscle relaxants is sedation. Particular attention should be paid to their concomitant use with opioids, TCAs, and SNRIs (Bair & Sanderson, 2011).

## Topical Capsaicin

Capsaicin is a substance found in chili peppers (Bolin, 2003). Capsaicin is available in a 0.025% or 0.075% cream form and an 8% patch form. The patch form is used in some types of neuropathic pain (Derry et al., 2016). The cream form is used in the treatment of arthritis (Abdulla et al., 2013). Capsaicin acts by binding to the nociceptors responsible for pain perception in the skin, especially TRPV1 receptors. TRPV1 receptors provide sodium and calcium ion passage control through the cell membrane. With the activation of TRPV1 receptors, itching, prickling and burning sensations occur (Derry et al., 2016). With the repeated use of capsaicin, desensitization of the calcium-dependent TRPV1 receptors develops, thereby desensitizing the channel to capsaicin and other painful stimuli (Iftinca et al., 2021). Erythema, warmth and a burning sensation are among the side effects, and especially the burning sensation that develops in the first week makes it difficult for patients to comply with the treatment (Bolin, 2003).

## CONCLUSION

In patients with musculoskeletal pain, drug therapy should be performed with a gradual clinical approach. The patient should be evaluated in a multi-faceted manner, and the most appropriate analgesic drugs should be selected according to the accompanying symptoms or factors. Nonsteroidal anti-inflammatory drugs, opioids and adjuvant analgesic drugs are used in the treatment of musculoskeletal pain. Efficacy and tolerability should be regularly re-evaluated, and if there is no reduction in pain, drug therapy should be rearranged.

## REFERENCES

Abdulla, A., Adams, N., Bone, M., Elliott, A. M., Gaffin, J., Jones, D., Knaggs, R., Martin, D., Sampson, L., Schofield, P., & British Geriatric Society. (2013). Guidance on the management of pain in older people. *Age and Ageing*, *42 Suppl 1*. https://doi.org/10. 1093/ageing/afs200.

Atkinson, T. J., & Fudin, J. (2020). Nonsteroidal Antiinflammatory Drugs for Acute and Chronic Pain. *Physical Medicine and Rehabilitation Clinics of North America*, *31*(2), 219–231. https:// doi.org/10.1016/j.pmr.2020.01.002.

Bair, M. J., & Sanderson, T. R. (2011). Coanalgesics for chronic pain therapy: A narrative review. *Postgraduate Medicine*, *123*(6), 140–150. https://doi.org/ 10.3810/pgm.2011.11.2504.

Banerjee, S., & Butcher, R. (2020). Pharmacological Interventions for Chronic Pain in Pediatric Patients: A Review of Guidelines. *Pharmacological Interventions for Chronic Pain in Pediatric Patients: A Review of Guidelines*. http://www.ncbi. nlm.nih.gov/ pubmed/33119240.

Benyamin, R., Singh, V., Parr, A. T., Conn, A., Diwan, S., & Abdi, S. (2009). Systematic review of the effectiveness of cervical epidurals in the management of chronic neck pain. In *Pain Physician* (Vol. 12, Issue 1, pp. 137–157). Centre for Reviews and Dissemination (UK). https://doi.org/10.36076/ppj.2009/12/137.

Bolin, D. J. (2003). Transdermal Approaches to Pain in Sports Injury Management. *Current Sports Medicine Reports*, *2*(6), 303–309. https://doi.org/10.1249/00149619-200312000-00004.

Boudreault, J., Desmeules, F., Roy, J. S., Dionne, C., Frémont, P., & MacDermid, J. C. (2014). The efficacy of oral non-steroidal anti-inflammatory drugs for rotator cuff tendinopathy: A systematic review and meta-analysis. *Journal of Rehabilitation Medicine*, *46*(4), 294–306. https://doi.org/10.2340/16501977-1800.

Brewer, A. R., McCarberg, B., & Argoff, C. E. (2010). Update on the use of topical NSAIDs for the treatment of soft tissue and musculoskeletal pain: A review of recent data and current treatment options. *Physician and Sportsmedicine*, *38*(2), 62–70. https://doi. org/10.3810/psm.2010.06.1784.

Bruyère, O., Honvo, G., Veronese, N., Arden, N. K., Branco, J., Curtis, E. M., Al-Daghri, N. M., Herrero-Beaumont, G., Martel-Pelletier, J., Pelletier, J. P., Rannou, F., Rizzoli, R., Roth, R., Uebelhart, D., Cooper, C., & Reginster, J. Y. (2019). An updated algorithm recommendation for the management of knee osteoarthritis from the European Society for Clinical and Economic Aspects of Osteoporosis, Osteoarthritis and Musculoskeletal Diseases (ESCEO). *Seminars in Arthritis and Rheumatism*, *49*(3), 337–350. https://doi. org/10.1016/j.semarthrit.2019.04.008.

Busse, J. W., Wang, L., Kamaleldin, M., Craigie, S., Riva, J. J., Montoya, L., Mulla, S. M., Lopes, L. C., Vogel, N., Chen, E., Kirmayr, K., De Oliveira, K., Olivieri, L., Kaushal, A., Chaparro, L. E., Oyberman, I., Agarwal, A., Couban, R., Tsoi, L., … Guyatt, G. H. (2018). Opioids for Chronic Noncancer Pain: A Systematic Review and Meta-analysis. In *JAMA - Journal of the American Medical Association* (Vol. 320, Issue 23, pp. 2448–2460). American Medical Association. https://doi.org/ 10.1001/jama.2018.18472.

Chou, R., Peterson, K., & Helfand, M. (2004). Comparative efficacy and safety of skeletal muscle relaxants for spasticity and musculoskeletal conditions: A systematic review. In *Journal of Pain and Symptom Management* (Vol. 28, Issue 2, pp. 140–175). J Pain Symptom Manage. https://doi.org/10.1016/j.jpainsymman.2004.05.002.

Cooper, C., Chapurlat, R., Al-Daghri, N., Herrero-Beaumont, G., Bruyère, O., Rannou, F., Roth, R., Uebelhart, D., & Reginster, J. Y. (2019). Safety of Oral Non-Selective Non-Steroidal Anti-Inflammatory Drugs in Osteoarthritis: What Does the Literature Say? *Drugs and Aging*, *36*(Suppl 1), 15–24. https://doi.org/10.1007/ s40266-019-00660-1.

Crofford, L. J. (2010). Adverse effects of chronic opioid therapy for chronic musculoskeletal pain. *Nature Reviews Rheumatology*, *6*(4), 191–197. https://doi.org/10.1038/nrrheum.2010.24.

Derry, S., Conaghan, P., Da Silva, J. A. P., Wiffen, P. J., & Moore, R. A. (2016). Topical NSAIDs for chronic musculoskeletal pain in adults. *Cochrane Database of Systematic Reviews*, *2016*(4). https://doi.org/ 10.1002/14651858.CD007400.pub3.

Eisenberg, E., River, Y., Shifrin, A., & Krivoy, N. (2007). Antiepileptic drugs in the treatment of neuropathic pain. In *Drugs* (Vol. 67, Issue 9, pp. 1265–1289). Drugs. https://doi.org/10.2165/00003495-200767090-00003.

El-Tallawy, S. N., Nalamasu, R., Salem, G. I., LeQuang, J. A. K., Pergolizzi, J. V., & Christo, P. J. (2021). Management of Musculoskeletal Pain: An Update with Emphasis on Chronic Musculoskeletal Pain. *Pain and Therapy*, *10*(1). https://doi.org/10. 1007/s40122-021-00235-2.

Eyichukwu, G. O. (2010). Non-Steroidal anti inflammatory drugs usage in orthopaedics and trauma practice. A guide and review. *Nigerian Journal of Medicine : Journal of the National Association of Resident Doctors of Nigeria*, *19*(4), 374–381. https://doi.org/10.4314/njm. v19i4.61959.

Finckh, A., Zufferey, P., Schurch, M. A., Balagué, F., Waldburger, M., & So, A. K. L. (2006). Short-term efficacy of intravenous pulse glucocorticoids in acute discogenic sciatica. A randomized controlled trial. *Spine*, *31*(4), 377–381. https://doi.org/ 10.1097/01.brs.0000199 917.04145.80.

Ghosh, N., Kolade, O. O., Shontz, E., Rosenthal, Y., Zuckerman, J. D., Bosco, J. A., & Virk, M. S. (2019). Nonsteroidal Anti-Inflammatory Drugs (NSAIDs) and Their Effect on Musculoskeletal Soft-Tissue Healing: A Scoping Review. *JBJS Reviews*, *7*(12). https://doi.org/ 10.2106/JBJS.RVW.19.00055.

Glazer, S., & Portenoy, R. K. (1991). Systemic local anesthetics in pain control. In *Journal of Pain and Symptom Management* (Vol. 6, Issue 1, pp. 30–39). *J Pain Symptom Manage*. https://doi.org/10.1016/ 0885-3924(91)90069-G.

Gottrup, H., Juhl, G., Kristensen, A. D., Lai, R., Chizh, B. A., Brown, J., Bach, F. W., & Jensen, T. S. (2004). Chronic oral gabapentin reduces elements of central sensitization in human experimental hyperalgesia. *Anesthesiology*, *101*(6), 1400–1408. https://doi.org/10.1097/0000 0542-200412000-00021.

Grond, S., Radbruch, L., Meuser, T., Sabatowski, R., Loick, G., & Lehmann, K. A. (1999). Assessment and treatment of neuropathic cancer pain following WHO guidelines. *Pain*, *79*(1), 15–20. https://doi.org/10.1016/S0304-3959(98)00138-9.

Iftinca, M., Defaye, M., & Altier, C. (2021). TRPV1-Targeted Drugs in Development for Human Pain Conditions. *Drugs*, *81*(1), 7–27. https://doi.org/10.1007/s40265-020-01429-2.

Kjaer, P., Kongsted, A., Hartvigsen, J., Isenberg-Jørgensen, A., Schiøttz-Christensen, B., Søborg, B., Krog, C., Møller, C. M., Halling, C. M. B., Lauridsen, H. H., Hansen, I. R., Nørregaard, J., Jørgensen, K. J., Hansen, L. V., Jakobsen, M., Jensen, M. B., Melbye, M., Duel, P., Christensen, S. W., & Povlsen, T. M. (2017). National clinical guidelines for non-surgical treatment of patients with recent onset neck pain or cervical radiculopathy. In *European Spine Journal* (Vol. 26, Issue 9, pp. 2242–2257). Springer Verlag. https://doi.org/10. 1007/s00586-017-5121-8.

Knotkova, H., & Pappagallo, M. (2007). Adjuvant Analgesics. In *Anesthesiology Clinics* (Vol. 25, Issue 4, pp. 775–786). Elsevier. https://doi.org/10.1016/j.anclin.2007.07.006.

Loveless, M. S., & Fry, A. L. (2016). Pharmacologic Therapies in Musculoskeletal Conditions. *Medical Clinics of North America*, *100*(4), 869–890. https://doi.org/10.1016/j.mcna.2016.03.015.

Lussier, D., Huskey, A. G., & Portenoy, R. K. (2004). Adjuvant Analgesics in Cancer Pain Management. *The Oncologist*, *9*(5), 571–591. https://doi.org/10.1634/theoncologist.9-5-571.

Magni, G. (1991). The Use of Antidepressants in the Treatment of Chronic Pain: A Review of the Current Evidence. In *Drugs* (Vol. 42, Issue 5, pp. 730–748). https://doi.org/10.2165/00003495-199142050-00002.

Max, M. B., Lynch, S. A., Muir, J., Shoaf, S. E., Smoller, B., & Dubner, R. (1992). Effects of Desipramine, Amitriptyline, and Fluoxetine on Pain in Diabetic Neuropathy. *New England Journal of Medicine*, *326*(19), 1250–1256. https://doi.org/10.1056/nejm199205073261904.

Moulin, D. E., Clark, A. J., Gilron, I., Ware, M. A., Watson, C. P. N., Sessle, B. J., Coderre, T., Morley-Forster, P. K., Stinson, J., Boulanger, A., Peng, P., Finley, G. A., Taenzer, P., Squire, P., Dion, D., Cholkan, A., Gilani, A., Gordon, A., Henry, J., … Velly, A. (2007). Pharmacological management of chronic neuropathic pain - Consensus statement and guidelines from the canadian pain society. *Pain Research and Management*, *12*(1), 13–21. https://doi.org/10. 1155/2007/730785.

*NICE | The National Institute for Health and Care Excellence*. (n.d.). NICE. Retrieved May 24, 2021, from https://www.nice.org.uk/.

*NSAIDs: Therapeutic use and variability of response in adults - UpToDate*. (n.d.). Retrieved May 24, 2021, from https://www. uptodate.com/contents/nsaids-therapeutic-use-and-variability-of-response-in-adults?csi=50adc123-bc87-4b20-9900-ff99c480246 0&source=contentShare.

Podichetty, V. K., Mazanec, D. J., & Biscup, R. S. (2003). Chronic non-malignant musculoskeletal pain in older adults: Clinical issues and opioid intervention. *Postgraduate Medical Journal*, *79*(937), 627–633. https://doi.org/10.1136/pmj.79.937.627.

Saba, R., Kaye, A. D., & Urman, R. D. (2017). Pharmacogenomics in Pain Management. *Anesthesiology Clinics*, *35*(2), 295–304. https:// doi.org/10.1016/j.anclin.2017.01.015.

Schwiebert, L. A., Beck, L. A., Stellato, C., Bickel, C. A., Bochner, B. S., & Schleimer, R. P. (1996). Glucocorticosteroid inhibition of cytokine production: Relevance to antiallergic actions. *Journal of Allergy and Clinical Immunology*, *97*(1 II), 143–152. https://doi.org/10.1016/ S0091-6749(96)80214-4.

See, S., & Ginzburg, R. (2008). Skeletal muscle relaxants. *Pharmacotherapy*, *28*(2), 207–213. https://doi.org/10.1592/phco.28. 2.207.

Shah, S., & Mehta, V. (2012). Controversies and advances in non-steroidal anti-inflammatory drug (NSAID) analgesia in chronic pain management. *Postgraduate Medical Journal*, *88*(1036), 73–78. https://doi.org/10.1136/postgradmedj-2011-130291.

Shaheed, C. A., Maher, C. G., Williams, K. A., Day R., McLachlan A. J. (2016, July 1). Efficacy, tolerability, and dose-dependent effects of opioid analgesics for low back pain a systematic review and meta-analysis. *JAMA Internal Medicine; American Medical Association.* https://doi.org/10.1001/jamainternmed.2016.1251.

Stahl, S. M., Grady, M. M., Moret, C., & Briley, M. (2005). SNRIs: The pharmacology, clinical efficacy, and tolerability in comparison with other classes of antidepressants. *CNS Spectrums*, *10*(9), 732–747. https://doi.org/10.1017/S1092852900019726.

Stanos, S. P. (2007). Topical Agents for the Management of Musculoskeletal Pain. *Journal of Pain and Symptom Management*, *33*(3), 342–355. https://doi.org/10.1016/j.jpainsymman.2006.11.005.

Sullivan, W. J., Panagos, A., Foye, P. M., Sable, A. W., Irwin, R. W., & Zuhosky, J. P. (2007). Industrial Medicine and Acute Musculoskeletal Rehabilitation. 2. Medications for the Treatment of Acute Musculoskeletal Pain. *Archives of Physical Medicine and Rehabilitation*, *88*(3 SUPPL.1). https://doi.org/10.1016/j.apmr.2006.12.009.

Toth, P. E., & Urtis, J. (2004). Commonly used muscle relaxant therapies for acute low back pain: A review of carisoprodol, cyclobenzaprine hydrochloride, and metaxalone. *Clinical Therapeutics*, *26*(9), 1355–1367. https://doi.org/10.1016/j.clinthera.2004.09.008.

Trescot, A. M., Datta, S., Lee, M., & Hans, H. (2008). Opioid pharmacology. In *Pain Physician* (Vol. 11, Issue SPEC. ISS. 2, pp. S133-53). https://doi.org/10.36076/ppj.2008/11/s133.

In: Musculoskeletal Pain (Common Clinical Presentations) ISBN: 978-1-68507-410-4
Editors: Mehmet Cenk Turgut and Serdar Toy 

*Chapter 27*

# PAIN MANAGEMENT AFTER SPORTS INJURIES

***Ali Erkan Yenigül*, MD***
Department of Orthopedics and Traumatology,
Bursa Uludağ University, Bursa, Turkey

## ABSTRACT

Sports injuries can be seen in millions of athletes every year, and therefore the pain caused by these injuries is treated. In these injuries, accurate and effective pain treatment is as important as correct diagnosis. As the athlete's return to sports can be shortened, activity losses due to pain are also prevented. There are many methods for pain management in sports injuries, from rest, medication and medical treatment to surgical interventions. Today, sports-related pain can be successfully treated with appropriate treatment methods.

## INTRODUCTION

Pain is defined in terms of "an unpleasant sensory and emotional experience associated with actual or potential tissue damage" by the International Society for Pain Studies (Merskey, 1994). For the detection of pain stimuli, action potentials must be formed after the activation of peripheral sensory organs (nociceptors) and their transmission to the central nervous system. Nociceptive afferents are widely distributed throughout the body (skin, muscle, joints, meninges) and contain both moderately slightly myelinated A-delta fibers and small-diameter, slow-conducting unmyelinated C fibers (Woolf, 2007). After sports injuries, depending on the severity of the trauma, the release

* Corresponding Author's E-mail: alierkanyenigul@uludag.edu.tr.

of cytokines, acute phase reactants, catecholamines, cortisol, growth hormone and adrenocorticotropic hormone increases. Anabolic hormone secretion such as insulin is reduced. Inadequate treatment of acute pain after injury increases morbidity (Anand, 1992).

Sports injuries are also problems that can be encountered in athletes of all ages and in all kinds of sports activities. After sports injuries, it is seen in chronic pain after prolonged activity as well as acute pain that concerns that time (Ready, 1992). Sports injuries are seen in 2.6 million young athletes annually. Acute injury to the epiphyseal region of the bone accounts for approximately 15% to 20% of all injuries to the long bones, most of which are caused by sports (Stanitski, 1994). Sports injuries can often cause pain in athletes. Generally, this pain is relieved with simple interventions or diaphoresis. However, some injuries can cause serious problems that may prevent short-term sports continuity and require medical or surgical intervention. In order to prevent sports-induced pain in the musculoskeletal system from turning into chronic pain, athletes should be treated correctly and effectively (Liu, 2019).

## Analgesic Agents

### Rice and Price

Conservative treatment is often the first choice in acute sports injuries (Iammarino, 2018). Conservative treatment can be summarized as RICE (rest, ice, compression, elevation) or PRICE (protection, rest, ice, compression, elevation). The response to pain by the body is proportional to the duration and size of the injury, which can have a significant impact on injury response (Liu, 2008). Early immobilization after injury reduces pain. While there are studies showing that ice application reduces pain, there are also studies showing that it does not contribute to immobilization (Koller, 2007). It has also been shown that early mobilization is effective in pain control in ankle injuries. Thanks to the cold applied to the injury area, the athlete can feel better psychologically and return to sports, and the cold reduces the blood flow to the injured area with vasoconstriction and reduces the pain and swelling. Cold application should be 15 minutes per hour and should not be directly in contact with the wound in cases of open wounds. Cooling sprays are used as local pain relievers in sports injuries. When applied to the skin, they affect a depth of approximately 3-4 mm and cause vasoconstriction in nearby vessels. The disadvantage is that their pain relief effects are temporary and they can cause cold injuries. Resting reduces the pain of the athlete in the early period and prevents additional injury due to overuse. In sports injuries, raising the extremity at an angle of approximately 45 degrees reduces bleeding and swelling. Therefore, there is a decrease in the patient's pain.

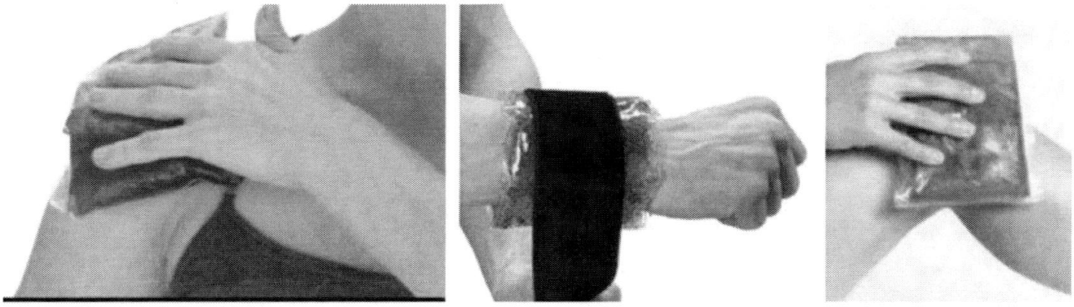

Figure 1. Examples of Cold Application.

## Thermotherapy

In sports injuries, the blood flow required for wound healing is increased with the heat applied after the early period (48 hours). In many cases, the elasticity and stretch of collagen fibers are increased by thermotherapy, which makes use of its pain-relieving properties (Petersen, 2000). When the tension in tendons, muscles and ligaments decreases, the pain is also reduced. Superficial heat treatment is supplied by whirlpools (hydromassage), hydrocollator packs, contrast baths (cool-heat), and synthetic materials that give a heat effect.

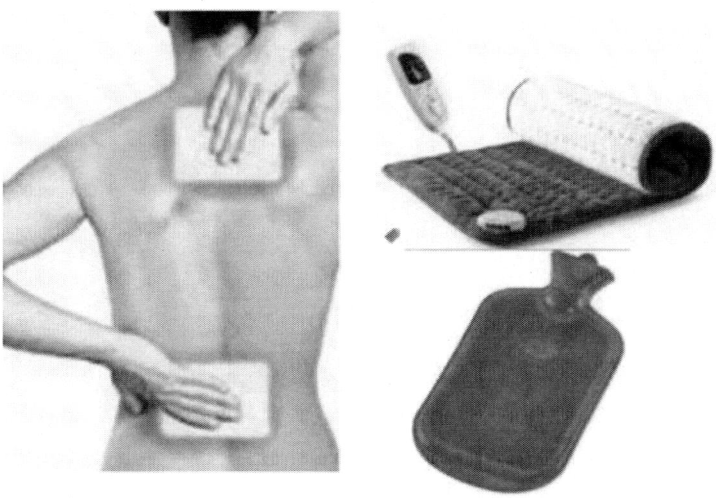

Figure 2. Examples of Thermotherapy.

## Electrical Stimulation

Pain is reduced by stimulating the sensory nerves subcutaneously with transcutaneous electrical nerve stimulation (TENS) (Petersen, 2000). The sensory pathway of pain is intervened with TENS, which is a weak electric current application method with electrons applied to the painful area. TENS is also used to strengthen the hypotrophy that may occur in the muscles after sports injury surgery.

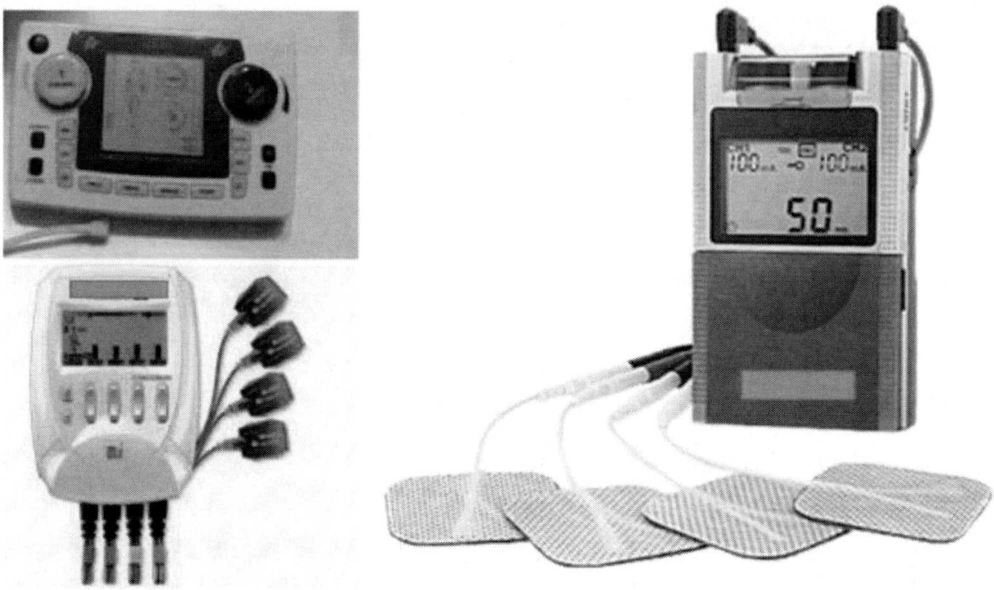

Figure 3. TENS application examples.

## PRP

Platelet-rich plasma (PRP) application in pain treatment; After whole blood coagulates, it is incubated with glass bubbles. After centrifugation, PRP is obtained by filtering. Thanks to the negative charges on the glass beads, thrombocytes are activated and growth factors are released. In addition, as IL-1 inhibitors increase, cartilage damage and pain are reduced (Wolters, 2011). PRP is used for musculoskeletal pain after sports, especially soft tissue damage due to continuous use. It is used to shorten the time to return to sports and to accelerate the healing process in degenerated tendons.

## Medication

There are many options available as medications for the treatment of acute or chronic sports injury pain. Treatment selection should be made considering the mechanism of action and side effects. Drug treatment should be determined after evaluating the athlete's age and comorbidities, the severity of the injury and the possibility of returning to sports. The drugs that we can use as analgesics are summarized in Table 1.

**Table 1. Analgesic drugs**

| | | |
|---|---|---|
| **Opioids** | Alkaloids | Codeine, Morphine, Opium |
| | Semi-synthetic derivatives | Acetylhydrocodeine, Desomorphine, Diamorphine |
| | Synthetics | Fentanyl, Tramadol |
| **Anilids** | | Paracetamol, Phenacetin |
| **Non-steroidal anti-inflammatory drugs** | Propionic acid derivatives | Naproxen, Ketoprofen, Ibuprofen |
| | Oxicams | Meloxicam, Piroxicam |
| | Acetic acid | Diklofenak, Indometazin |
| | Cox-2 | Celecoxib, Rofecoxib |
| | Salicylate | Aspirin (Acetylsalicylic acid) |
| | Others | Nabumeton, Meklofenomat |
| **Atypical** | | Gabapentin, Trazodon |

Paracetamol (acetaminophen) is one of the first-choice drugs in sports injuries and the most widely used analgesic. It is especially preferred in those who find it inconvenient to take NSAIDS, those with bronchial asthma, those who are sensitive to salicylates, those with peptic ulcer disease, children under 12 years of age, and pregnant women. Serious side effects are seen in cases where it is not used properly or in high doses (> 4 g/day) (34).

NSAIDS are often used in sports injuries to take advantage of their pain relief and anti-inflammatory effects. Since they act by inhibiting Cox-1 and Cox-2, they can have positive or negative effects on most tissues and activities. Therefore, Cox-2 selective NSAIDs have fewer side effects. The most commonly used are diclofenac, naproxen, ibuprofen, celecoxib, and dexketoprofen. They have been shown in animal studies to cause problems in fracture healing as they inhibit prostaglandins, which play a role in bone healing (Beck et al., 2003, Altman et al., 1995). Some physicians criticize the use of ibuprofen for fear that it will adversely affect bone healing (Dodwell et al., 2010). Reuben and Ekman found that Cox-2 selective inhibitors did not affect the spinal fusion rate (Reuben, 2005). NSAIDS reduce pain in tendon strain and ligament strain and shorten the time to return to sports. Considering the side effects, the recommended use of NSAIDS is at the lowest effective dose and for a short time. There are fewer systemic side effects of topically applied NSAIDS. In their study, Galer et al., applied a diclofenac patch and placebo to the group with 222 minor sports injuries to investigate their effectiveness. As a result, there was no significant difference between the topical diclofenac patch and placebo in terms of safety and side effects. Therefore, we can safely use the topical diclofenac patch as pain relief in minor sports injuries (Galer et al., 2000). Topical capsaicin, transdermal opioid, topical lidocaine and topical NSAI drugs are used in the treatment of pain in sports-induced injuries, but there are no prospective studies investigating the efficacy of these drugs.

Opioids are drugs that have morphine-like effects that are used for analgesia in the body. They act by binding to opioid receptors in the central nervous system and peripheral nervous system. When used for pain relief, they have a very strong effect and are safe. Constipation, drowsiness, nausea and vomiting can be seen as side effects. Intranasal administration of ketamine has similar effects as an analgesic effect as intranasal phenytoin (Graudins et al., 2015).

## Invasive Agents

Epidural anesthesia, intravenous drug applications, nerve blocks and local anesthesia can be given as examples. Lower extremity nerve blocks are femoral nerve, adductor canal nerve block, sciatic nerve and epidural blocks. It has been shown that nerve blocks performed in anterior cruciate ligament surgeries significantly reduce pain and increase graft removal (Farid, 2010). Postoperative pain is reduced with the application of a local anesthesia pump placed under the fascia (Bulut et al., 2011). The peripheral nerve block catheter applied postoperatively reduces the number of days of hospitalization. In a study of patients with limb fractures, intravenous lidocaine was found to have a more effective analgesic effect than intravenous morphine (Forouzan et al., 2017). It is effective in reducing regional anesthesia and acute pain in acute extremity injuries. Nerve blocks (ulnar nerve, median nerve, radial nerve with low dose lidocaine) performed for regional anesthesia to reduce pain in emergency departments are effective and reduce the need for opioids. Compartment syndrome examination should be done carefully in high-energy sports injuries, and regional anesthesia should be applied after compartment syndrome is ruled out. Although some studies claim that regional anesthesia does not obscure the diagnosis of compartment syndrome, we should not let go of caution. Pain intensity is higher in displaced fractures than non-displaced fractures. Therefore, non-enteral pain relievers are needed in these patients. No statistically significant difference was found between steroid, clonidine, gabapentin and muscle relaxants in the treatment of acute pain.

## Pediatric Age Group

Injuries, especially in young athletes, cause physical and psychological problems for athletes and their families. When adult and adolescent athletes are compared, it is seen that anxiety and pain are higher in the adolescent group. In the use of analgesics in children, choices should be made so that side effects are minimal. The primary choice of non-opioid drugs and other conservative treatment methods is recommended for acute sports injury-related pain in young people (Liu, 2019). The most common causes of sports-related pain in children are sprains, contusions and fractures (Damore et al., 2003). Sports injuries requiring surgical intervention were found in 7.1% of the pediatric age group. Ibuprofen, naproxen, acetaminophen, codeine, oxycodone and morphine can be used as enteral pain relievers in children. It has been stated that the use of tramadol and codeine in children under the age of 12 can cause breathing difficulties and death. No significant difference was found between acetaminophen and naproxen in terms of pain relief in children with soft tissue injuries (Cukiernik, 2007). Ibuprofen has been shown to reduce musculoskeletal pain faster than acetaminophen and codeine (Clark, 2007). In the study conducted by May et al., the groups treated with ibuprofen and codeine, and ibuprofen and placebo were compared in terms of pain response and no statistically significant difference was found (May et al., 2013). In injuries involving fractures, patients experience a lot of pain during radiological examination. Patients should be comfortable for quality and appropriate radiological examination. This situation creates a problem especially in pediatric patients. Analgesic (oxycodone, codeine) can be given to provide relief during shooting. Wille et al., showed that sublingual midazolam or oral morphine did not significantly change pain scores (Wille et al., 2011). Saunders et al., showed in their study that intranasal administration of phenytoin was effective in acute fracture pain in children (Saunders, 2010). In addition, Borland et al., demonstrated that intranasal phenytoin is as effective as intravenous morphine (Borland et al., 2007). Mahar et al., demonstrated that oral transmucosal administration of phenytoin is superior in reducing pain compared to intravenous morphine (Mahar et al., 2007). Intra-articular bupivacaine reduces the need for postoperative opioids in distal humeral fractures (Georgoulos et al., 2012). After the operation, diazepam or dexamethasone can be used as analgesic drugs in children. Kay et al., showed in their study that the use of ibuprofen or ketorolac did not cause non-unions in children with fractures (Kay et al., 2010). WHO guidelines recommend non-opioid drugs such as acetaminophen and ibuprofen for mild pain in children. Again, low-dose morphine is recommended for moderate pain in children.

## Conclusion

As it can be understood from the data above, there are many methods in the management of sports-induced pain. This process should be managed by specialist doctors according to the athlete's injury type, duration and need to return to sports. As a result, improved pain management has not only increased the comfort of patients with sports injuries, but has also been shown to reduce morbidity and improve long-term outcomes. We must accurately analyze injuries and effectively treat pain at every stage of life and in all types of sports.

## REFERENCES

Altman, R. D., Latta, L. L., Keer, R., Renfree, K., Hornicek, F. J., & Banovac, K. (1995). Effect of nonsteroidal antiinflammatory drugs on fracture healing: a laboratory study in rats. *Journal of orthopaedic trauma*, 9(5), 392-400.

Anand, K. J. S., & Hickey, P. R. (1992). Halothane–morphine compared with high-dose sufentanil for anesthesia and postoperative analgesia in neonatal cardiac surgery. *New England Journal of Medicine*, 326(1), 1-9.

Borland M, Jacobs I, King B, et al. A randomized controlled trialcomparing intranasal fentanyl to intravenous morphine for managing acute pain in children in the emergency department. *Ann. Emerg. Med.* 2007;49:335–340.

Beck, A., Krischak, G., Sorg, T., Augat, P., Farker, K., Merkel, U., ... & Claes, L. (2003). Influence of diclofenac (group of nonsteroidal anti-inflammatory drugs) on fracture healing. *Archives of orthopaedic and trauma surgery*, 123(7), 327-332.

Bulut, T., Yilmazlar, A. H. M. E. T., Yavascaoglu, B., & Sarisozen, B. (2011). The effect of local anaesthetic on post-operative pain with wound instillation via a catheter for paediatric orthopaedic extremity surgery. *Journal of children's orthopaedics*, 5(3), 179-185.

Clark, E., Plint, A. C., Correll, R., Gaboury, I., & Passi, B. (2007). A randomized, controlled trial of acetaminophen, ibuprofen, and codeine for acute pain relief in children with musculoskeletal trauma. *Pediatrics*, 119(3), 460-467.

Cukiernik, V. A., Lim, R., Warren, D., Seabrook, J. A., Matsui, D., & Rieder, M. J. (2007). Naproxen versus acetaminophen for therapy of soft tissue injuries to the ankle in children. *Annals of Pharmacotherapy*, 41(9), 1368-1374.

Damore, D. T., Metzl, J. D., Ramundo, M., Pan, S., & Van Amerongen, R. (2003). Patterns in childhood sports injury. *Pediatric emergency care*, 19(2), 65-67.

Dodwell ER, Latorre JG, Parisini E, et al. NSAID exposure and risk of nonunion: a meta-analysis of case-control and cohort studies. *Calcif. Tissue Int.* 2010;87:193–202.

Farid, I. S., Heiner, E. J., & Fleissner, P. R. (2010). Comparison of femoral nerve block and fascia iliaca block for analgesia following reconstructive knee surgery in adolescents. *Journal of clinical anesthesia*, 22(4), 256-259.

Forouzan, A., Barzegari, H., Motamed, H., Khavanin, A., & Shiri, H. (2017). Intravenous lidocaine versus morphine sulfate in pain management for extremity fractures; a clinical trial. *Emergency*, 5(1).

Galer, B. S., Rowbotham, M., Perander, J., Devers, A., & Friedman, E. (2000). Topical diclofenac patch relieves minor sports injury pain: results of a multicenter controlled clinical trial. *Journal of pain and symptom management*, 19(4), 287-294.

Georgopoulos, G., Carry, P., Pan, Z., Chang, F., Heare, T., Rhodes, J., ... & Erickson, M. (2012). The efficacy of intra-articular injections for pain control following the closed reduction and percutaneous pinning of pediatric supracondylar humeral fractures: a randomized controlled trial. *The Journal of bone and joint surgery. American volume*, 94(18), 1633.

Graudins, A., Meek, R., Egerton-Warburton, D., Oakley, E., & Seith, R. (2015). The PICHFORK (Pain in Children Fentanyl or Ketamine) trial: a randomized controlled trial comparing intranasal ketamine and fentanyl for the relief of moderate to severe pain in children with limb injuries. *Annals of emergency medicine*, 65(3), 248-254.

Iammarino, K., Marrie, J., Selhorst, M., & Lowes, L. P. (2018). Efficacy of the stretch band Ankle traction technique in the treatment of pediatric patients with acute ankle sprains: a randomized control trial. *International journal of sports physical therapy*, 13(1), 1.

Jóźwiak-Bebenista, M., & Nowak, J. Z. (2014). Paracetamol: mechanism of action, applications and safety concern. *Acta poloniae pharmaceutica*, 71(1), 11-23.

Kay, R. M., Directo, M. P., Leathers, M., Myung, K., & Skaggs, D. L. (2010). Complications of ketorolac use in children undergoing operative fracture care. *Journal of Pediatric Orthopaedics*, 30(7), 655-658.

Kehlet, H., & Dahl, J. B. (2003). Anaesthesia, surgery, and challenges in postoperative recovery. *The Lancet*, 362(9399), 1921-1928.

Koller, D. M., Myers, A. B., Lorenz, D., & Godambe, S. A. (2007). Effectiveness of oxycodone, ibuprofen, or the combination in the initial management of orthopedic injury-related pain in children. *Pediatric emergency care*, 23(9), 627-633.

Le May, S., Gouin, S., Fortin, C., Messier, A., Robert, M. A., & Julien, M. (2013). Efficacy of an ibuprofen/codeine combination for pain management in children presenting to the emergency department with a limb injury: a pilot study. *The Journal of emergency medicine*, 44(2), 536-542.

Liu S S & Wu C L (2008) Neural blockade: impact on outcome. In: *Neural Blockade in Clinical Anesthesia and Pain Medicine 4th edn*. Cousins M J, Bridenbaugh PO, Carr D and Horlocker T (eds). Philadelphia.

Liu, D. V., & Lin, Y. C. (2019). Current evidence for acute pain management of musculoskeletal injuries and postoperative pain in pediatric and adolescent athletes. *Clinical Journal of Sport Medicine*, 29(5), 430-438.

Mahar, P. J., Rana, J. A., Kennedy, C. S., & Christopher, N. C. (2007). A randomized clinical trial of oral transmucosal fentanyl citrate versus intravenous morphine sulfate for initial control of pain in children with extremity injuries. *Pediatric emergency care*, 23(8), 544-548.

Merskey H & Bogduk N (1994) *Classification of Chronic Pain, IASP Task Force on Taxonomy*. Seattle, IASP Press.

Peterson L., Renstrom P. - Sports injuries. *Their prevention and treatment-Informa Healthcare* (2000).

Ready L B & Edwards W T (1992) Management of Acute Pain: a Practical Guide. *Taskforce on Acute Pain*. Seattle, IASP Publications.

Reuben, S. S., & Ekman, E. F. (2005). The effect of cyclooxygenase-2 inhibition on analgesia and spinal fusion. *JBJS*, 87(3), 536-542.

Saunders, M., Adelgais, K., & Nelson, D. (2010). Use of intranasal fentanyl for the relief of pediatric orthopedic trauma pain. *Academic emergency medicine*, 17(11), 1155-1161.

Stanitski, C. L., DeLee, J. C., & Drez Jr, D. (1994). Meniscal lesions. *Pediatric and Adolescent Sports Medicine*. Philadelphia, WB Saunders, 371-386.

The National Federation of State High School Associations. *2017–18 High School Athletics Participation Survey*. Available at: http://www.nfhs.org/Participation Statistics/PDF/2017-18%20High%20School%20
Athletics%20Participation%20Survey.pdf. Accessed January 28, 2018.

Wolters Kluwer, Lippincott, Williams & Wilkins.Hraha, T. H., Doremus, K. M., McIlwraith, C. W., & Frisbie, D. D. (2011). Autologous conditioned serum: the comparative cytokine profiles of two commercial methods (IRAP and IRAP II) using equine blood. *Equine veterinary journal*, 43(5), 516-521.

Woolf CJ & Ma Q (2007) Nociceptors–noxious stimulus detectors. *Neuron* 55(3): 353–64.

Wille-Ledon, C., Chappuy, H., Giraud, C., Tréluyer, J. M., & Chéron, G. (2011). Comparison of a morphine and midazolam combination with morphine alone for paediatric displaced fractures: a randomized study. *Acta Paediatrica,* 100(11), e203-e207.

In: Musculoskeletal Pain (Common Clinical Presentations) ISBN: 978-1-68507-410-4
Editors: Mehmet Cenk Turgut and Serdar Toy 

*Chapter 28*

# POSTOPERATIVE ANALGESIA IN ORTHOPEDIC SURGERY

***Mesut Öterkuş*[*], MD***
Department of Anesthesiology and Reanimation,
Malatya Turgut Özal University, Malatya, Turkey

## ABSTRACT

Postoperative analgesia is an important part of the healing process. Adequate analgesia allows early mobilization, reducing complications such as thromboembolism and allowing patients to start their daily lives. Many pharmacological and non-pharmacological (peripheral nerve blocks and neuraxial blocks) methods are used to provide postoperative analgesia.

In this chapter, we aim to discuss the postoperative analgesia methods in general terms.

## INTRODUCTION

Pain is defined by the International Association for the Study of Pain as "an unpleasant special sensation originating from any part of the body, including all the past experiences of a person with or without an organic cause" (International Pain Research Association 2016). Pain is part of the body's defense mechanisms. Tissue damage due to internal causes (perforations, septic arthritis, otitis, myocardial infarction, etc.) and external factors (trauma, burn, etc.) triggers pain. This pain is one of the main reasons

[*] Corresponding Author's E-mail: mesut.oterkus@ozal.edu.tr.

why patients apply to a healthcare facility. The response to pain (pain threshold) varies. Factors such as psychological status, education, sex, religious beliefs, etc., determine the pain threshold.

Determining the type of pain plays an important role in treatment planning. Postoperative pain is usually acute pain that develops due to tissue and/or nerve damage at the surgical site. This pain in the postoperative period can cause many complications and prolong the treatment process. Emotional stress caused by pain activates the sympathetic system and causes many symptoms or complications such as tachycardia, hypertension, muscle spasms, thrombosis due to immobility, cardiac ischemia, atelectasis, infection, and decreased bowel movements. It is an important part of respiratory therapy to maintain and/or increase the functional capacity of the lungs in patients undergoing major surgery such as thoracic surgery (Üçel 2009).

## Postoperative Pain

This develops due to tissue and/or nerve damage during surgery. Although it is usually acute, it can become chronic, like phantom pain that may develop as a result of amputation. Pain that develops after orthopedic surgery is usually acute somatic pain. Although pharmacological treatment is the priority in postoperative pain management, non-pharmacological methods such as epidural catheters and nerve blocks can be added to the treatment protocol. Nowadays, regional anesthesia is used as a method of anesthesia in a significant number of orthopedic surgeries. Depending on the duration of action of drugs, less analgesia is needed in the first hours postoperatively in patients undergoing regional anesthesia (Erdem 2011).

## Pharmacological Treatment

Pharmacological treatment is the first applied method of postoperative analgesia. The main aim is to provide the best analgesia with the lowest effective dose of the agent(s) and the least side effects. Analgesics can be used as a single agent, or by using more than one analgesic agent, the amount of the required dose and the incidence of side effects can be reduced. It is necessary to comply with the basic principles in the use of analgesia. These principles are as follows:

1. Stepped therapy: the treatment is determined, starting from weaker analgesics (non-opioids) to the most potent analgesics.

2. Determining the analgesic according to the nature of the pain. For example, if the pain is of inflammatory origin, non-steroidal agents should be preferred.
3. Analgesic drugs should primarily be given orally.
4. They should be given before the onset of pain and at regular time intervals.
5. The dose of analgesia should be determined individually for each patient.

It is possible to examine the analgesics used in two parts as opioids and non-opioid analgesics.

## Opioids

These are powerful analgesic agents. Morphine and codeine, which are natural opioids, were obtained for the first time from a plant of the Papaver somniferum genus from the Papaveraceae family (Kılıç 2017). After morphine and codeine, semi-synthetic opioids such as heroin and synthetic derivatives with stronger effects such as meperidine, fentanyl, alfentanil, and remifentanil were obtained. They reduce the perception of pain by inhibiting the release of neurotransmitters in the nervous system (Çevik 2011). Three main receptors were identified: μ (mu), κ (kappa), and δ (delta). Generally, μ (mu) receptors are responsible for the analgesic effect and the addiction effect. All opioids have a more or less addictive potential. They are used orally, intravenously, intramuscularly, rectally, intrathecally, and transdermally. Opioids have dose-dependent side effects such as nausea-vomiting, emotional disorders, constipation, urinary retention, itching, hypotension, and respiratory depression (Kayhan et al. 2013). Another problem with opioid use is tolerance. The need for opioids increases gradually in patients using long-term opioids, such as cancer patients. In the perioperative and/or intraoperative use of short-acting opioids such as remifentanil, this tolerance may develop in a short time. In this condition, known as *acute opioid tolerance*, the patient develops hyperalgesia. Patients need additional analgesia earlier. Patients will benefit from additional analgesics to be administered close to the end of surgery.

## Non-Opioid Analgesics

Non-steroidal anti-inflammatory drugs, local anesthetics, adjuvant drugs, and paracetamol are in this group.

a. *Non-steroidal anti-inflammatory drugs (NSAIDs):* These are analgesic, antipyretic, and anti-inflammatory drugs that are widely used around the world. Basically, they inhibit the cyclooxygenase enzyme (COX-1 and COX-2), which provides the synthesis of prostaglandin from arachidonic acid. Their analgesic effects are achieved by inhibiting the synthesis of prostaglandins, which are hyperalgesic mediators. Furthermore, they provide central analgesic effects by inhibiting the synthesis of prostaglandins in the central nervous system, as they easily pass the blood-brain barrier due to their lipophilic structure (Dural 2002). These are drugs with a high potential for side effects. They have many side effects such as indigestion, dyspepsia, peptic ulcer, decrease in renal blood flow, decrease in glomerular filtration rate, prolongation of bleeding time (with thromboxane A2 inhibition) and triggering of asthma attacks. Nowadays, selective (meloxicam, nimesulide, etc.) or specific (celecoxib, rofecoxib) COX-2 inhibitor drugs have started to be used to reduce the incidence of side effects. They interact with many drugs. Some of these interactions are as follows:

- They increase the effect of anticoagulants (thromboxane A2 inhibition, platelet aggregation inhibition, etc.).
- Due to their high binding to plasma proteins, they increase the effect of antiabetics.
- They reduce the effect of diuretic drugs (prostaglandin inhibition).
- While they cause an increase in the plasma level of drugs such as phenytoin and digoxin, they cause a slowdown in lithium excretion.

Due to the incidence of side effects and drug interactions, care should be taken in their use, and long-term use should be avoided.

b. *Paracetamol:* This is an antipyretic and analgesic agent that has been widely used in the world for many years. Paracetamol, which is used in the oral form for mild and moderate pain, started to be used successfully in severe postoperative pain with the introduction of the intravenous form (Çelik et al. 2005). Although its mechanism of action is not fully understood, pathways such as the inhibition of cyclooxygenase (COX), the L-arginine/nitric oxide (NO) pathway, its effect on cannabinoid (CB)-vanilloid receptors and its effect on the descending inhibitory serotonergic pathway are thought to play a role in its analgesic effect (Karataş et al. 2013). The treatment dose is 10 - 15mg/kg every 6 hours and a maximum of 4g (titck.gov.tr. 2019). Although it is quite safe, there is a risk of developing acute liver injury, renal failure and encephalopathy at toxic doses (more than 250mg/kg for adults or 12g or more in 24 hours) (Emet and Yayla 2016). Activated charcoal (1g/kg max: 50g, first 2 - 3 hours) and N-acetyl cysteine (150mg/kg IV 15 minutes, 50 mg/kg for the first 4 hours and 100 mg/kg for the next 16 hours) are given in the treatment. However, in cases with acute liver failure, the treatment should be transplantation (Craig et al. 2010).

## Local Anesthetics

With the development of regional anesthesia techniques, the use of local anesthetics has become quite common. In a significant number of orthopedic surgeries, regional anesthesia techniques are used as a method of anesthesia and postoperative analgesia. Local anesthetics inhibit the passage of sodium, causing nerve membrane stabilization and temporarily and reversibly inhibiting nerve conduction. According to their structures, they are divided into two as the ester type (cocaine, tetracaine, etc.) and amide type (lidocaine, prilocaine, bupivacaine, etc.). According to their duration of action, they are divided into three groups: short-acting (cocaine, chloroprocaine, etc.), medium-acting (lidocaine, prilocaine, etc.) and long-acting (bupivacaine, tetracaine, levobupivacaine, etc.). Ester-type local anesthetics are metabolized by plasma pseudocholinesterases, while amide-type local anesthetics are metabolized in the liver. Factors such as lipophilicity of the agent, administration dose and concentration, solubility constant (pKa), tissue vascularity and protein binding rate are the factors responsible for the potency and toxic effect of local anesthetics (Karasu et al. 2016). Vasoconstrictor agents can be added to local anesthetics to prolong the duration of action and obtain better vision by reducing the blood build-up in surgical patients. However, it is contraindicated to apply to end organs such as fingertips and penis. Another problem with local anesthetics is toxicity. Complications such as ischemic necrosis, paresthesia (perioral and facial), tinnitus, tachycardia, bradycardia, hypertension, respiratory depression, allergic reactions (ester-type local anesthetics), seizures, severe cardiac toxicity (bupivacaine, lidocaine) and methemoglobinemia (prilocaine, tetracaine) can be observed (Cherobin and Tavares 2020). In treatment, first of all, airway safety should be ensured, circulatory support should be provided (epinephrine, norepinephrine, etc.), and benzodiazepines should be administered if seizures develop. It is an effective treatment for the neurological and cardiac toxicity of lipid emulsion (1.5mL/kg bolus 20% lipid emulsion and maintenance 0.25ml/kg/min per minute). If methemoglobinemia develops, 1 - 2mg/kg 1% methylene blue can be administered intravenously (Ok et al. 2018).

## Adjuvant Drugs

Nowadays, adjuvant agents are produced to increase the analgesic effectiveness in pain treatment and increase the incidence of side effects by reducing the effective dose. Most of these drugs are in the research phase or animal testing phase. Although agents such as anticonvulsants, conotoxins, $Na^+$ channel blockers, $Ca^{++}$ channel blockers (SNX-111, a synthetic analog of ω-conotoxin, ω-grammotoxin SIA, SNX-482, etc.), neurotensin receptor antagonists (Contulakin-G), etc., have been shown to provide analgesia with different mechanisms, most of them are in the animal testing phase (Kelle

2006). Although the analgesic efficacy of low-dose ketamine is known, it is not used for this purpose. However, its perioperative use reduces the dose of analgesic needed with a synergistic effect.

## NON-PHARMACOLOGICAL METHODS

Orthopedic surgeries are surgeries in which regional anesthesia techniques are frequently used. They reduce the need for analgesics in the early postoperative period. The early mobilization of patients thus shortens the recovery period and reduces the risk of thromboembolism. Peripheral nerve blocks and intrathecal applications can be considered in this group. If it is desired to provide a longer block and postoperative analgesia, a catheter is placed and an analgesic and/or anesthetic agent can be administered continuously or intermittently. Furthermore, this catheter allows patient-controlled analgesia. These are procedures that require more experience compared to pharmacological methods.

### Peripheral Nerve Block

This is the most commonly used anesthesia method in orthopedic interventions in the lower and upper extremities. It is aimed to provide adequate anesthesia and analgesia by administering a local anesthetic to the innervating motor and sensory nerve at the surgical site. It can be used as a stand-alone anesthesia method, or it can be used to provide analgesia after general anesthesia. Attention should be paid to overdose when performing a nerve blockade. The presence of symptoms such as nausea-vomiting, headache, paresthesia, and tinnitus in the mouth and face of the patient may be the first indication of overdose. In their meta-analysis, Guay et al. showed that peripheral nerve blocks provided better analgesia than systemic analgesic agents (Guay et al. 2017). With the introduction of ultrasonography into anesthesia practice, the blockade can be performed with lower doses and volumes. Furthermore, the use of ultrasonography enabled the *differential blockade* (sensory block without motor block) (Balaban 2018). Since there is no motor blockade in the differential blockade, it allows the intraoperative monitoring of finger and tendon movements in operations such as tendon incision and carpal tunnel. The duration of anesthesia and analgesia varies according to the agent used, its dose and concentration, and vascularization. Adjuvant agents such as opioids (morphine, fentanyl, tramadol) and dexmedetomidine can be added to prolong the block duration and have a more effective postoperative effect (Kılıç et al. 2014; Küçükay et al. 2006).

### *Upper Extremity Blocks*

The brachial plexus blockade, intravenous regional block (RIVA) and blockade of digital nerves are defined as upper extremity blocks. There are four approaches to brachial plexus blocks, including the interscalene block, infraclavicular block, supraclavicular block and axillary block. The interscalene block is preferred in shoulder and upper arm operations. However, it cannot be used in hand surgery because it does not block the C8 and T1 roots. Supraclavicular and infraclavicular blocks are preferred in arm and hand surgery. However, the risk of pneumothorax, intravascular injection, and hematoma is higher in the infraclavicular block. The axillary block can be used in elbow and hand surgery.

### *Lower Extremity Blocks*

A significant number of patients who undergo lower extremity surgery are geriatric patients. They are accompanied by many comorbidities such as coronary artery disease, heart failure, COPD, hypertension, and diabetes. There are many studies stating that peripheral nerve blocks are more reliable than neuraxial blocks in these patients (Öztürk et al. 2016; Özkalaycı et al. 2019). The femoral block, sciatic nerve block, popliteal block, adductor block (saphenous nerve block), and digital blocks are examined with this group. In general, the combined femoral and sciatic nerve blockade is performed for anesthesia and postoperative analgesia. Many studies compared the combined femoral-sciatic block with the adductor nerve block. The combined femoral-sciatic block provides better results in terms of postoperative analgesia, but the adductor block only creates the sensory block and allows early rehabilitation (Borys et al. 2019). The popliteal block can be used as a method of anesthesia and postoperative analgesia in below-knee surgery without a tourniquet.

## Neuraxial Blocks

Spinal, epidural, and caudal blocks are included in this group. The caudal block is a reliable method used for postoperative analgesia in lower extremity surgeries in pediatric cases (Wu 2020; Suresh et al. 2015).

A successful caudal block was shown to reduce the need for additional postoperative analgesia in major surgical procedures such as hip surgery in adolescent children (Suresh et al. 2015; Villalobos et al. 2019). Spinal and epidural anesthesia methods are applied separately or in combination. Although spinal anesthesia has an onset time, it makes it possible to provide a longer period of analgesic effect in epidural anesthesia applications. Spinal anesthesia application is not a suitable option for long-term anesthesia with a catheter because of risks such as respiratory depression, bradycardia and cardiac arrest due to rise in level. In the literature, only one patient had a successful use of long-term analgesics by the spinal route (McKenzie and Sherwood 2009). Local anesthetics, and opioids such as morphine and clonidine are used alone or in combination to prolong the duration of analgesia by the epidural route. Epidural anesthesia with the use of opioids causes less itching compared to peripheral blocks (Guay et al. 2017).

Although it demonstrates effective analgesia with an epidural catheter in the literature, the failure rate seems to be higher. The requirement of experience and dislocation of the catheter (insufficient fixation) are factors increasing the failure rate (Suksompong et al. 2020).

### Patient-Controlled Analgesia

Patient-controlled analgesia is a method that allows patients to determine their own analgesic needs. Infusion pumps are used, where dose limits and minimum administration time can be adjusted to avoid frequent use. These pumps allow patients to administer bolus doses when they need analgesics. It can be administered intravenously, through a catheter placed for peripheral nerve blockade, and epidurally.

Opioids (morphine, tramadol) and local anesthetics (used in epidural and peripheral nerve blockades) can be used alone or in combination as analgesics.

It reduces the amount of opioid used and provides effective analgesia compared to traditional methods (Atım et al. 2009). In many studies, patient satisfaction was found to be higher than in traditional methods (Alon et al. 2003).

## Conclusion

Appropriate and adequate postoperative analgesia is very important in the rehabilitation process, as it provides early mobilization, reduces possible complications, and provides psychological relief to the patient due to the reduction or complete disappearance of the pain sensation, as well as being a part of the surgery.

## References

Alon, E., Jaquenod, M., Schaeppi, B. Post-operative epidural versus intravenous patient-controlled analgesia. *Minerva Anestesiol.,* 2003 May; 69(5):443 - 6. PMID: 12768181.

Atım, A., Deniz, S., Orhan, M. E. Ali Sızlan, A., Kurt, E. A clinic's experiences in postoperative patient controlled analgesia. *Pain,* 2009; 21(4):155 - 160.

Balaban, O. Ultrasound-Guided Differential Upper Extremity Block Experience: Retrospective Observational Research. *Sakarya Medical Journal,* 2018; 8 (3): 650 - 656.

Borys, M., Domagała, M., Wencław, K., Jarczyńska-Domagała, J., Czuczwar, M. Continuous femoral nerve block is more effective than continuous adductor canal block for treating pain after total knee arthroplasty: A randomized, double-blind, controlled trial. *Medicine,* (Baltimore). 2019; 98(39): e17358. doi:10.1097/ MD.0000000000017358.

Cherobin, A. C. F. P., Tavares, G. T. Safety of local anesthetics. *An. Bras. Dermatol.,* 2020; 95(1):82 - 90. doi:10.1016/j.abd.2019.09.025.

Çelik, M., Saricaoglu, F., Canbay, O., Dal, D., Uzumcigil, A., Leblebicioglu, G., Aypar, U. 2005. The analgesic effect of paracetamol when added to lidocaine for intravenous regional anesthesia. *Akush. Ginekol.*, (Sofiia). 2005; 44: 50 - 54.

Çevik, Ş. E., Yeşil, O., Öztürk, T. C., Güneysel, Ö. Opioid use in the treatment of acute pain in Emergency Room. *Sakaryamj,* 2011(2):39 - 4.

Craig, D. G., Lee, A., Hayes, P. C., Simpson, K. J. Review article: the current management of acute liver failure. *Aliment Pharmacol. Ther.,* 2010; 31 (3):345 - 58.

Dural, E. A. O. *Pharmacology.* 3rd Edition. 2002. Nobel Medical Bookstores. s: 264 - 305.

Emet, M., Yayla, M. Acetaminophen (paracetamol) intoxication. *Turkey Clinics J. Emerg. Med.-Special Topics,* 2016; 2 (1):51 - 57.

Erdem, D., Ugiş, C. M., Albayrak, D., Akan, B., Aksoy, E., Göğüş, E. The effect of anesthesia methods used in patients undergoing perianal surgery on preoperative and postoperative anxiety and pain levels. *Bakırköy Medical Journal,* 2011; 7: 11 - 16.

Guay, J., Johnson, R. L., Kopp, S. Nerve blocks or no nerve blocks for pain control after elective hip replacement (arthroplasty) surgery in adults. *Cochrane Database Syst. Rev.*, 2017; 10(10):CD011608. doi:10.1002/14651858.CD011608.pub2.

https://titck.gov.tr/storage/Archive/2019/dynamicModulesAttachment/Parasetamol sendika%20dernek%20duyurusu_24042019.pdf_1aaed18f-63d2-443d-9021-54dc27749dc6.pdf.

International Pain Research Association website. http://www.iasp-pain.org/Taxonomy Date of access: 06.09.2016.

Karakuş, O., İlkaya, F., Yılmaz, M. Paracetamol and cyclooxygenase enzyme inhibition. *Journal of Experimental and Clinical Medicine,* 2013; 30 (1s): 9 - 14.

Karasu, D., Yılmaz, C., Özgünay, Ş. E., Dayıoğlu, M., Baytar, Ç., Korfalı, G. Knowledge of the Research Assistants Regarding Local Anaesthetics and Toxicity. *Turk J. Anaesthesiol. Reanim.,* 2016; 44: 201 - 205.

Kayhan, G. E., Gülha, Ç. N., Aslan, A., Durmu, Ç. M. Management of treatment and complications in cancer patients applied to our algology outpatient clinic: A retrospective evaluation. *J. Turgut Ozal Med. Cent.,* 2013; 20(1):50 – 54. DOI: 10.7247/jtomc.20.1.11.

Kelle, İ. Alternative Medicines in Pain Management. *Dicle Medical Journal,* 2006; 33(3):192 - 200.

Kılıç, F. Opipdis, Pain, Abuse and Misuse of Opioids. *Osmangazi Medical Journal,* 2017; 39(3):125 - 129.

Kılınç, E., Özbek, H. T., Güzeldağ, S., İnigel, M. T., İnigel, Ş. Effects of Dexamethasone Added to Levobupivacaine during USG-Guided Infraclavicular Brachial Plexus Block. *Turkiye Klinikleri J. Med. Sci.,* 2014; 34(3):307 - 12.

Küçükay, S., Çeliker, T., Aşık, M., Salioğlu, F. Comparison of the effects of perineural and systemic morphine applications on postoperative analgesia after axillary block. *Acta Orthopaedica et Traumatologica Turcica,* 2006; 30 (4): 352 - 354.

McKenzie, A., Sherwood, M. Continuous spinal analgesia after extensive lumbar spine surgery. *Anaesth. Intensive Care,* 2009; 37:473 - 476.

Ok, S. H., Hong, J. M., Lee, S. H., Sohn, J. T. Lipid Emulsion for Treating Local Anesthetic Systemic Toxicity. *Int. J. Med. Sci.,* 2018; 15(7):713 - 722. doi:10.7150/ijms.22643.

Özkalaycı, Ö., Seçil Çetin, S., Muhammet Ahmet Karakaya, Aytekin Ünlükaplan, Agah Rauf İşgüzar, Yavuz Gürkan. Ultrasound guided popliteal and saphenous nerve blocks for diabetic foot surgery in a morbidly obese patient. *JARSS,* 2019; 27(3): 232 - 234.

Öztürk, T., Çevikkalp, E., Nizamoglu, F., Özbakkaloğlu, A., Topcu, İ. The Efficacy of Femoral Block and Unilateral Spinal Anaesthesia on Analgesia, Haemodynamics and Mobilization in Patients undergoing Endovenous Ablation in the Lower Extremity. *Turk J. Anaesth. Reanim.,* 2016; 44: 91 – 5. DOI: 10.5152/TJAR.2015.66933.

Suksompong, S., von Bormann, S., von Bormann, B. Regional Catheters for Postoperative Pain Control: Review and Observational Data. *Anesth. Pain Med.,* 2020; 10(1):e99745. Published 2020, Feb. 19. doi:10.5812/aapm.99745.

Suresh, S., Long, J., Birmingham, P. K. Are caudal blocks for pain control safe in children? An analysis of 18,650 caudal blocks from the Pediatric Regional Anesthesia Network (PRAN) database. *Anesth. Analg.,* 2015; 120(1):151 - 156.

Üçel, A. Postoperative Analgesia. *J. Exp. Clin. Med.,* 2009; 10(3 - 4): 127 - 132.

Villalobos, M. A., Veneziano, G., Miller, R. et al. Evaluation of postoperative analgesia in pediatric patients after hip surgery: Lumbar plexus versus caudal epidural analgesia. *J. Pain Res.,* 2019; 12:997 - 1001. Published 2019, Mar. 18. doi:10.2147/JPR.S191945.

Wu, J. P. Pediatric Anesthesia Concerns and Management for Orthopedic Procedures. *Pediatr. Clin. North Am.,* 2020; 67 (1): 71 - 84. doi: 10.1016/j.pcl.2019.09.006.

In: Musculoskeletal Pain (Common Clinical Presentations) ISBN: 978-1-68507-410-4
Editors: Mehmet Cenk Turgut and Serdar Toy 

*Chapter 29*

# IMAGING METHODS IN MUSCULOSKELETAL SYSTEM PAIN

***Mehmet Akçiçek**, MD***
Department of Radiology, Malatya Turgut Özal University Medicine Faculty, Malatya, Turkey

## ABSTRACT

Musculoskeletal system pain frequency increases with the aging population. Taking a detailed history and physical examination are the most important things for a correct diagnosis. Imaging should be considered as a tool to confirm the diagnosis. A number of imaging modalities are used to evaluate musculoskeletal system diseases.

Despite the emergence of new imaging techniques for the assessment of musculoskeletal system pain, conventional radiology remains the cornerstone of diagnostic imaging. Radiography is the most advantageous and cheapest method in evaluating bone abnormalities such as fractures, dislocations, and osteoarthritis. Computed tomography can provide high-resolution, two- and three-dimensional images. Nuclear medicine applications are used in investigating stress fractures, occult fractures, bone tumors, or infections. Magnetic resonance imaging is used to evaluate soft tissue disorders, including ligaments, tendons, cartilage tissue, and masses. Ultrasonography is effective in evaluating effusions, cysts, ligaments, muscles, and tendons. Vascularization can also be identified with the use of Doppler. There is also the possibility to perform aspirations and injections under ultrasonography guidance.

It is important to choose the most appropriate imaging method to accelerate the diagnosis and treatment. The imaging method to be preferred also changes depending on the structure of each joint and region investigated and the characteristics of the diseases considered in the differential diagnosis.

* Corresponding Author's E-mail: mehmet.akcicek@ozal.edu.tr.

# INTRODUCTION

Musculoskeletal system (MSK) pain is a common reason among patients for consulting physicians (Aagesen & Melek, 2013), and its frequency increases in the aging population (Tang & Aggarwal, 2013). Taking a detailed history and physical examination is essential for a correct diagnosis. Imaging should be considered as an instrument for confirming or ruling out a diagnosis considered in the differential diagnosis. It is crucial to select the most suitable imaging test for the purpose of accelerating the patient's diagnosis and treatment and limiting the health cost (Aagesen & Melek, 2013; Tang & Aggarwal, 2013). A number of imaging modalities are utilized for the evaluation of MSK diseases, including radiography, ultrasonography (USG), computed tomography (CT), and magnetic resonance imaging (MRI) (Tang & Aggarwal, 2013) (Table 1).

Despite the emergence of new imaging techniques to assess regional MSK pain, conventional radiology remains the cornerstone of diagnostic imaging (Grassi et al., 2003). Radiography is the most advantageous and cheapest method in evaluating bone abnormalities, including dislocations, fractures, and osteoarthritis. However, it is difficult to evaluate stress fractures, complex fractures, and soft tissue structures on radiography (Seidenberg & Howe, 2014). CT, which uses much higher doses of radiation but can provide high-resolution, two- and three-dimensional images (Buckwalter et al., 2001), is beneficial in their evaluation (Seidenberg & Howe, 2014).

Bone scintigraphy represents a nuclear medicine application utilized to investigate occult fractures, stress fractures, infections, or bone tumors (Wheeless, 2013). In fluorine-18 2-deoxy-D-glucose (FDG) positron emission tomography (PET), it is very important to know that occult fractures have a significant metabolic uptake that can cause false positivity for metastatic disease (Ravenel et al., 2004). Integrated hybrid single-photon emission computed tomography (SPECT) is an application that combines the detection of abnormal bone metabolism with scrupulous anatomical details at high resolution (Jarraya et al., 2013).

MRI is used with the aim of evaluating soft tissue disorders, including tendons, ligaments, cartilage tissue, and masses (Kumar & Hayashi, 2016; Levin et al., 2012). Moreover, it is efficient in the further characterization of occult and subtle fractures (Hakkarinen et al., 2012).

USG is effective in evaluating effusions, cysts, ligaments, muscles, and tendons (Yim & Corrado, 2012). Vascularization can also be identified with the use of Doppler. Although it depends on the sonographer, there is also the possibility to perform aspirations and injections under USG guidance (Seidenberg & Howe, 2014).

**Table 1. Basic imaging methods preferred in some indications**

| Indication | Imaging Method |
|---|---|
| Fracture, Dislocation, Osteoarthritis | Radiography |
| Stress fractures, Complex fractures, Soft tissue calcification, Bone tumors | CT |
| Effusion, Cyst, Soft tissue disorders, Aspiration and injection | USG |
| Soft tissue disorders, Occult and subtle fractures, Bone tumors, Infections | MRI |
| Stress fractures, Occult and subtle fractures, Bone tumors, Infections | NUCLEAR MEDICINE |

Although these stated methods and more can be used by clinicians, it should not be forgotten that MSK imaging cannot substitute for a detailed history and physical examination but is a method used to confirm the suspected diagnosis.

## SHOULDER

The shoulder joint's complex anatomy makes selecting diagnostic imaging tests difficult (Aagesen & Melek, 2013). Anterior-posterior (AP) radiographs in external and internal rotation and lateral radiographs are imaging methods that are used most commonly to evaluate the shoulder joint (Kumar & Hayashi, 2016).

According to the type of trauma and the pain location in traumas, special radiography may be required for a comprehensive evaluation (Aagesen & Melek, 2013). For example, AP, AP radiograph with internal rotation, axillary, West Point axillary, and scapular Y radiographs may be useful in the preliminary diagnosis of glenohumeral joint dislocation (Seidenberg & Howe, 2014; Manaster et al., 2008). However, routine radiographs rarely identify clinically significant abnormalities, except in the case of trauma or in the absence of a deformity (Fraenkel et al., 2000).

CT is mainly used to evaluate complex fractures and demonstrates the association of fracture fragments more clearly (Akhtar & Robinson, 2010). Furthermore, CT can evaluate bone tumors and soft tissue calcifications (Aagesen & Melek, 2013). A CT arthrogram constitutes a good option to assess labral damage in people in whom MRI cannot be performed (Manaster et al., 2008).

Both MRI and USG are the most appropriate and complementary imaging modalities to evaluate shoulder pain (Levine et al., 2012). Ultrasound represents a dynamic investigation that is capable of showing subluxation of the biceps tendon, or subacromial impingement (Aagesen & Melek, 2013). Moreover, USG has advantages in detecting foreign bodies, when a dynamic maneuver is required, and in guiding interventional procedures (Levine et al., 2012). There is an indication for MRI in the case of an abnormality in the articular cartilage, labrum, deep soft tissues, or bone marrow (Levine et al., 2012). MRI is utilized to detect bone contusions, occult fractures that cannot be detected using other methods, and tendon, ligament, and labral tears (Kumar & Hayashi, 2016). A better identification of labral injury is provided with an MR arthrogram (MRA) and MRI (Teefey et al., 2004).

An axillary nerve injury constitutes a known complication of glenohumeral dislocation (Avis & Power, 2018). The nerve may also be compressed by ganglion cysts, paralabral cysts, or tumors (Cothran & Helms, 2005). Paralabral cysts typically occur adjacent to a torn glenoid labrum. MRI shows them as well-circumscribed, uni-multilocular, non-contrast-enhancing, fluid-filled masses (O'Connor et al., 2004). It is possible to easily visualize hyperintense ganglion cysts on coronal, sagittal, and axial T2W images (Murray & Shaffer, 2009).

There is a possibility for confusing brachial neuritis clinically with rotator cuff or labral pathologies. In MRI, it is possible to observe a significant signal increase in the muscles that are innervated by the relevant nerves on T2W images and atrophy and fatty infiltration showing an increased signal in the relevant muscles on T1W images in subjects with a long-term follow-up (Gaskin & Helms, 2006).

In adhesive capsulitis, while MRI shows effusion in the glenohumeral joint during the early inflammatory period (Murray & Shaffer, 2009), MRI and MRA results in the later phases involve an increase in the capsule thickness in the axillary recess, obliteration of the fat triangle between the coracohumeral ligament and the coracoid process, and a decrease in the axillary recess volume (Mengiardi et al., 2004; Lefevre-Colau et al., 2005).

A lipoma, which is an occasional cause of application due to pain, is the most common soft tissue tumor in adulthood. They are non-contrast homogeneous masses that usually have the same signal on MRI (O'Connor et al., 2004). Soft tissue sarcomas usually exhibit low signal intensity on T1W images and high signal intensity on T2W images and are heavily contrasted following the administration of IV gadolinium. Malignant fibrous histiocytoma and liposarcoma represent the most frequently observed malignant soft tissue tumors of the shoulder (O'Connor et al., 2004).

## ELBOW

AP and lateral radiographs are the most frequently preferred imaging modalities to evaluate the elbow joint (Kumar & Hayashi, 2016). In acute traumas, the fracture may not be obvious at first. However, it can be detected by evaluating clues about its presence (Goswami, 2002). If there is a joint effusion that is confined by the synovial capsule, there are elevated extra synovial fat pads, resulting in signs of a visible posterior fat pad and an elevation of the anterior fat pad (Fowler & Chung, 2004). In patients with acute or chronic pain who are skeletally immature, radiographs of the contralateral elbow must also be taken for an epiphyseal injury that may be disregarded (Seidenberg & Howe,

2014). CT is used to evaluate complex fractures and assess them with three-dimensional images, as in other joints (Kumar & Hayashi, 2016).

The MRI assessment of the elbow should also involve the careful investigation of the medial, lateral, anterior and posterior major group muscles and tendons (Sampath et al., 2013). Repetitive valgus stress that involves the medial muscle group may cause tendinopathy, a partial tear, or a complete tear of the common flexor tendon. MRI presents this as alterations in the tendon diameter, an increase in signal on fat-suppressed T2W images of the tendon or adjacent medial epicondyle (Kijowski et al., 2005; Sampath et al., 2013). Likewise, repetitive varus stress that involves the proximal tendon of the lateral muscle group originating from the lateral epicondyle of the humerus may cause tendinopathy or tear (lateral epicondylitis) (Kijowski et al., 2005; Kotnis et al., 2012). The distal biceps tendon rupture is rare. The lack of a low-signal tendon at the radial insertion site or varying degrees of retraction of the tendon's proximal part indicate this (Sampath et al., 2013). An injury of the triceps tendon, which is the major tendon of the posterior muscle group, occurs rarely and, like the biceps tendon, both partial and complete tears may be observed. On MRI, tendon damage may occur as an alteration in the bone marrow signal at the insertion site instead of the tendon itself on fat-suppressed T2W images (Sampath et al., 2013).

In ulnar (cubital tunnel syndrome) and radial nerve pathologies, findings such as an increased diameter in the affected nerve and a high T2 signal on MRI can be detected (Bäumer et al., 2011).

In the case of synovitis, which may emerge due to inflammatory or post-traumatic conditions, MRI is not specific, and hyperintense effusion in the joint, synovial hypertrophy and a marked contrast enhancement after intravenous contrast can usually be detected on T2W images (Jbara et al., 2006). Bone erosions and hyperintense pannus on T2W images can be observed in people with rheumatoid arthritis. The joint fluid in an uncomplicated effusion is usually hypointense on T1W images but can become isointense or complex in the case of a superinfection (Jbara et al., 2006).

Several bursae may occur around the elbow, involving the olecranon and cubital bursae. The cubital bursae involve the bicipitoradial bursa and the interosseous bursa (Fowler & Chung, 2006). It may include infection with an intermediate signal on T1W images and variable signals on T2W images (Sampath et al., 2013).

## Hand and Wrist

It is necessary to start the imaging of acute and chronic hand and wrist pain with routine radiographs (Aagesen & Melek, 2013). Basic radiographic assessments involve posteroanterior (PA), oblique, and lateral views (Kumar & Hayashi, 2016).

Hand and wrist fractures are observed very frequently. Distal radius and ulna fractures are the most common, while phalangeal and metacarpal fractures come after them (Karl et al., 2015). Radiographs are useful in assessing these fractures (Kumar & Hayashi, 2016). CT can also be used to help in preoperative planning with the characterization of known fractures and evaluate the healing of fractures poorly demonstrated on radiographs (Lisle et al., 2009; Sundaram et al., 2013).

It has been demonstrated that CT arthrography provides at least as accurate results as MRA in diagnosing intrinsic ligament and triangular fibrocartilage complex (TFCC) tears (Lisle et al., 2009).

Dual-energy CT (DECT) musculoskeletal applications include the creation of virtual non-calcium images, the reduction of a metal artifact, the creation of iodine maps in contrast studies, and the determination of monosodium urate accumulation in gout (Fukuda & Fukuda, 2018).

Cone beam CT is an alternative method for detecting carpal region fractures and monitoring fracture healing with its advantage of a lower radiation dose compared to conventional CT (Edlund et al., 2016; Tiegs-Heiden & Howe, 2020).

MRI is employed for the purpose of evaluating TFCC tears, ligament and tendon pathologies, and complicated ganglion cysts (Seidenberg & Howe, 2014). The scapholunate and TFCC represent the most frequently observed ligament injuries and are defined as the loss of fiber integrity and increased T2 signal on MRI (Wessely & Grenier, 2007). MRA represents the least invasive technique providing higher sensitivity than MRI in detecting scapholunate and TFCC injuries (Cockenpot et al., 2016). However, since the sensitivity of MRA is lower than that of arthroscopy, it may not be indicated in cases in which injury is amenable to arthroscopic treatment (Manaster et al., 2008; Mack et al., 2003).

Furthermore, MRI is indicated for radiographically undetectable occult carpal fractures, soft tissue injury, mass, osteonecrosis, or synovitis (Berquist, 2006; Manaster et al., 2008). MRI shows an acute fracture as a line with a low signal intensity that extends along the bone in all sequences with a surrounding bone marrow edema (Hayter et al., 2013).

Avascular necrosis (AVN) is observed most frequently at the scaphoid's proximal pole following a scaphoid fracture. Although radiography or CT is adequate for establishing diagnosis and treatment planning, the diagnosis can be established earlier with MRI. On MRI, bone marrow edema is observed in the acute phase, and bone fragmentation and collapse are observed in the advanced process (Lisle et al., 2009).

Osteophyte formation, joint space narrowing and irregularity, cysts, and subchondral sclerosis are among the radiographic and CT findings of osteoarthritis. MRI is beneficial to show the related chondral damage, bone marrow edema, and synovitis (Feydy et al., 2009).

USG can be used to identify tendons, cysts, peripheral nerves, and radiolucent foreign bodies (Olubaniyi et al., 2013). Moreover, USG can be utilized with the aim of detecting joint space narrowing, synovitis, and joint effusions. It can also safely guide interventional procedures such as aspiration or injection (Olubaniyi et al., 2013). On USG, while tendinopathy emerges as the enlargement, thickening and hypoechogenicity of the related tendon, tenosynovitis refers to the hypoechoic or anechoic fluid that surrounds the tendon (Olubaniyi et al., 2013). Thickening and an increase in T2 signal are MRI signs of tendinopathy. An increase in the fluid surrounding the tendon, which is hyperintense in fluid-sensitive knees, indicates tenosynovitis (Olubaniyi et al., 2013). USG and MRI are also beneficial for confirming the clinical diagnosis of entrapment neuropathy and detecting any cause of neuropathy, including bone or soft tissue abnormality. The nerve's focal compression, enlargement of the nerve that is proximal to the compression region, the increase in signal in the nerve on MRI, and hypoechoic signal in the nerve on USG are guiding (Miller & Reinus, 2010).

## SPINE

The routine radiographic assessment of the cervical spine involves AP, lateral, oblique, and open-mouth views. The anterior and posterior vertebral line, the spinolaminar line, and the posterior spinous line must be continuous on lateral radiographs (Kumar & Hayashi, 2016).

Indications for imaging in the thoracic spine include the assessment of trauma and degenerative disc diseases, as well as scoliosis, compression fractures, and juvenile kyphosis. In scoliosis, radiography is useful to determine the etiology and monitor treatment (Kumar & Hayashi, 2016). The Cobb angle refers to a measurement, which is commonly used for the purpose of assessing the severity of scoliosis and in which the limit is 10 degrees (Horng et al., 2019).

Although lumbar spine radiography performed with AP and lateral projcctions does not provide a specific diagnosis, it can exclude vertebral fractures that may occur due to minor traumas (Patrick et al., 2016).

Spondylolysis is a pars interarticularis defect that generally occurs secondary to repetitive loading or traumatic events. Accordingly, it causes varying degrees of slippage of the vertebral body on the lower vertebra, which is called spondylolisthesis (Shamrock et al., 2020).

CT must be considered for subjects without an indication for MRI or with the requirement of anatomical bone details (Becker & Stumbo 2013). Furthermore, it is possible to easily detect a narrowing of the spinal canal and neural foramen, leading to the compressed spinal cord and nerve roots (Klein, 2015).

Although it is no longer used frequently, myelography represents a valuable method for evaluating spinal canal stenosis, nerve root compression in the lateral recess and neural foramina (Bartynski & Lin, 2003; Siemund et al., 2015). CT myelography has many benefits in the postoperative assessment of the spine and has fewer artifacts than surgical hardware-related MRI. Additionally, myelography or CT myelography are methods that can be preferred in evaluating patients for whom MRI is not possible in terms of safety (Siemund et al., 2015).

MRI constitutes the method preferred to investigate intervertebral discs, ligaments and spinal cord and paravertebral soft tissue. To evaluate the spine, standard MRI sequences should involve sagittal and axial T1 and T2 weighted images and sagittal STIR (short TI inversion recovery) (Siemund et al., 2015).

Vertebral collapse is mostly the result of trauma, but it can also be observed in pathological processes that weaken the bone structure, including osteoporosis, osteomyelitis, and primary or metastatic tumors. This can cause the compression of nerve structures and an unstable vertebral column (Klein, 2015). MRI is the most commonly used imaging technique to examine compression fractures since it enables the evaluation of the spinal canal and its contents along with the vertebral bodies (Siemund et al., 2015). When spinal tumors and infectious, inflammatory or demyelinating diseases are investigated and it is desired to differentiate between scar and recurrent disc herniation in patients after surgery, T1W sagittal and axial images are needed following intravenous contrast (Siemund et al., 2015). It has been suggested that imaging techniques, e.g., diffusion-weighted imaging and perfusion MRI, are helpful in detecting and distinguishing benign and pathological vertebral compression fractures (Biffar et al., 2010; Siemund et al., 2015).

MRI is the technique with the highest sensitivity for spinal infection, which allows the direct visualization of bone marrow edema with increased T2 signal intensity (Prodi et al., 2016). Contrast agent application also enables the detection of paravertebral abscesses and allows differential diagnosis with other pathologies that can mimic spondylodiscitis, particularly degenerative changes at the early stages (Prodi et al., 2016).

Rheumatoid arthritis (RA) mainly influences the cervical and, at a lower frequency, the thoracic and lumbosacral spine. Cervical instability and bone and ligament erosions occur after involvement in the ligamentous structures around the occipito-atlantoaxial joints at the cervical level (Jurik, 2011). More rarely, inflammatory changes can also be observed in the thoracolumbar spine and sacroiliac joints (Mattar et al., 2013).

Synovial cysts related to facet joint arthritis and degenerative spondylolisthesis have been recorded as the possible causes of unilateral radicular pain, low back pain, and cauda equina syndrome (Siemund et al., 2015). The mentioned cysts are diffuse intraspinal extradural masses with a posterior-lateral location to the thecal sac and are most frequently observed in the L4-L5 region (Eipstein, 2004). MRI signal characteristics vary according to the presence of hemorrhagic debris or calcification in the cysts (Siemund et al., 2015).

Another important cause of spinal pain is spinal tumors. The most frequently encountered spinal tumors originate from the spinal cord, vertebral bone column, paravertebral tissues, or dorsal roots (Erlemann 2006). Morphological signs such as the involvement of posterior elements and epidural or paraspinal masses may be utilized with the aim of predicting metastatic disease (Siemund et al., 2015).

Nuclear medicine applications such as SPECT and PET are mostly useful in distinguishing benign vertebral fractures from neoplastic ones (Becker and Stumbo, 2013).

## PELVIS, HIP AND SACROILIAC JOINT

The complex hip and pelvic anatomy and potentially radicular symptoms that originate from spinal pathologies can make hip and pelvic pain difficult to diagnose (Aagesen & Melek, 2013). The routine assessment of the pelvis is performed with AP, hip AP, and lateral views (Kumar & Hayashi, 2016).

The degenerative joint disease of the hip occurs frequently and is characterized by decreased joint space, sclerosis, and marginal osteophytes (Guermazi et al., 2013). The dysplastic or impingement (pincer, cam, or combined) status of the hip can be evaluated on radiography, and it is also possible to identify pathological processes such as infection, inflammatory diseases, or tumors (Ruiz Santiago et al., 2016).

MRI has high sensitivity and specificity for hip and pelvis injuries. It is the preferred imaging method when radiography may be negative, such as a nondisplaced femoral neck fracture (Aagesen & Melek, 2013; Manaster et al., 2008). MRI is also used to differentiate transient synovitis from septic arthritis or osteomyelitis, diagnose inflammatory joint disease and bone tumors, and establish the early diagnosis and follow up Perthes disease (Ruiz Santiago et al., 2016; Yang et al., 2006).

The causes of intra-articular bone pain include conditions such as transient osteoporosis of the hip, avascular necrosis (AVN), tumors, and insufficiency or stress fractures. In all the above-mentioned pathologies, it is possible to detect a pattern of bone marrow edema that is characterized by a decrease in signal intensity on T1W images and an increase in signal intensity on fat-suppressed T2W or STIR sequences (Ruiz Santiago et al., 2016).

MRA is accepted as the most suitable technique for evaluating the labrum (Ruiz Santiago et al., 2016). Therapeutic joint injections can also be performed during MRA (Aagesen & Melek, 2013).

USG is the technique of first choice in diagnosing neonatal hip dysplasia (Schwend et al., 2007). It may also show synovial thickening, hip joint effusion, and cartilage damage in septic arthritis, but the findings are not specific (Zamzam, 2006).

In patients with hip pain, bone scanning is used as a complement to other imaging studies to clarify whether indistinct bone lesions with abnormal radiotracer deposition are active lesions (Ruiz Santiago et al., 2016).

Sacroiliac joint (SIJ) disorders frequently lead to low back pain, and lumbar spine evaluation must always be performed in the case of negative relevant examinations (Kumar and Hayashi, 2016). Radiographs are suggested as the initial imaging test for subjects with SIJ pain (Inanc et al., 2005). Although the main clinical indication for SIJ imaging is excluding or confirming inflammatory sacroiliitis, it must not be forgotten that a lot of diseases or stress reactions may also influence the sacroiliac joints (Tsoi et al., 2019). Anterior marginal osteophytes, joint space narrowing, minimal subchondral sclerosis, and cyst and articular surface irregularity are observed in SIJ osteoarthritis (Tsoi et al., 2019). Sacral insufficiency fracture frequently causes low back pain in older adults with osteoporosis, and accompanying insufficiency fractures are usually observed in the pubic bones' parasymphyseal regions. MRI and, to a lesser extent, CT have higher sensitivity than radiography in the detection of sacral insufficiency fractures (Tsoi et al., 2019).

SIJ inflammation can result from inflammatory bowel disease, ankylosing spondylitis, infections, and rheumatoid arthritis. Erosions, joint space enlargement in the early phases, followed by narrowing, and sclerosis are among the signs of sacroiliitis (Kumar & Hayashi, 2016). Bone marrow edema is the diagnostic MRI finding of active sacroiliitis with the highest reliability. Bone marrow edema represents an inflammation marker and must be of great importance before the diagnosis of sacroiliitis is established (Tsoi et al., 2019). Different disease processes causing sacroiliitis can be distinguished with their specific findings together with the clinical history. The detection of findings such as bilateral involvement and bamboo spine due to fusion in ankylosing spondylitis can be shown as an example (Tuite, 2008).

Some research has demonstrated that CT has higher sensitivity and specificity in the diagnosis of early erosions of sacroiliitis and sclerosis (Puhakka et al., 2003). MRI represents the preferred imaging modality for the characterization of SIJ disease and the evaluation of the disease severity and activity (Tsoi et al., 2019). Moreover, some research has indicated that MRI has higher sensitivity and specificity in comparison with scintigraphy (İnanç et al., 2005). Intravenous non-contrast and contrast-enhanced MRI is the suggested method for imaging subjects with clinically suspected sacroiliitis and negative or suspicious radiographs (Puhakka et al., 2003).

## Knee

Radiographs are usually the first step in evaluating knee pain (Koplas et al., 2008). AP and lateral radiographs represent the primary examinations suggested to evaluate the tibiofemoral joints (Kumar & Hayashi, 2016). Knee radiographs are superior to MRI in detecting joint space narrowing since they are taken with the patient standing up (Seidenberg & Howe, 2014).

Radiographs are sufficient to evaluate osteoarthritis, and joint space narrowing is a pathognomonic feature (Ridley & Ridley, 2020). Osteophytes, subchondral sclerosis, and cystic changes are among the other basic findings associated with degenerative change (Johnson, 2004). MRI is generally not helpful in diagnosing osteoarthritis changes (Koplas et al., 2008). Advanced imaging to diagnose osteoarthritis depends on the presence of conditions that suggest complications such as subchondral insufficiency fractures and avascular necrosis (Fox et al., 2018).

MRI is preferred because it can identify pathological features that cannot be directly observed on radiography, namely non-bone pathologies including cartilage damage, a torn meniscus, bone marrow edema, ligament injuries, and synovitis (Hayashi et al., 2014). The sensitivity of MRI in detecting meniscus and cruciate ligament injury varies between 75% and 88% (Jackson et al., 2003). It may also be helpful in evaluating other injuries for which radiography does not provide benefits, e.g., stress or insufficiency fractures, synovitis, osteonecrosis, and osteochondral defects (Koplas et al., 2008). An anterior cruciate ligament tear is among the most frequently encountered knee traumatic injuries, and there is generally an association between this and medial meniscus and medial collateral ligament injuries. On MRI, it is possible to identify a focal defect in the ACL fibers with soft tissue and bone marrow edema (Naraghi & White, 2014).

In the diagnosis of Osgood-Schlatter disease, a chronic avulsion injury that is considered to be caused by repetitive microtrauma and traction on the tibial tubercle, a radiological assessment can demonstrate a superficial ossicle in the patellar tendon, soft tissue swelling in front of the tibial tuberosity, and patellar ligament thickening (Circi et al., 2017). Jumper's knee, which is also known under the name of patellar tendinopathy, represents a painful knee condition induced by small tears in the patellar tendon, resulting in localized patellar tendon tenderness. Currently, a gold standard diagnostic technique that is commonly accepted is not available (Owoeye et al., 2018), and abnormalities in the patellar tendon can be detected using both USG and MRI (Santana & AI, 2018).

CT constitutes the preferred imaging modality in the case of knee traumas in patients and includes a rapid procedure that is capable of better identifying fractures visible on conventional radiographs (Koplas et al., 2008).

USG, which is also used for guiding interventional procedures, may be beneficial to assess the rupture of the quadriceps and patellar tendon or the postoperative tendon.

Moreover, it represents a fast and reliable method to identify the presence of joint effusions and popliteal cysts (Koplas et al., 2008).

Different forms of arthritis may present as acute monoarticular arthritis. A differential diagnosis includes gout, septic arthritis, osteoarthritis, rheumatoid arthritis, and pseudogout (Ma et al., 2009). In rheumatoid arthritis, bone marrow edema and bone erosions together with synovial proliferation and synovitis will be observed. While bone erosions and periarticular osteopenia with radiographic changes generally emerge at later stages, USG and MRI may demonstrate synovial proliferation before erosions develop. Bone marrow edema represents another significant feature of rheumatoid arthritis on MRI and is predictive of erosive progression (Colebatch et al., 2013). Septic arthritis constitutes a rare but important condition, which must be evaluated in monoarthritis all the time. MRI usually shows an effusion. There is also bone erosion in severe cases. When a septic joint is suspected, synovial fluid aspiration is needed to make a diagnosis (Clerc et al., 2011).

## Ankle and Foot

In the case of chronic ankle or foot pain, radiographs are routinely the first study. AP and lateral, ankle mortise radiographs represent the routine radiographs of the foot and ankle (Aagesen & Melek, 2013). Radiographs are suitable for the detection of fractures and misalignment (Kumar & Hayashi, 2016). CT is used to detect subtle fractures and to better evaluate the intra-articular extensions of complex fractures (Kumar & Hayashi, 2016).

If it is not possible to determine chronic foot or ankle pain during the examination, MRI is usually the recommended method because pathologies such as edema in tendons, ligaments, soft tissues, and bone can be detected (Aagesen & Melek, 2013; Kumar & Hayashi, 2016).

Osteochondritis dissecans (OCD) represents a term that describes subchondral osteonecrosis of the talar dome's medial corner. This condition is considered to be caused by repetitive trauma. Subchondral lucency or focal sclerosis can be observed on direct radiographs (Ostlere, 2003). MRI is useful in staging OCD lesions (Park et al., 2012).

Stress and insufficiency fractures of the ankle usually emerge in the immediate vicinity of the distal fibula, calcaneus, and medial malleolus. It is possible that the said lesions are not visible on the radiograph (Ostlere, 2003). The typical appearance on MRI is an edema surrounding the linear hypointense line (Kiuru et al., 2002). A linear sclerotic lesion and periosteal reaction are detected on CT (Ostlere, 2003).

Ankle impingement syndromes constitute painful conditions induced by the friction of joint tissues (Cerezal et al., 2003). Anterior impingement syndrome is a relatively frequent cause of chronic ankle pain. Radiographs mostly demonstrate anterior osteophytes (Robinson & White, 2002). MRI provides benefits in evaluating the degree of cartilage damage and identifying synovitis and bone marrow edema in the anterior capsular recess (Robinson & White, 2002).

It is easy to evaluate tendon injuries in the foot and ankle using USG techniques (Seidenberg & Howe, 2014).

Tarsal tunnel syndrome and Morton's neuroma are common neuropathic conditions in the ankle and foot. Trauma, space-occupying lesions, and foot deformities can cause the compression of the posterior tibial nerve and its branches in the tarsal tunnel. MRI represents a perfect method to image the tarsal tunnel and identify possible causes of nerve entrapment. An increase in signal intensity, and an increase in size, and displacement can be observed due to nerve damage (Donovan et al., 2010). Morton's neuroma is actually a process of perineural fibrosis caused by the compression of an interdigital nerve. On MRI, it is observed as a small lesion located between the metatarsal heads with moderate signal intensity on T1W images and low signal intensity on T2W images (Torres-Claramunt et al., 2012).

Ganglion cysts are lesions associated with an adjacent joint or tendon sheath or completely separate lesions, and regardless of their anatomical location, they are observed as hypointense masses on T1W images and hyperintense masses on T2W images in MRI (Rosenberg et al., 2000).

In infectious processes, radiographs are usually normal in the early phases of the disease. Periarticular osteopenia, loss of joint space, bone erosion, and periosteal reaction are among the characteristic late properties. Ultrasound is beneficial for the purpose of confirming the presence of effusion and guiding aspiration. MRI has benefits in evaluating the degree of bone involvement and detecting an intraosseous abscess, which can require drainage (Ostlere, 2003).

The MRI findings of gout involve bone erosion as well as inflammatory alterations such as joint effusion, periarticular edema, articular or periarticular nodules, and thickened synovium. Lesions are especially frequently observed in the first metatarsophalangeal joint. Nodules are typically hypointense on T1W and T2W images, possibly because of their fibrous composition and the presence of urate crystals (Rosenberg et al., 2000).

There is a high possibility of the association of plantar fasciitis with repetitive trauma and mechanical stress, causing microtears and inflammation of the fascia and perifacial soft tissues. While calcaneal spurs are frequently observed on lateral radiographs, MRI is useful in demonstrating a plantar fascia tear. In the presence of inflammatory changes, the plantar fascia is thickened, and isointense on T1W and proton-density-weighted images, and hyperintense on T2W images. The said alterations are most evident at or close to the plantar fascia's location over the calcaneus (Rosenberg et al., 2000).

Malignant bone tumors are rarely observed in the ankle. It is necessary to always think of osteoid osteoma as a cause of ongoing pain. Lesions can be observed in all bones. It can appear as a well-circumscribed lucency on the radiograph. The most evident MRI finding is usually perilesional edema and reactive effusion. It is possible to employ CT with the aim of confirming the diagnosis and guiding percutaneous treatment (Ostlere, 2003).

## CONCLUSION

A detailed anamnesis and physical examination are the two most valuable methods for an accurate diagnosis of MSK diseases. Imaging should be considered as a tool used to confirm the diagnosis or exclude a pathology considered in the differential diagnosis. It is crucial to select the most suitable imaging method to accelerate the patient's diagnosis and treatment.

Conventional radiographs are the cornerstone and first step of diagnostic imaging in evaluating MSK pain, and some imaging modalities, such as CT, USG, MRI, and bone scans, are used. The preferred imaging method also changes depending on the structure of each joint and region investigated and the characteristics of the diseases considered in the differential diagnosis.

## REFERENCES

Aagesen, A. L., & Melek, M. (2013). Choosing the right diagnostic imaging modality in musculoskeletal diagnosis. *Primary Care: Clinics in Office Practice*, *40*(4), 849-861.

Akhtar, M. A., & Robinson, C. M. (2010). Computed tomography scan evaluation for recurrent shoulder dislocations after sports injuries. *British Journal of Sports Medicine*, *44*(14), i1-i1.

Avis, D., & Power, D. (2018). Axillary nerve injury associated with glenohumeral dislocation: a review and algorithm for management. *EFORT open reviews*, *3*(3), 70-77.

Bäumer, P., Dombert, T., Staub, F., et al. (2011). Ulnar neuropathy at the elbow: MR neurography—nerve T2 signal increase and caliber. *Radiology*, *260*(1), 199-206.

Bartynski, W. S., & Lin, L. (2003). Lumbar root compression in the lateral recess: MR imaging, conventional myelography, and CT myelography comparison with surgical confirmation. *American journal of neuroradiology*, *24*(3), 348-360.

Becker, J. A., & Stumbo, J. R. (2013). Back pain in adults. *Primary Care: Clinics in Office Practice*, *40*(2), 271-288.

Berquist, T. H. (2006). *Musculoskeletal imaging companion*. Lippincott Williams & Wilkins.

Biffar, A., Sourbron, S., Schmidt, et al. (2010). Measurement of perfusion and permeability from dynamic contrast-enhanced MRI in normal and pathological vertebral bone marrow. *Magnetic resonance in medicine*, *64*(1), 115-124.

Bredella, M. A., Steinbach, L. S., Morgan, S., et al. (2006). MRI of the sacroiliac joints in patients with moderate to severe ankylosing spondylitis. *American Journal of Roentgenology*, *187*(6), 1420-1426.

Buckwalter, K. A., Rydberg, J., Kopecky, K. K., et al. (2001). Musculoskeletal imaging with multislice CT. *American Journal of Roentgenology*, *176*(4), 979-986.

Cerezal, L., Abascal, F., Canga, A., et al. (2003). MR imaging of ankle impingement syndromes. *American Journal of Roentgenology*, *181*(2), 551-559.

Circi, E., Atalay, Y., & Beyzadeoglu, T. (2017). Treatment of Osgood–Schlatter disease: review of the literature. *Musculoskeletal surgery*, *101*(3), 195-200.

Clerc, O., Prod'hom, G., Greub, G., et al. (2011). Adult native septic arthritis: a review of 10 years of experience and lessons for empirical antibiotic therapy. *Journal of antimicrobial chemotherapy*, *66*(5), 1168-1173.

Cockenpot, E., Lefebvre, G., Demondion, X., et al. (2016). Imaging of sports-related hand and wrist injuries: sports imaging series. *Radiology*, *279*(3), 674-692.

Colebatch, A. N., Edwards, C. J., Østergaard, M., et al. (2013). EULAR recommendations for the use of imaging of the joints in the clinical management of rheumatoid arthritis. *Annals of the rheumatic diseases*, *72*(6), 804-814.

Cothran Jr, R. L., & Helms, C. (2005). Quadrilateral space syndrome: incidence of imaging findings in a population referred for MRI of the shoulder. *American Journal of Roentgenology*, *184*(3), 989-992.

Donovan, A., Rosenberg, Z. S., & Cavalcanti, C. F. (2010). MR imaging of entrapment neuropathies of the lower extremity: part 2. the knee, leg, ankle, and foot. *Radiographics*, *30*(4), 1001-1019.

Edlund, R., Skorpil, M., Lapidus, G., & Bäcklund, J. (2016). Cone-beam CT in diagnosis of scaphoid fractures. *Skeletal radiology*, *45*(2), 197-204.

Erlemann, R. (2006). Imaging and differential diagnosis of primary bone tumors and tumor-like lesions of the spine. *European journal of radiology*, *58*(1), 48-67.

Feydy, A., Pluot, E., Guerini, H., & Drapé, J. L. (2009). Role of imaging in spine, hand, and wrist osteoarthritis. *Rheumatic Disease Clinics*, *35*(3), 605-649.

Fowler, K. A., & Chung, C. B. (2006). Normal MR imaging anatomy of the elbow. *Radiologic Clinics*, *44*(4), 553-567.

Fraenkel, L. I. A. N. A., Shearer, P. E. T. E. R., Mitchell, P. A. T. R. I. C. I. A., et al. (2000). Improving the selective use of plain radiographs in the initial evaluation of shoulder pain. *The Journal of rheumatology*, *27*(1), 200-204.

Fox, M. G., Chang, E. Y., Amini, B., et al. (2018). ACR appropriateness Criteria® chronic knee pain. *Journal of the American College of Radiology*, *15*(11), S302-S312.

Fukuda, T., & Fukuda, K. (2018). The role of dual-energy computed tomography in musculoskeletal imaging. *PET clinics*, *13*(4), 567-578.

Gaskin, C. M., & Helms, C. A. (2006). Parsonage-Turner syndrome: MR imaging findings and clinical information of 27 patients. *Radiology*, *240*(2), 501-507.

Grassi, W., Filippucci, E., Carotti, M., & Salaffi, F. (2003). Imaging modalities for identifying the origin of regional musculoskeletal pain. *Best Practice & Research Clinical Rheumatology*, *17*(1), 17-32.

Goswami, G. K. (2002). The fat pad sign. *Radiology*, *222*(2), 419-420.

Guermazi, A., Hayashi, D., Eckstein, F., et al. (2013). Imaging of osteoarthritis. *Rheumatic Disease Clinics*, *39*(1), 67-105.

Hakkarinen, D. K., Banh, K. V., & Hendey, G. W. (2012). Magnetic resonance imaging identifies occult hip fractures missed by 64-slice computed tomography. *The Journal of emergency medicine*, *43*(2), 303-307.

Hayashi, D., Guermazi, A., & Kwoh, C. K. (2014). Clinical and translational potential of MRI evaluation in knee osteoarthritis. *Current rheumatology reports*, *16*(1), 391.

Hayter, C. L., Gold, S. L., & Potter, H. G. (2013). Magnetic resonance imaging of the wrist: bone and cartilage injury. *Journal of Magnetic Resonance Imaging*, *37*(5), 1005-1019.

Horng, M. H., Kuok, C. P., Fu, M. J., et al. (2019). Cobb angle measurement of spine from X-ray images using convolutional neural network. *Computational and mathematical methods in medicine*, *2019*.

Inanc, N., Atagündüz, P., Şen, F., Biren, T., et al. (2005). The investigation of sacroiliitis with different imaging techniques in spondyloarthropathies. *Rheumatology international*, *25*(8), 591-594.

Jackson, J. L., O'Malley, P. G., & Kroenke, K. (2003). Evaluation of acute knee pain in primary care. *Annals of internal medicine*, *139*(7), 575-588.

Jarraya, M., Hayashi, D., Roemer, F. W., et al. (2013). Radiographically occult and subtle fractures: a pictorial review. *Radiology research and practice*, *2013*.

Jbara, M., Patnana, M., Kazmi, F., & Beltran, J. (2006). MR imaging: arthropathies and infectious conditions of the elbow, wrist, and hand. *Radiologic Clinics*, *44*(4), 625-642.

Joseph, S. Y., Dardani, M., & Fischer, R. A. (2000). MR observations of posttraumatic osteolysis of the distal clavicle after traumatic separation of the acromioclavicular joint. *Journal of computer assisted tomography*, *24*(1), 159-164.

Jurik, A. G. (2011). Imaging the spine in arthritis—a pictorial review. *Insights into imaging*, *2*(2), 177-191.

Karl, J. W., Olson, P. R., & Rosenwasser, M. P. (2015). The epidemiology of upper extremity fractures in the United States, 2009. *Journal of orthopaedic trauma*, *29*(8), e242-e244.

Kijowski, R., Tuite, M., & Sanford, M. (2005). Magnetic resonance imaging of the elbow. Part II: abnormalities of the ligaments, tendons, and nerves. *Skeletal radiology*, *34*(1), 1-18.

Kiuru, M. J., Pihlajamaki, H. K., Hietanen, H. J., & Ahovuo, J. A. (2002). MR imaging, bone scintigraphy, and radiography in bone stress injuries of the pelvis and the lower extremity. *Acta Radiologica*, *43*(2), 207-212.

Klein, J. P. (2015). A practical approach to spine imaging. *Continuum: Lifelong Learning in Neurology*, *21*(1), 36-51.

Koplas, M., Schils, J., & Sundaram, M. (2008). The painful knee: choosing the right imaging test. *Cleveland Clinic journal of medicine*, *75*(5), 377.

Kotnis, N. A., Chiavaras, M. M., & Harish, S. (2012). Lateral epicondylitis and beyond: imaging of lateral elbow pain with clinical-radiologic correlation. *Skeletal radiology*, *41*(4), 369-386.

Kumar, Y., & Hayashi, D. (2016). Role of Imaging in musculoskeletal care. *Current Physical Medicine and Rehabilitation Reports*, *4*(1), 28-36.

Lefevre-Colau, M. M., Drapé, J. L., Fayad, F., et al. (2005). Magnetic resonance imaging of shoulders with idiopathic adhesive capsulitis: reliability of measures. *European radiology*, *15*(12), 2415-2422.

Levine, B. D., Motamedi, K., & Seeger, L. L. (2012). Imaging of the shoulder: a comparison of MRI and ultrasound. *Current sports medicine reports*, *11*(5), 239-243.

Lisle, D. A., Shepherd, G. J., Cowderoy, G. A., & O'Connell, P. T. (2009). MR imaging of traumatic and overuse injuries of the wrist and hand in athletes. *Magnetic Resonance Imaging Clinics*, *17*(4), 639-654.

Ma, L., Cranney, A., & Holroyd-Leduc, J. M. (2009). Acute monoarthritis: What is the cause of my patient's painful swollen joint?. *Cmaj*, *180*(1), 59-65.

Mack, M. G., Keim, S., Balzer, J. O., et al. (2003). Clinical impact of MRI in acute wrist fractures. *European radiology*, *13*(3), 612-617.

Manaster, B. J., Andrews, C. L., Crim, J., et al. (2008). Diagnostic and Surgical Imaging Anatomy: Musculoskeletal. *Journal of Medical Imaging and Radiation Sciences*, *39*(1), 50.

Mattar, M., Salonen, D., & Inman, R. D. (2013). Imaging of spondyloarthropathies. *Rheumatic diseases clinics of North America*, *39*(3), 645-667.

Mengiardi, B., Pfirrmann, C. W., Gerber, C., et al. (2004). Frozen shoulder: MR arthrographic findings. *Radiology*, *233*(2), 486-492.

Miller, T. T., & Reinus, W. R. (2010). Nerve entrapment syndromes of the elbow, forearm, and wrist. *American Journal of Roentgenology*, *195*(3), 585-594.

Murray, P. J., & Shaffer, B. S. (2009). Clinical update: MR imaging of the shoulder. *Sports medicine and arthroscopy review*, *17*(1), 40-48.

Naraghi, A., & White, L. M. (2014). MR imaging of cruciate ligaments. *Magnetic Resonance Imaging Clinics*, *22*(4), 557-580.

O'Connor, E. E., Dixon, L. B., Peabody, T., & Stacy, G. S. (2004). MRI of cystic and soft-tissue masses of the shoulder joint. *American Journal of Roentgenology*, *183*(1), 39-47.

Olubaniyi, B. O., Bhatnagar, G., Vardhanabhuti, V., et al. (2013). Comprehensive musculoskeletal sonographic evaluation of the hand and wrist. *Journal of Ultrasound in Medicine*, *32*(6), 901-914.

Ostlere, S. (2003). Imaging the ankle and foot. *Imaging*, *15*(4), 242-269.

Owoeye, O. B., Wiley, J. P., Walker, R. E., et al. (2018). Diagnostic accuracy of a self-report measure of patellar tendinopathy in youth basketball. *Journal of orthopaedic & sports physical therapy*, *48*(10), 758-766.

Park, H. J., Cha, S. D., Kim, S. S., et al. (2012). Accuracy of MRI findings in chronic lateral ankle ligament injury: comparison with surgical findings. *Clinical radiology*, *67*(4), 313-318.

Patrick, N., Emanski, E., & Knaub, M. A. (2016). Acute and chronic low back pain. *Medical Clinics*, *100*(1), 169-181.

Prodi, E., Grassi, R., Iacobellis, F., & Cianfoni, A. (2016). Imaging in Spondylodiskitis. *Magnetic resonance imaging clinics of North America*, *24*(3), 581-600.

Puhakka, K. B., Jurik, A. G., Egund, N., et al. (2003). Imaging of sacroiliitis in early seronegative spondylarthropathy: assessment of abnormalities by MR in comparison with radiography and CT. *Acta Radiologica*, *44*(2), 218-229.

Ravenel, J. G., Gordon, L. L., Pope, T. L., & Reed, C. E. (2004). FDG-PET uptake in occult acute pelvic fracture. *Skeletal radiology*, *33*(2), 99-101.

Ridley, U., & Ridley, L. (2020). Imaging of the knee: 'Common acute presentations to general practice'. *Australian Journal of General Practice*, *49*(6), 344.

Robinson, P., & White, L. M. (2002). Soft-tissue and osseous impingement syndromes of the ankle: role of imaging in diagnosis and management. *Radiographics*, *22*(6), 1457-1469.

Rosenberg, Z. S., Beltran, J., & Bencardino, J. T. (2000). MR imaging of the ankle and foot. *Radiographics*, *20*(suppl_1), S153-S179.

Ruiz Santiago, F., Santiago Chinchilla, A., Ansari, A., et al. (2016). Imaging of hip pain: From radiography to cross-sectional imaging techniques. *Radiology research and practice*, *2016*.

Sampath, S. C., Sampath, S. C., & Bredella, M. A. (2013). Magnetic resonance imaging of the elbow: a structured approach. *Sports health*, *5*(1), 34-49.

Santana, J. A., & Al, S. (2018). *Jumpers knee*.

Schwend, R. M., Schoenecker, P., Richards, B. S., et al. (2007). Screening the newborn for developmental dysplasia of the hip: now what do we do?. *Journal of Pediatric Orthopaedics*, *27*(6), 607-610.

Shamrock, A. G., Donnally III, C. J., & Varacallo, M. (2020). Lumbar spondylolysis and spondylolisthesis. *StatPearls [Internet]*.

Siemund, R., Thurnher, M., & Sundgren, P. C. (2015). How to image patients with spine pain. *European journal of radiology*, *84*(5), 757-764.

Seidenberg, P. H., & Howe, A. H. (2014). Musculoskeletal imaging: types and indications. *Medical Clinics*, *98*(4), 895-914.

Sundaram, N., Bosley, J., & Stacy, G. S. (2013). Conventional radiographic evaluation of athletic injuries to the hand. *Radiologic Clinics of North America*, *51*(2), 239-255.

Tang, C., & Aggarwal, R. (2013). Imaging for musculoskeletal problems. *InnovAiT*, *6*(11), 735-738.

Teefey, S. A., Rubin, D. A., Middleton, W. D., et al. (2004). Detection and quantification of rotator cuff tears: comparison of ultrasonographic, magnetic resonance imaging, and arthroscopic findings in seventy-one consecutive cases. *JBJS*, *86*(4), 708-716.

Tiegs-Heiden, C. A., & Howe, B. M. (2020). Imaging of the Hand and Wrist. *Clinics in sports medicine*, *39*(2), 223-245.

Torres-Claramunt, R., Ginés, A., Pidemunt, G., et al. (2012). MRI and ultrasonography in Morton's neuroma: diagnostic accuracy and correlation. *Indian journal of orthopaedics*, *46*, 321-325.

Tsoi, C., Griffith, J. F., Lee, R. K. L., et al. (2019). Imaging of sacroiliitis: Current status, limitations and pitfalls. *Quantitative imaging in medicine and surgery*, *9*(2), 318.

Tuite, M. J. (2008, March). Sacroiliac joint imaging. In *Seminars in musculoskeletal radiology* (Vol. 12, No. 01, pp. 072-082). © Thieme Medical Publishers.

Wessely, M. A., & Grenier, J. M. (2007). MR imaging of the wrist and hand—A review of the normal imaging appearance with an illustration of common disorders affecting the wrist and hand. *Clinical Chiropractic*, *10*(3), 156-164.

Wheeless, C. R. (2013). Triphasic bone scan. *Wheeless' textbook of orthopaedics.* Available at: http://www. wheelessonline.com/ortho/triphasic_bone_scan. Accessed November, 16.

Yang, W. J., Im, S. A., Lim, G. Y., et al. (2006). MR imaging of transient synovitis: differentiation from septic arthritis. *Pediatric radiology*, *36*(11), 1154-1158.

Yim, E. S., & Corrado, G. (2012). Ultrasound in athletes: emerging techniques in point-of-care practice. *Current sports medicine reports*, *11*(6), 298-303.

Zamzam, M. M. (2006). The role of ultrasound in differentiating septic arthritis from transient synovitis of the hip in children. *Journal of Pediatric Orthopaedics B*, *15*(6), 418-422.

In: Musculoskeletal Pain (Common Clinical Presentations) ISBN: 978-1-68507-410-4
Editors: Mehmet Cenk Turgut and Serdar Toy 

*Chapter 30*

# POLYNEUROPATHY

***Onur Yıldız[1,*], MD and Hamit Çelik[2], MD***
[1]Department of Neurology, Health Sciences University,
Erzurum Regional Health Application and Research Hospital,
Erzurum, Turkey
[2]Department of Neurology, Private Buhara Hospital,
Erzurum, Turkey

## ABSTRACT

Polyneuropathies, especially diabetic polyneuropathy, are the most common peripheral nervous system disease that affects adults. Polyneuropathies can be classified in many ways, and axonal damage is a common result of this disease. In many neuropathies, the sensory fibers are primarily affected, and if the damage continues, motor weakness develops.

Some neuropathies cause severe pain and are due to damage of the small fibers. The most common cause of this type of pain is distal symmetrical polyneuropathy due to diabetes. Anamnesis and examination findings should be noted in a patient with suspected polyneuropathy. Laboratory findings, electrodiagnostic tests and, if necessary, lumbar puncture or genetic tests are helpful in identifying diagnostic and etiological factors.

## INTRODUCTION

Polyneuropathy is a peripheral nervous system disease that affects more than one nerve in the body and causes sensory or motor symptoms. Neuropathies have many

* Corresponding Author's E-mail: dronuryildiz@hotmail.com.

etiological causes and may be metabolic, toxic, inflammatory, or genetic. Some neuropathies may present with only sensory complaints, while others may present with only motor findings. Electrodiagnostic tests can diagnose most polyneuropathies and provide information about the primary physiopathology. If the etiologic cause of polyneuropathy is found, it can be completely cured, or the progression of the disease can be reduced. In this section, I discuss the anatomy of the peripheral nervous system, diagnostic tests used in the diagnosis of polyneuropathies, and common causes of painful polyneuropathies.

## ANATOMICAL CHARACTERISTICS

The peripheral nervous system includes anterior horn cells, dorsal root ganglia, peripheral nerves, primary sensory receptors, neuromuscular junctions, and muscles. Many peripheral nerves functionally contain three types of fibers: sensory, motor, and autonomic. Sensory fibers transmit information from peripheral receptors to the dorsal root ganglion with myelinated and unmyelinated fibers. Motor axons originate from anterior horn cells in the ventral root of the spinal cord. These axons combine with the sensory nerves to form the mixed spinal nerve. Peripheral nerves classify according to the myelin structure. Large myelinated fibers (A alpha and beta) provide rapid conduction and can be measured in standard nerve conduction studies. Small myelinated (A gamma and B) and unmyelinated fibers (C) transport pain, heat sensation, and autonomic information. Positive (pain, burning, and tingling) and negative (numbness and imbalance) symptoms can occur with sensory nerve damage. Unlike sensory nerves, all motor axons are myelinated and terminate at the neuromuscular junction. Weakness, fasciculation, and atrophy occur in the damage of motor neurons and axons.

## CLASSIFICATION

Polyneuropathies can be classified in many ways: Acute-subacute-chronic according to the onset of symptoms; symmetrical-asymmetrical according to the involvement pattern; and axonal-demyelinating according to the primary physiopathology. The onset of polyneuropathy can be determined by anamnesis, the involvement pattern by physical examination, and the primary pathophysiology by nerve conduction studies. Polyneuropathies divide into axonal damage and demyelination according to physiopathology. This classification is of great importance in clinical evaluation (Donofrio and Albers 1990). Polyneuropathies with primary axonal damage are observed more frequently and metabolic, nutritional deficiency, and toxic causes are the main causes in the etiology. The most common polyneuropathies with demyelination are acute and chronic inflammatory demyelinating polyneuropathies, and hereditary motor and sensory neuropathies (HMSN).

## Clinical Evaluation in Polyneuropathy

In a patient with suspected polyneuropathy, the symptoms should be carefully listened to, previous diseases and family history should be questioned, and finally, the examination findings should be noted. With these findings, the necessary diagnostic tests should be requested. In a patient diagnosed with polyneuropathy with clinical and laboratory findings, the main purpose is to determine the etiological factors and a polyneuropathy that it is possible to treat.

### Clinical Signs

Many peripheral neuropathies begin symmetrically in the distal extremities because the transport from the cell body to the distal axon becomes more difficult as the length increases. This damage, which starts from the distal and spreads to the proximal part, is called "dying-back" neuropathy (Spencer and Schaumburg 1977). The sural nerve is the longest nerve of the peripheral nervous system and is usually the first nerve to be affected by peripheral neuropathies. Accordingly, the first sensory symptoms begin, and paresthesia, pain, and numbness occur in the distal lower extremities. With the progression of neuropathy, weakness begins in the distal lower extremities due to motor axon damage. Polyneuropathies due to metabolic (diabetes mellitus, uremia), toxic (chemotherapy), and nutritional (vitamin B12 deficiency) causes are the best examples of this clinic. In small nerve fiber neuropathies, pain and loss of heat sensation, painful paresthesias, and autonomic dysfunctions are observed in the distal lower extremities. The most common cause of this type of pain is distal symmetrical polyneuropathy due to diabetes (Marchettini et al. 2006). Common causes of painful peripheral neuropathies are given in Table 1.

In many sensory or sensory-motor polyneuropathies, significant sensory defects are found in the distal extremities on examination. This examination finding is called "glove and stocking" hypoesthesia. Sensory examination findings in neuropathies vary according to the involved fibers. For example, in neuropathies in which small myelinated fibers are primarily involved, findings such as loss of pain and thermal sensation in the distal extremities and orthostatic hypotension are observed. On the other hand, in the involvement of large myelinated fibers, loss of vibration and position sense, hypo- or areflexia, sensory ataxia, and Romberg sign are prominent. If motor findings are present, this is due to second motor neuron involvement and symptoms such as weakness, atrophy, and fasciculation may be observed.

**Table 1. Painful peripheral neuropathies**

| |
|---|
| Diabetic neuropathy |
| Uremic neuropathy |
| Toxic neuropathy |
| Vasculitis |
| Guillain-Barré syndrome |
| Amyloidosis |
| Alcoholic neuropathy |
| HIV related neuropathy |
| Fabry disease |
| Cryptogenic sensory neuropathy |

HIV: Human immunodeficiency virus.

In addition to a neurological examination, a detailed system examination should be performed. Although skeletal deformities are common in hereditary neuropathies, they are not a specific examination finding. Spinal abnormalities such as kyphosis and scoliosis and foot deformities can be clues for hereditary neuropathies. Foot deformities can be seen as pes cavus and pes planus deformities.

## Laboratory

The majority of polyneuropathies are distal, symmetrical, and length-dependent sensory-motor polyneuropathies. First, laboratory examination should be performed for metabolic and nutritional causes, the most common causes of these. Then, rarer causes should be investigated. Laboratory investigations to investigate the etiology in these patients are summarized in Table 2 (Levine and Saperstein 2013).

## Electrodiagnostic Tests

Nerve conduction tests are widely used for diagnostic purposes in polyneuropathies because they are easily accessible.

These tests measure large myelinated nerves and are often found to be normal in small fiber neuropathies. Therefore, normal nerve conduction tests in patients with neuropathic pain do not indicate the absence of polyneuropathy. Electrodiagnostic tests also show whether the primary pathology in polyneuropathy is demyelination or axonal degeneration. Thus, etiological causes can be reduced. In axonal polyneuropathies, decreased sensory and compound muscle action potential amplitudes are evident, and nerve conduction velocities are in the normal range or slightly slow. In demyelinating polyneuropathies, the most prominent finding is a marked slowing of nerve conduction velocities and a prolongation of distal latencies (Johnsen and Fuglsang-Frederiksen 2000).

**Table 2. Laboratory evaluation of peripheral neuropathy**

| *Primarily* | *Secondarily* |
|---|---|
| Hemogram | Serum and urine immunofixation tests |
| Fasting glucose, HgbA1c | ANA, anti-dsDNA, SS-A, SS-B |
| 2-h oral glucose tolerance test | Anti-ganglioside antibodies |
| Renal functions tests | Paraneoplastic antibodies |
| Thyroid function tests | HIV serology |
| Vitamin B12 levels | Serum a-galactosidase levels |
| ESR | |

ANA: Antinuclear antibodies, ESR: Erythrocyte sedimentation rate, HgbA1c: hemoglobin A1c, HIV: Human immunodeficiency virus.

## Lumbar Puncture

Analysis of cerebrospinal fluid (CSF) by lumbar puncture can provide important information. In cases with polyradiculopathy such as inflammatory demyelinating polyneuropathies and meningeal carcinomatosis due to nerve root involvement, protein levels increase in the CSF. In inflammatory polyneuropathies, cellular components are either absent or scarcely visible. This finding is called "albuminocytological dissociation". Malignant cells can be seen in the CSF in patients with meningeal carcinomatosis.

## Nerve Biopsy

Peripheral nerve biopsies are required to diagnose very few neuropathies and are most commonly performed in vasculitic and amyloid neuropathies. The sural nerve is most commonly used for a nerve biopsy. Performing the biopsy as a muscle-nerve biopsy may provide additional information. The examination of epidermal nerve fiber density by punch biopsy from the skin is helpful in the diagnosis of small fiber neuropathies (England et al. 2009).

## Genetic Tests

Genetic testing for hereditary neuropathies is usually ordered based on clinical phenotype, transition pattern, and electrophysiological features (axonal or demyelinating). Duplication of the PMP22 gene is most common in HMSN and presents the CMT-1A phenotype (Holmberg 1993).

# Common Causes of Painful Neuropathies

## Diabetic Polyneuropathies

Diabetic polyneuropathy is the most common cause of peripheral neuropathies. About half of diabetic patients develop neuropathy during the illness which can lead to neuropathy in many different ways (Dyck et al. 1993). The most effective method in preventing and treating diabetic neuropathy is to keep the blood glucose level under good control. Distal symmetrical polyneuropathy (DSP) is the most common form of diabetic neuropathy. DSP damages the distal axons of long peripheral nerves and "length-dependent" symptoms thus occur. Since small myelinated fibers are first affected, pain complaints are common. Therefore, the first complaints are positive symptoms increasing at night in the distal lower extremities, such as pain, tingling, burning, and an electric shock-like feeling. Sometimes patients experience allodynia, which is severe pain with an ordinarily non-painful stimulus (Galer et al. 2000). Small fiber neuropathy can be seen in the impaired glucose tolerance or early stages of diabetes and nerve conduction tests may be normal during this period (Tesfaye 2011). Diabetic polyradiculoneuropathy (diabetic amyotrophy) affects nerve roots and peripheral nerves simultaneously and is often seen in uncontrolled type 2 DM patients. It is possibly a vasculitis caused by autoimmune mechanisms. The lower extremity is most commonly involved, and the most common initial symptom is severe pain in the lower back, hips, and thigh. Asymmetric weakness and atrophy of the proximal thigh muscles are added to the symptoms within days to weeks. Pain and weakness are most commonly seen in the femoral nerve innervation area.

Diabetic neuropathic cachexia is an acute onset clinical condition independent of disease duration which sometimes occurs after tight glycemic control. Small fiber involvement is more prominent in the disease, and following significant weight loss, a burning sensation, severe pain, and allodynia develop in the lower extremities, being pronounced at night. Motor involvement is not expected (Knopp et al. 2013).

Insulin neuritis is a form of therapy-related neuropathy which occurs in patients starting insulin or having an insulin dose increment during treatment. Small myelinated or unmyelinated fibers are involved. Severe pain in the distal lower extremities is accompanied by autonomic dysfunction (Knopp et al. 2013).

## Hereditary Motor and Sensory Neuropathy

HMSNs are the most common hereditary neuropathies, having a prevalence between 20 and 28/100.000 (Combarros et al. 1987; Holmberg 1993). Instead of HMSN, it is also called Charcot-Marie-Tooth disease, dedicated to its definers. Symptoms usually begin in the first decade and progress slowly. Especially, foot dorsiflexors are weak and neuropathic pain may be evident in the feet. Hammertoe, pes cavus, or pes planus deformity becomes evident during adolescence. CMT1A due to duplication in the PMP22 gene constitutes 50% of all HMSNs, and these patients have the classic CMT phenotype. There is still no proven treatment option for the disease. Strengthening training programs, passive stretching movements, and ankle orthoses are recommended in the treatment, and surgical methods (plantar fasciotomy, tendon transfer, osteotomy, arthrodesis) can be applied for symptomatic joint deformities.

## Inflammatory Neuropathy

Guillain-Barré Syndrome (GBS) is an acute, monophasic, and immune-mediated polyradiculoneuropathy with an incidence of 1.1-1.8/100.000 (McGrogan et al. 2009). Acute inflammatory demyelinating polyneuropathy (AIDP) is the most common form of classical GBS, and axonal variants may be seen less frequently. The most common initial symptom is tingling and paresthesias in the distal extremities. In addition, there may be severe radicular pain due to inflammation of the roots. Low back pain may be the first symptom which may start before muscle weakness in some patients. However, 90% of patients complain of pain, which may persist for months in many cases. Symmetrical weakness starting from the lower extremity ascends in spread, and mechanical ventilation may be required due to the involvement of respiratory muscles. Furthermore, hypo- or areflexia is seen on physical examination. Proven immunological treatments for AIDP are plasmapheresis and IVIG, showing greater efficacy with the treatment initiation within the first two weeks ("Randomised trial of plasma exchange, intravenous immunoglobulin, and combined treatments in Guillain-Barré syndrome. Plasma Exchange/Sandoglobulin Guillain-Barré Syndrome Trial Group" 1997).

Chronic inflammatory demyelinating polyneuropathy develops due to an autoimmune mechanism similar to AIDP and progresses with multifocal demyelination in peripheral nerves. In general, there is muscle weakness involving the distal and proximal extremities that is quite symmetrical. Unlike AIDP, muscle weakness develops slowly over months, with remitting or exacerbating symptoms. Most patients complain of numbness and paresthesias in the hands and feet, and there is albuminocytological dissociation in most cases. Nerve conduction tests show non-uniform pathologies of focal demyelination in different nerves and different regions of the same nerve.

Steroids, IVIG, plasmapheresis, and cytostatic drugs are used in the treatment.

## Toxic Neuropathy

Drug-induced polyneuropathies are the most common cause of toxic neuropathies. They most commonly cause length-dependent axonal neuropathy, and symmetrical sensory or sensory-motor findings are observed in the distal extremities. Pain is a common symptom, and when persistent axonal degeneration develops, symptoms may not completely resolve even if the drug is not discontinued. Even in some patients, clinical findings may show a progression for weeks despite discontinuation of the responsible drug.

**Table 3. Drug-induced peripheral neuropathy**

| |
|---|
| Chemotherapy (vincristine, cisplatin, paclitaxel) |
| Amiodarone |
| Metronidazole, Chloramphenicol |
| Colchicine |
| Isoniazid, Ethambutol |
| Chloroquine |

The drugs that can cause neuropathy are given in Table 3 (Vilholm et al. 2014).

## Vasculitic Neuropathy

Vasculitis-related polyneuropathies can be seen during the course of primary systemic vasculitis (polyarteritis nodosa, Wegener granulomatosis, Churg-Strauss disease, microscopic polyangiitis) or secondary systemic vasculitis (systemic lupus erythematosus, Sjogren's syndrome, rheumatoid arthritis). Vasculitis causes a mononeuritis multiplex picture characterized by the asymmetric involvement of peripheral nerves as well as DSP. These patients present with severe pain and asymmetric weakness in the affected nerve area.

While vasculitis can cause pain due to many organ involvements, it can also cause pain by causing peripheral neuropathy.

### Cryptogenic Sensory Polyneuropathy

In one group of patients, a cause of polyneuropathy cannot be determined (10 - 25%), despite all researches. These patients are generally over 60 years old and complain of burning pain in the distal extremities at night. Nerve conduction tests include normal or minimal sensory abnormalities. Cryptogenic sensory neuropathy is an exclusion diagnosis and all causes of sensory axonal neuropathy should be investigated in detail before making this diagnosis (Pasnoor et al. 2013).

## Conclusion

In a patient with suspected polyneuropathy, the symptoms should be carefully listened to, previous diseases and family history should be questioned, and finally, the examination findings should be noted. In a patient diagnosed with polyneuropathy with clinical and laboratory findings, the main purpose is to determine the etiological factors and a polyneuropathy that it is possible to treat.

## References

Combarros, O., Calleja, J., Polo, J. M. and Berciano, J. (1987, Jan.). Prevalence of hereditary motor and sensory neuropathy in Cantabria. *Acta Neurol. Scand.,* 75(1), 9 - 12. https://doi.org/10.1111/j.1600-0404.1987.tb07882.x.

Donofrio, P. D., and Albers, J. W. (1990, Oct.). AAEM minimonograph #34: polyneuropathy: Classification by nerve conduction studies and electromyography. *Muscle Nerve,* 13(10), 889 - 903. https://doi.org/ 10.1002/mus.880131002.

Dyck, P. J., Kratz, K. M., Karnes, J. L., Litchy, W. J., Klein, R., Pach, J. M., Wilson, D. M., O'Brien, P. C., Melton, L. J. 3rd and Service, F. J. (1993, Apr.). The prevalence by staged severity of various types of diabetic neuropathy, retinopathy, and nephropathy in a population-based cohort: The Rochester Diabetic Neuropathy Study. *Neurology,* 43(4), 817 - 824. https://doi.org/10.1212/wnl.43.4.817.

England, J. D., Gronseth, G. S., Franklin, G., Carter, G. T., Kinsella, L. J., Cohen, J. A., Asbury, A. K., Szigeti, K., Lupski, J. R., Latov, N., Lewis, R. A., Low, P. A., Fisher, M. A., Herrmann, D., Howard, J. F., Lauria, G., Miller, R. G., Polydefkis, M. and Sumner, A. J. (2009, Jan.). Practice parameter: The evaluation of distal symmetric polyneuropathy: the role of autonomic testing, nerve biopsy, and skin biopsy (an evidence-based review). Report of the American Academy of Neurology, the American Association of Neuromuscular and Electrodiagnostic Medicine, and the

American Academy of Physical Medicine and Rehabilitation. *Pm R,* 1(1), 14 - 22. https://doi.org/ 10.1016/j.pmrj.2008.11.011.

Galer, B. S., Gianas, A. and Jensen, M. P. (2000, Feb). Painful diabetic polyneuropathy: Epidemiology, pain description, and quality of life. *Diabetes Res. Clin. Pract.,* 47(2), 123 - 128. https://doi.org/10.1016/ s0168-8227(99)00112-6.

Holmberg, B. H. (1993, May). Charcot-Marie-Tooth disease in northern Sweden: An epidemiological and clinical study. *Acta Neurol. Scand.,* 87(5), 416 - 422. https://doi.org/10.1111/j.1600-0404.1993.tb04127.x.

Johnsen, B. and Fuglsang-Frederiksen, A. (2000, Dec.). Electrodiagnosis of polyneuropathy. *Neurophysiol. Clin.,* 30(6), 339 - 351. https:// doi.org/10.1016/ s0987-7053(00)00237-9.

Knopp, M., Srikantha, M. and Rajabally, Y. A. (2013, May). Insulin neuritis and diabetic cachectic neuropathy: A review. *Curr. Diabetes Rev.,* 9(3), 267 - 274. https://doi.org/10.2174/15733998113090300007.

Levine, T. D. and Saperstein, D. S. (2013, May). Laboratory evaluation of peripheral neuropathy. *Neurol. Clin.,* 31(2), 363 - 376. https://doi.org/ 10.1016/j.ncl. 2013.01.004.

Marchettini, P., Lacerenza, M., Mauri, E. and Marangoni, C. (2006, Jul.). Painful peripheral neuropathies. *Curr. Neuropharmacol.,* 4(3), 175 - 181. https://doi.org/10.2174/157015906778019536.

McGrogan, A., Madle, G. C., Seaman, H. E. and de Vries, C. S. (2009). The epidemiology of Guillain-Barré syndrome worldwide. A systematic literature review. *Neuroepidemiology,* 32(2), 150 - 163. https://doi.org/10.1159/000184748.

Pasnoor, M., Dimachkie, M. M. and Barohn, R. J. (2013, May). Cryptogenic sensory polyneuropathy. *Neurol. Clin.,* 31(2), 463 - 476. https://doi.org/10.1016/ j.ncl.2013.01.008.

Randomised trial of plasma exchange, intravenous immunoglobulin, and combined treatments in Guillain-Barré syndrome. Plasma Exchange/Sandoglobulin Guillain-Barré Syndrome Trial Group. (1997, Jan. 25). *Lancet,* 349(9047), 225 - 230.

Spencer, P. S. and Schaumburg, H. H. (1977, Mar.-Apr.). Ultrastructural studies of the dying-back process. III. The evolution of experimental peripheral giant axonal degeneration. *J. Neuropathol. Exp. Neurol.,* 36(2), 276 - 299. https://doi.org/10. 1097/00005072-197703000-00005.

Tesfaye, S. (2011, Jan. 24). Recent advances in the management of diabetic distal symmetrical polyneuropathy. *J. Diabetes Investig,* 2(1), 33 - 42. https://doi.org/ 10.1111/j.2040-1124.2010.00083.x.

Vilholm, O. J., Christensen, A. A., Zedan, A. H. and Itani, M. (2014, Aug.). Drug-induced peripheral neuropathy. *Basic Clin. Pharmacol. Toxicol.,* 115(2), 185 - 192. https://doi.org/10.1111/bcpt.12261.

In: Musculoskeletal Pain (Common Clinical Presentations) ISBN: 978-1-68507-410-4
Editors: Mehmet Cenk Turgut and Serdar Toy 

*Chapter 31*

# INHERITED MUSCULAR DISORDERS

***Gözde Öztan**, PhD***
Department of Medicine, Istanbul University,
Istanbul, Turkey

## ABSTRACT

In muscle diseases, muscle weakness, thinning and sometimes pain or cramps are seen due to the disease of the muscle fibers. Hereditary muscle diseases can be classified into seven categories. Disease forms consist of "Duchenne and Becker; myotonic dystrophy; facioscapulohumeral; Emery-Dreifuss; oculopharyngeal; distal; and limb-girdle." They occur due to mutations in various genes.

Although the disorder that causes hereditary muscle diseases is present from birth, the age at which it manifests itself is variable. Some appear from birth, while others begin at a later age. Congenital deficiency of proteins necessary for the proper functioning of the muscles leads to disorders and diseases in the muscles. Muscle diseases that show familial characteristics and cause progressive weakness are called "dystrophy." In some of these, the disease is passed from mother to son (X-linked), and in others, from mother or father to children (autosomal dominant). In others, both the mother and father must be carriers. In this type, the disease occurs in children who inherit the disease gene from both parents, while the parents don't show the disease characteristics (autosomal recessive).

In this chapter, hereditary muscle diseases were classified and their phenotypic findings and gene mutations were defined. The genotype-phenotype relationship was revealed and the criteria that could guide the diagnosis were expressed.

* Corresponding Author's E-mail: gozdeoztan@yahoo.com.

## INTRODUCTION

Hereditary muscular disorders are a variety of muscle disease groups that present with common signs and physical symptoms. Myopathies are induced by genetic deficiency in the contraction appliance of the muscle and expressed as pronounced histochemical alterations in muscle biopsy. Muscular dystrophies (MDs) are muscle membrane diseases described by the pathological demonstration of muscle degeneration and regeneration (Cardamone et al., 2008).

**Table 1. Gene loci in the most common types of MD**

| Disorder | Gene locus |
|---|---|
| Congenital (AR) | 6q |
| | 12q |
| | 9q |
| | 1p |
| | 1p |
| Duchenne and Becker (XR) | Xp21 |
| Emery-Dreifuss (XR) | Xq28 |
| Emery-Dreifuss (AD/AR) | 1q |
| Distal (AD) | 14q, 2q |
| Distal (AR) | 2p |
| Facioscapulohumeral (AD) | 4q |
| Oculopharyngeal (AD) | 14q |
| Limb-girdle (AD) | |
| 1A | 5q |
| 1B | 1q |
| 1C | 3p |
| 1D | 6q |
| 1E | 7q |
| 1F | 2q |
| Limb-girdle (AR) | |
| 2A | 15q |
| 2B | 2p |
| 2C | 13q |
| 2D | 17q |
| 2E | 4q |
| 2F | 5q |
| 2G | 17q |
| 2H | 9q |
| 2I | 19q |

Inheritance: AR = autosomal recessive; AD = autosomal dominant; XR = X-linked recessive.

MDs are inherited myogenic disorders described by increasing muscle loss and feebleness of unstable intensity. According to the dispersion of predominant muscle feebleness, division into different groups is possible, including congenital forms; Duchenne and Becker; myotonic dystrophy; facioscapulohumeral; Emery-Dreifuss; oculopharyngeal; distal; and limb-girdle. Seven main forms of congenital dystrophy can be classified according to the distribution of dominant muscle weakness (Table 1) (Emery, 2002).

## Duchenne Muscular Dystrophy (DMD) and Becker Muscular Dystrophy (BMD) (Dystrophinopathies)

DMD is one of the most widespread neuromuscular diseases in childhood, with an incidence of 10.71 to 27.78 per 100,000 men. DMD, resulting from out-of-frame mutations of the dystrophin gene and a lack of protein expression, is inherited as X-linked. Reading frame-keeping mutations in the dystrophin gene are seen in BMD, which has a milder phenotype (Brusa et al., 2020). DMD shows a progressive manifestation that begins at the average age of three years. The first sign of disease seen in male patients with DMD is the use of their hands and arms while trying to lift their bodies from the squatting position. On the other hand, patients have difficulty running, jumping, an unusual gait, and pseudohypertrophy of the calf muscles. The high level of serum creatine kinase enzyme in the blood leaking from the damaged muscle mediates the diagnosis of muscular dystrophy with clinical examination (Barthélémy & Wein, 2018).

The DMD gene has 79 exons of 2.2 Mb, with a high mutation rate and a de novo mutation-induced DMD is seen in one in 3 cases. Although most patients have deletions (68%) or duplications (11%) of one or more exons, minor mutations are also present (20% of patients). DMD gene deletions and duplications occur anywhere in the gene, while deletions are more common in exons 45-55 and duplications in exons 2-10 (Aartsma-Rus et al., 2016). Dystrophin binds the inner cytoskeleton to the extracellular matrix and has an important structural function in muscle. The amino terminal of dystrophin is attached to F-actin in sarcoma and the carboxyl terminal of dystrophin to the dystrophin-associated protein complex (Figure 1). The dystrophin-related protein complex includes dystroglycans, sarcoglycans, integrins and caveolin. Mutations that can occur in any of these components cause autosomal hereditary muscular dystrophies. In the deficiency of dystrophin, the dystrophin-related protein complex becomes unbalanced and the levels of member proteins decrease (Nowak & Davies, 2004).

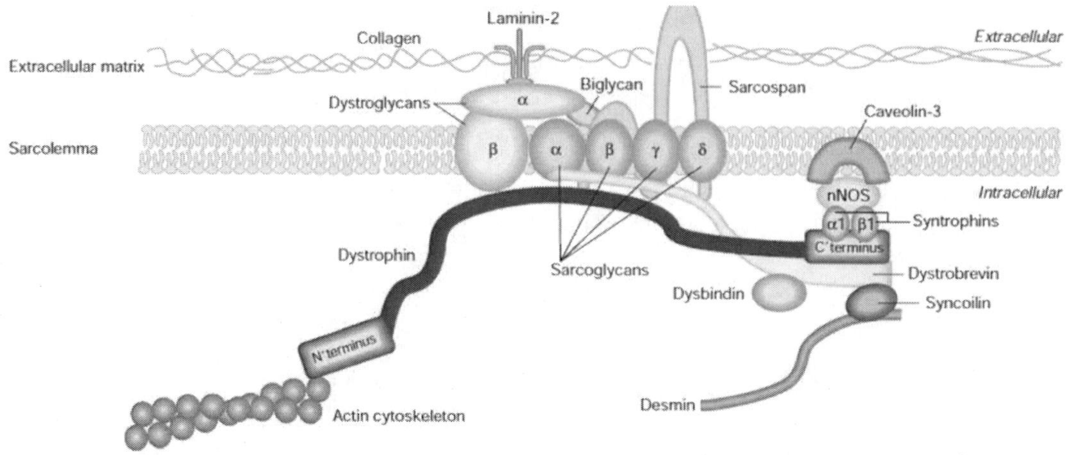


Figure 1. Protein complex associated with dystrophin in muscle connecting the inner cytoskeleton to the extracellular matrix. NOS, nitric oxide synthase.

## MYOTONIC DYSTROPHY

Myotonic dystrophies (DMs) are a group of AD multiple systemic diseases with changeable phenotypes, defined by the International Myotonic Dystrophy Consortium as a clinical syndrome that contains different subtypes defined as DM type 1, DM type 2, DM type 3, and so on (Huang & Kuo, 2005). DM is one of the most common muscular dystrophies seen in 1 in 8,000 people worldwide. Patients may have heterogeneous multisystemic symptoms with myotonia, development of cataracts, progressive muscle feebleness, and heart defects (Cho, & Tapscott, 2007).

It has been determined that DM1 is caused by the expansion of the "CTG" repeat in the DM protein kinase gene on chromosome (chr) 19, while DM2 is caused by the expansion of the "CCTG" repeat in the zinc finger protein 9 gene on chr 3. Since DM1 and DM2 have similar clinical results, the diagnosis of these 2 diseases must be approved by genetic analysis methods (Huang & Kuo, 2005). Unlike DM2, the DM1 locus has a congenital form (Cho & Tapscott, 2007). DM3 is a multisystem myotonic disease by frontotemporal dementia and involves a link to chr 15q21-24 (Huang & Kuo, 2005). DM1 and DM2 are associated with the separation of RNA binding proteins and a re-expansion due to misregulated alternative splicing. Misregulation of alternative placement is the root cause of symptoms observed in DM1 and DM2. Myotonia and cataracts accompanying muscle weakness can be seen in DM1 and DM2. The clinical findings of myotonic DM1 and DM2 are given in Table 2 (Johnson, 2019).

**Table 2. Comparison of Myotonic Dystrophies**

| | DM1 | DM2 |
|---|---|---|
| Prevalence | 1 per 2500 | Unknown |
| Gene mutation | CTG repeat in 3' UTR of the DMPK gene | Intronic CCTG repeat in the CNBP gene |
| Age of onset | Birth to adulthood | Early to late adulthood |
| Pattern of weakness | Distal muscles, face | Proximal muscles |
| Myotonia/pain | Prominent myotonia | Prominent pain |

## Fasioscapulohumeral Muscular Dystrophy (FSHD)

FSHD is the most common inherited myopathy and predicted to affect 1 in 8333 people worldwide. According to the linkage analysis results, the FSHD genetic locus on chromosome 4q35 was identified. FSHD1 and FSHD2 constitute two forms of the disease. According to recent studies, it has been revealed that genes related to FSHD2 may have disease-modifying effects on FSHD1 and it may be necessary to examine FSHD2 genes in FSHD1 patients. The classical form of the disease (FSHD1) has been demonstrated to be associated with DNA rearrangements in this region, which consists of a sequence of tandem units known as D4Z4. It is called FSHD2, the alternative form of the disease, and can be said to occur much less commonly than the different and classical type (Zampatt et al., 2019).

FSHD1 and FSHD2 encompass a disease process in which genetic defects (e.g., D4Z4 constriction in the chromosome) and epigenetic defects (e.g., mutations in D4Z4 suppressing factors such as SMCHD1 and DNMT3B) are determined by a combination. All forms of FSHD are associated with the epigenetic irregularity of the D4Z4 macrosatellite sequence at 4q35, resulting in abnormal expression of the DUX4 retrogene in skeletal muscle and pathology. DUX4 is a leading transcription factor that activates gene expression during early human development, with most DUX4 expression silenced in the somatic cell. FSHD asymptomatic individuals resist increased epigenetic stress and activation at the FSHD locus. D4Z4/DUX4 upstream regulators can offer selective therapeutic targets, reducing the likelihood of deleterious off-target effects (Himeda & Jones, 2019).

## Emery-Dreifuss Muscular Dystrophy (EDMD)

Laminopathies caused by mutations in the LMNA gene are defined as a continuous spectrum of sequential phenotypes. The frequency of EDMD is 0.13:100,000-0.2:100,000. Most of the variants that cause EDMD show an AD inheritance. Single nucleotide mutations, insertions and deletions occur in one of the 2 LMNA alleles. Some of the patients have been found to have an X-linked EDMD associated with mutations in the EMD gene encoding emerin on the X chromosome. EDMD manifests itself as slow progressive muscle weakness, joint contractures and heart disease in patients in the middle of childhood (Bianchi et al., 2018).

Germinal mosaicism in the LMNA gene is possible and should be differentiated in terms of a recessive trait in families with several affected siblings. In the case of XL-EDMD, the complete deletion of the gene may be due to an inversion within the Xq28 region, and almost a quarter of the cases carry this inversion. Almost all mutations are null mutations (stop, splice site mutation or out-of-frame deletion/insertion) and rare cases (due to a rare missense mutation) with a small amount of protein may have a milder phenotype. FHL1 mutations mainly lead to truncated proteins and the absence or high reduction of FHL1 proteins (Bonne & Quijano-Roy, 2013). Pathogenetic mechanisms leading to variability in clinical phenotypes of EDMD are unclear. For patients with frameshift mutations, it is anticipated that late onset phenotypes may result from the secondary loss of function of haplotype deficiency, whereas the dominant negative or toxic gain of function in these early onset phenotypes is associated with increased severity. At histological and histochemical levels, both X-EDMD and AD-EDMD are similar in the degree of muscle-related changes (Brown et al., 2008).

## Oculopharyngeal Muscular Dystrophy (OPMD)

OPMD is a late-onset muscle disease associated with progressive ptosis of the eyelids and unique tubulopathy lamentous intranuclear inclusions in skeletal muscle and belongs to the autosomal dominant myopathy group. Identification of PABPN1 mutations is important in the pathophysiology of OPMD. When looking at OPMD cases in the community, there is a high mutation diversity that reveals the presence of large independent original mutations. AD and AR OPMD were found to be allelic. According to the cloning strategy, the (GCN) 12-17 expansion of the PABPN1 gene was demonstrated in all predominant cases of OPMD (Brais, 2009). The age of onset and severity of the OPMD phenotype are determined by gene dosage. The most severe OPMD phenotype remains valid for individuals who are homozygous for 2 dominant OPMD mutations.

PABPN1 contains a polyalanine tract; a coil-coiled domain important for the stimulation of the poly(A) polymerase, a ribonucleoprotein-motif RNA-binding domain essential for self-interaction, a nuclear localization signal and two oligomerization regions that overlap the RNA-binding domain and the NLS (Brais, 2011). AD OPMD occurs due to GCG triple replacements in the polyadenylation binding protein 2 gene localized on 14q11, while AR OPMD occurs due to a double dose of the GCG 7 PABP2 allele. OPMD patients with clinical and pathological evidence of neuropathy associated with muscle pathology were also seen. Understanding the spectrum of neurophysiological changes associated with OPMD, distinguishing them from other neuromuscular disorders and making an accurate genetic examination in atypical cases may contribute (Luigetti et al., 2015).

## Distal Muscular Dystrophy

Distal myopathies are genetic disorders with progressive loss of muscle tissue called distal muscular dystrophies. Distal dystrophies have a distal onset and are found to be more distal than proximal throughout the course of the disease. Some distal dystrophies (such as myosynopathy) start very early. In the early forms, the defects in the muscles are mostly congenital; signs such as drop foot occur when patients start walking (Udd, 2007).

As a result of advances in molecular genetics and immunohistochemical techniques, genetics have identified many distal dystrophies related to the underlying cause. Although the specific chromosomal localization has been clarified, it is also possible to understand the molecular pathophysiology early in some. The defect gene is present in Miyoshi myopathy, distal myopathy with edged vacuoles, tibial muscular dystrophy and early onset distal myopathy. The majority of genes that cause distal muscular dystrophy encode protein components of the sarcomere, many of which cause defects in sarcolemmal proteins (Udd, 2009).

## Limb-Girdle Muscular Dystrophy (LGMD)

LGMD is defined as non-congenital genetic muscle disorders that cause weakness of proximal limb muscles in the first stage, and vary in the age of onset. There are 8 AD subtypes and 26 AR subtypes of LGMD. Many subtypes of LGMD may have associated cardiac manifestations. LGMD may arise from pathogenic genetic variants that cause abnormal protein synthesis in various areas of the muscle fiber including the nucleus, sarcoplasma, and extracellular matrix. The low estimated incidence of LGMD is 1 to 6 per 100,000 (Chu & Moran, 2018). It is known that the average prevalence of LGMD is

1-6 per 100,000 people. More than 30 genes are associated with the condition, and it is expected that the number of associated genes will increase as the number of genetic tests becomes more frequent. Although clinical symptoms vary according to subtypes, many of them are present as congenital disorders. Present symptoms may include myoglobinuria and hyperemia, and distal limb weakness. Symptomatic cardiopulmonary involvement is seen in about half of the subtypes of the disease (Hunter, et al., 2019).

## CONCLUSION

Hereditary muscular dystrophies are a group of hereditary diseases characterized by progressive weakness and loss of muscle mass. It is a clinically and genetically heterogeneous group of diseases. In muscle diseases, creatine kinase (CK) is usually found to be high, but there are also muscle diseases in which it is normal. If it is too high, it has more diagnostic value and may indicate certain muscle diseases. Some of the muscle diseases can be treated, and the patient can lead a completely normal life. These are usually acquired diseases. Treatment possibilities have also started to emerge in genetics. Physiotherapy is of great importance in all muscle diseases.

Duchenne and Becker muscular dystrophies are X-linked recessive neuromuscular diseases characterized by progressive muscle weakness. They begin with a similar presentation in BMD; however, the clinical course is milder, and muscle weakness is milder and less progressive. In molecular genetic studies conducted in Duchenne and Becker muscular dystrophies, deletion was found in 60-65% of patients, partial gene duplication was found in 5% of the patients, while no deletion or duplication was found in 30-35% of them. Point mutations, which are difficult to detect due to the large size of the dystrophin gene, are thought to be the cause of the disease in this 30-35% group, and an increasing number of point mutations are reported. As a result of dystrophin gene mutations, dystrophin protein can't be fully synthesized and sarcolemmal stability is impaired, causing muscle cell necrosis. When mutations were examined in patients with DMD and BMD, no difference was found in terms of the size and location of the deletion (Darras, 1990).

Myotonic dystrophy Type 1 (DM1) is caused by an increase in the number of cytosine-thymine-guanine (CTG) trinucleotide repeats in the 3' untranslated region (3'-UTR) of the dystrophia myotonica-protein kinase (DMPK) gene, which is encoded at locus 13.32 in the long leg of chromosome 19. It is the most common form of autosomal dominant adult muscular dystrophy. Clinical findings are polymorphic; It progresses with central nervous system findings together with myotonia of varying severity, amyotrophy, cataract, endocrine disorders and cardiac myopathy. Mental retardation is seen in congenital cases, and behavioral disorders such as obsessive compulsive disorder, schizotypal personality disorder, lack of empathy and cognitive loss are seen in the adult form (Sistiaga et al., 2010).

Fasioscapulohumeral muscular dystrophy; this is a muscular dystrophy with autosomal dominant inheritance, weakness and atrophy of facial muscles, and periscapular-perihumeral muscles. It is known that the disease shows a connection with the 4q35 region (Zouvelou et al., 2009). Emery-Dreifuss muscular dystrophy (EDMD) is an inherited disease characterized by contracture that occurs in early childhood, mild muscle weakness that manifests later, and cardiac involvement in all adult patients. X-linked recessive, autosomal dominant and autosomal recessive mutations have been detected on four different genes so far (emerin, lamin A/C, nesprin, domain genes) (Holaska et al., 2006). The onset in Emery-Dreifuss muscular dystrophies is between the neonatal period and the third decade. The clinical picture varies even within the same family. In laboratory examinations; While the CK level may be found to be normal or elevated, electroneuromyography (EMG) may also reveal neurogenic potentials as well as myogenic changes (Alzira et al., 2000).

Oculopharyngodistal myopathy (OPDM) is an extremely rare hereditary myopathy with early adult onset, inherited autosomal dominant (AD). It has also been shown genetically that the disease is a different myopathy. Progressive oculopharyngeal and distal muscle weakness are the most prominent features of the disease. The genetic defect that causes the disease is GCG repeat increases in the nuclear poly(A) binding protein-1 (PABN-1; PABP2) gene in the 14q11.2-q13 region. The worst OPDM phenotype was observed in patients homozygous for the AD mutation in PABPN1. CK is slightly elevated. EMG is myopathic. Muscle biopsy has red-rimmed vacuoles. Electron microscopically, very thin filaments are shown in muscle fibers and nuclei and are diagnostic. The definitive diagnosis is made by demonstrating the mutation in genetic examination (Abu-Baker & Rouleau, 2007). Limb-girdle muscular dystrophies (LGMD) are a subgroup of autosomal dominant or recessive, highly heterogeneous muscular dystrophies. These progress with limb-extremity type involvement. In this group of diseases, the symptoms of which begin in childhood or adulthood, there are diseases that have clinically similar characteristics. There are eighteen variants of limb-girdle muscular dystrophies. Seven of them show autosomal dominant inheritance and eleven show autosomal recessive inheritance. One of the limb-girdle muscular dystrophies is LGMD2B. LGMD2B arises as a result of disruption of the structure of the dysferlin protein and its presence in the cell (Bansal & Campbell, 2004).

In this chapter, it is important to decide which gene to examine in the clinical diagnosis of patients and to determine the genetic disorder that causes the disease. Despite this genotypic difference, phenotypic features are similar in many of the diseases and differential diagnosis is very difficult, and sometimes impossible in the clinical plan. Therefore, differential diagnosis requires DNA analysis. However, due to the troublesome and expensive mutation screening of many known genes today, immunohistochemical examination for the relevant protein in muscle tissue or revealing the protein quality with Western blot and confirming the diagnosis by genetic examination for the existing protein defect have become the gold standard in these dystrophies. The use of genetic tests in the clinic has provided the clarification of the etiology-pathogenesis relationship of hereditary muscular dystrophies and opened new horizons in diagnosis and treatment. A better understanding of the pathological mechanisms leading to hereditary muscle diseases has paved the way for specific treatment options for the disorders. These developments in the field of treatment have increased the importance of making a definitive diagnosis with genetic evaluations based on clinical clues.

## REFERENCES

Aartsma-Rus, A., Ginjaar, I. B., & Bushby, K. (2016). The importance of genetic diagnosis for Duchenne muscular dystrophy. *Journal of Medical Genetics*, 53(3), 145-51.

Abu-Baker, A., Rouleau, G. A. (2007). Oculopharyngeal muscular dystrophy: Recent advances in the understanding of the molecular pathogenic mechanisms and treatment strategies. *Biochimica et Biophysica Acta*, 1772, 173–185.

Alzira, A. C., Jose, A. L., Paulo, G., Suely, N. M., Eduardo, A. S., Maurícıo, S. (2000). Emery-Dreifuss muscular dystrophy anotomical-clinical corelation. *Arq. Neuropsiquiatr.*, 58 (4), 1123-27.

Bansal, D., Campbell, K. (2004). Dysferlin and the plasma membrane repair in muscle dystrophy. *Trends Cell Biol.*, 14 (4):206-213.

Barthélémy, F., & Wein, N. (2018). Personalized gene and cell therapy for Duchenne Muscular Dystrophy. *Neuromuscular Disorders*, 28(10), 803-824.

Bianchi, A., Manti, P. G., Lucini, F., Lanzuolo, C. (2018). Mechanotransduction, nuclear architecture and epigenetics in Emery Dreifuss Muscular Dystrophy: tous pour un, un pour tous. *Nucleus*, 9(1), 276–290.

Bonne, G., & Quijano-Roy, S. (2013). Emery-Dreifuss muscular dystrophy, laminopathies, and other nuclear envelopathies. *Handbook of Clinical Neurology*, 113, 1367-76.

Brais, B. (2009). Oculopharyngeal muscular dystrophy: a polyalanine myopathy. *Current Neurology and Neuroscience Reports*, 9(1), 76-82.

Brais, B. (2011). Oculopharyngeal muscular dystrophy. *Handbook of Clinical Neurology*, 101, 181-92.

Brown, S. C., Piercy, R. J., Muntoni, F., Sewry, C. A. (2008). Investigating the pathology of Emery–Dreifuss muscular dystrophy. *Biochemical Society Transactions*, 36 (6), 1335–1338.

Brusa, R., Magri, F., Bresolin, N., Comi, G. P., & Corti, S. (2020). Noncoding RNAs in Duchenne and Becker muscular dystrophies: role in pathogenesis and future prognostic and therapeutic perspectives. *Cellular and Molecular Life Sciences*, 77(21), 4299-4313.

Cardamone, M., Darras, B. T., Ryan, M. M. (2008). Inherited myopathies and muscular dystrophies. *Seminars in Neurology*, 28(2):250-9.

Cho, D. H., & Tapscott, S. J. (2007). Myotonic dystrophy: Emerging mechanisms for DM1 and DM2. *Biochimica et Biophysica Acta*, 1772(2), 195-204.

Chu, M. L., & Moran, E. (2018). The Limb–Girdle Muscular Dystrophies: Is Treatment on the Horizon? *Neurotherapeutics*, 15(4):849-862.

Darras, B. T. (1990). Molecular genetics of Duchenne and Becker muscular dystrophy. *The Journal of Pediatrics*, 117(1), 1-15.

Emery, A. E. H. (2002). The muscular dystrophies. *Lancet*, 359(9307), 687-95.

Himeda, L. C., & Jones, P. L. (2019). The Genetics and Epigenetics of Facioscapulohumeral Muscular Dystrophy. *Annual Review of Genomics and Human Genetics*, 20, 265-291.

Holaska, J. M., & Wilson, K. L. (2006). Multiple roles for emerin: implications for Emery-Dreifuss muscular dystrophy. *Anat. Rec. A Discov. Mol. Cell Evol. Biol.*, 288 (7), 676–80.

Huang, C. C., & Kuo, H. C. (2005). Myotonic Dystrophies. *Chang Gung Medical Journal*, 28(8), 517-26.

Hunter, M., Heatwole, C., Wicklund, M., Weihl, C. C., Mozaffar, T., Statland, J. M., Johnson, N. E. (2019). Limb-girdle muscular dystrophy: A perspective from adult patients on what matters most. *Muscle & Nerve*, 60(4):419-424.

Johnson, N. E. (2019). Myotonic Muscular Dystrophies. *Continuum*, 25(6), 1682-1695.

Luigetti, M., Lo Monaco, M., Mirabella, M., Primiano, G., Lucchini, M., Monforte, M., Servidei, S. (2015). Oculopharyngeal muscular dystrophy: Clinical and neurophysiological features. *Clinical Neurophysiology*, 126(12), 1-2.

Udd, B. (2009). Genetics and Pathogenesis of Distal Muscular Dystrophies. *Advances in Experimental Medicine and Biology*, 652:23-38.

Udd, B. (2007). Molecular biology of distal muscular dystrophies—Sarcomeric proteins on top. *Biochimica et Biophysica Acta*, 1772(2):145-58.

Nowak, K. J., & Davies, K. E. (2004). Duchenne muscular dystrophy and dystrophin: pathogenesis and opportunities for treatment. *EMBO reports*, 5(9), 872–876.

Sistiaga, A., Urreta, I., Jodar, M., Cobo, A. M., Emparanza, J., Otaegui, D., Poza, J. J., Merino, J. J., Imaz, H., Martí-Massó, J. F., López de Munain, A. (2010). Cognitive/personality pattern and triplet expansion size in adult myotonic dystrophy type 1 (DM1):CTG repeats, cognition and personality in DM1. *Psychol. Med.*, 40 (3), 487-495.

Zampatt, S., Colantoni, L., Strafella, C., Galota, R. M., Caputo, V., Campoli, G., Pagliaroli, G., Carboni, S., Mela, J., Peconi, C., Gambardella, S., Cascella, R., Giardina, E. (2019). Facioscapulohumeral muscular dystrophy (FSHD) molecular diagnosis: from traditional technology to the NGS era. *Neurogenetics*, 20(2), 57-64.

Zouvelou, V., Manta, P., Kalfakis, N., Evdokimidis, I., Vassilopoulos, D. (2009). Asymptomatic elevation of serum creatine kinase leading to the diagnosis of 4q35 facioscapulohumeral muscular dystrophy. *J. Clin. Neurosci.*, 16 (9), 1218-1219.

In: Musculoskeletal Pain (Common Clinical Presentations) ISBN: 978-1-68507-410-4
Editors: Mehmet Cenk Turgut and Serdar Toy 

*Chapter 32*

# PAIN IN MUSCULOSKELETAL TUMORS

***Ali Erkan Yenigül, MD and Erhan Okay*, MD***
[1]Department of Orthopedics and Traumatology,
Uludağ University Faculty of Medicine, Bursa, Turkey
[2]Department of Orthopedics and Traumatology,
Istanbul Göztepe Prof. Dr. Suleyman Yalcin City Hospital, Istanbul, Turkey

## ABSTRACT

Pain is the most common complaint in musculoskeletal tumors. It should be addressed appropriately to increase the health quality of life of these patients. There are operative and medical treatment options. The treatment should be individualized according to the patient's general status, stage of the disease, and estimated life expectancy. This chapter will give an overview of the management of pain in musculoskeletal tumors.

## INTRODUCTION

Bone is a common site for metastasis. In metastatic bone disease, the health quality of life of the patient is disturbed. Pain in musculoskeletal tumors is a devastating symptom. Various studies stated that pain in cancer patients had an overall prevalence of 52-72% (Kuo et al., 2011). Therefore, the alleviation of pain by medical or interventional treatment directly affects the well-being of this patient group.

* Corresponding Author's E-mail: erhanokay@ yahoo.com.

In pathogenesis, nerve fibers innervating bone are sensitive to cancer/stromal cells. Stromal cells produce pain-generating molecules like bradykinin, endothelins, prostaglandins, and proteases. When tumor cells have metastasized to the skeleton, there is a dull, constant, and gradually increasing pain. Peripheral nociceptors innervate to the periosteum, which is responsible for pain development (Mercadante, 1997). Pain is the most common symptom in patients with musculoskeletal tumors. Pain can develop episodically or immediately (Glithero, 2020). It is essential to differentiate carcinogenic pain from other pain-related diseases like fibromyalgia, arthritis and osteoporosis (Krajnik & Zylicz, 2013). Patients with musculoskeletal tumors can have swelling, restricted motion, and pathologic fracture in the metastatic region. The most critical step in pain evaluation is the duration and characteristics of the pain, whether the pain is intense at night or a history of trauma is present. Minimal physical activity and tenderness with palpation are indicative of malignancy (Mantyh, 2013).

The most common primary bone malignancies are osteosarcoma, chondrosarcoma, and Ewing sarcoma. These tumors are located mainly in the upper and lower extremities. The diagnosis can be delayed until the patient becomes symptomatic. These rapidly growing tumors can invade adjacent soft tissues. Chondrogenic and osteogenic cells can proliferate and destroy the periosteal structures.

Pain is present mainly in the affected limb. The emergence of symptoms varies depending on various types of tumors. The lag time in osteosarcoma and Ewing sarcoma is 56 and 72 days, respectively (Pollock et al., 1991). In soft tissue tumors, symptoms are not observed quickly compared to bone tumors. In these tumors, the limp is the most frequent complaint, and the lesions grow gradually. Pain can present or not. In managing pain in musculoskeletal tumors, an improved understanding of the biological process of cancer pain has supported the treatment strategy so far.

The treatment can be pharmacological, surgical, and minimally invasive techniques. Pharmacological options include opioids, NSAIDs, steroids, bone-directed therapies, chemotherapeutic agents, and hormonal therapy. External beam radiation, tumor ablative techniques, and intrathecal analgesics are invasive approaches. Surgical treatments aim to stabilize an impending fracture (Ahmad et al., 2018; Smith & Mohsin, 2013). The type of pain determines the therapeutic option. The pain can be nociceptive due to tissue damage, or somatic or visceral due to disturbance in the nervous system. Paracetamol and NSAIDs are used in mild pain. When pain intensity increases to mild to moderate, codeine, tramadol, dihydrocodeine, and non-opioid analgesics should be considered. In moderate to severe pain, potent opioids like morphine, methadone, oxycodone, hydromorphone, fentanyl, and buprenorphine are preferred. Corticosteroids, antiepileptic, and antidepressant drugs can be prescribed for every patient. If pain has a persistent or breakthrough course, percutaneous techniques, surgical techniques, neuromodulation, and intrathecal drug delivery should be considered (Ripamonti et al., 2012; Schweiger et al., 2013).

Medical treatment should begin with non-opioids. NSAIDs and paracetamol are the first choices. These drugs should be given in periodic intervals. The duration of analgesics should be planned to determine the period. The period can be diminished according to pain intensity. The response to NSAIDs is variable. Thus, there is no optimal dosage. Side effects should be taken into account during dosage increases (Vargas-Schaffer, 2010). Corticosteroids have a supportive role in neuropathic and bone pain treatment. Their efficacy is not apparent (Leppert & Buss, 2012). A recent meta-analysis stated that corticosteroids could provide moderate pain relief and a protective analgesic effect after radiotherapy-induced pain. The adverse effects should be considered (Lim et al., 2017). Bisphosphonates are effective in pain relief. Where pain is resistant to analgesics or radiotherapy, the use of bisphosphonates is the next step (Wong & Wiffen, 2002). There is evidence to support the effectiveness of bisphosphonates in providing some pain relief for bone metastases (D'Oronzo et al., 2021). Rosen et al., found that treatment with 4 mg of zoledronic acid also delayed the onset of skeletal complications and pain (Rosen et al., 2004). Osteoclastic and osteoblastic activities cause mechanical instability. A compression fracture can develop in vertebral metastasis. In this situation, cementation and augmentation of the vertebra are necessary. When there is a fracture with neurological compromise and severe pain, surgical stabilization is necessary. When the expected survival is beyond 6 months, durable implants such as endoprosthesis should be performed in pathologic fractures. When the expected survival is less than six months, a less invasive approach like intramedullary nailing, plate fixation, or radiotherapy is considered. Adjuvant radiotherapy is complementary after stabilization of a complete pathologic fracture or an impending fracture. Radiofrequency ablation (RFA) is another invasive option. It provides pain relief in the short term. Di Staso obtained more pain relief at 12 weeks after radiofrequency ablation with or without radiotherapy (Di Staso et al., 2011). The performance status and cancer type determine the analgesic effect of radiotherapy (Habberstadvd, 2021).

## Conclusion

The management of pain in musculoskeletal tumors needs collaboration between algology, physical therapy and rehabilitation, and oncology, radiation oncology, and surgical departments. The risks and benefits of each treatment should be analyzed for every patient.

## REFERENCES


Ahmad, I., Ahmed, M. M., Ahsraf, M. F., Naeem, A., Tasleem, A., Ahmed, M., & Farooqi, M. S. (2018). Pain Management in Metastatic Bone Disease: A Literature Review. *Cureus*, *10*(9), e3286-e3286. PubMed. https://doi.org/10.7759/cureus.3286.

Di Staso, M., Zugaro, L., Gravina, G., Bonfili, P., Marampon, F., Di Nicola, L., Conchiglia, A., Ventura, L., Franzese, P., & Gallucci, M. (2011). A feasibility study of percutaneous radiofrequency ablation followed by radiotherapy in the management of painful osteolytic bone metastases. *European radiology*, *21*(9), 2004-2010.

D'Oronzo, S., Wood, S., & Brown, J. (2021). The use of bisphosphonates to treat skeletal complications in solid tumours. *Bone*, *147*, 115907.

Glithero, C. (2020). The Challenges of Managing Bone Pain in Cancer. *The Ulster Medical Journal*, *89*(1), 7-10. PubMed.

Habberstad, R., Frøseth, T. C. S., Aass, N., Bjerkeset, E., Abramova, T., Garcia-Alonso, E., Caputo, M., Rossi, R., Boland, J. W., Brunelli, C., Lund, J.-Å., Kaasa, S., & Klepstad, P. (2021). Clinical Predictors for Analgesic Response to Radiotherapy in Patients with Painful Bone Metastases. *Journal of Pain and Symptom Management*. https://doi.org/10.1016/j.jpainsymman.2021.03.022.

Krajnik, M., & Zylicz, Z. B. (2013). Pain assessment, recognising clinical patterns, and cancer pain syndromes. İçinde *Cancer Pain* (ss. 95-108). Springer.

Kuo, P., Yen, J., Parker, G., Chapman, S., Kandikattu, S., Sohanpal, I., Barbachano, Y., & Williams, J. (2011). The prevalence of pain in patients attending sarcoma outpatient clinics. *Sarcoma*, *2011*.

Leppert, W., & Buss, T. (2012). The role of corticosteroids in the treatment of pain in cancer patients. *Current Pain and Headache Reports*, *16*(4), 307-313. PubMed. https://doi.org/10.1007/s11916-012-0273-z.

Lim, F. M., Bobrowski, A., Agarwal, A., & Silva, M. F. (2017). Use of corticosteroids for pain control in cancer patients with bone metastases: A comprehensive literature review. *Current opinion in supportive and palliative care*, *11*(2), 78-87.

Mantyh, P. (2013). Bone cancer pain: Causes, consequences, and therapeutic opportunities. *PAIN®*, *154*, S54-S62.

Mercadante, S. (1997). Malignant bone pain: Pathophysiology and treatment. *Pain*, *69*(1-2), 1-18.

Pollock, B. H., Krischer, J. P., & Vietti, T. J. (1991). Interval between symptom onset and diagnosis of pediatric solid tumors. *The Journal of pediatrics*, *119*(5), 725-732.

Ripamonti, C., Santini, D., Maranzano, E., Berti, M., & Roila, F. (2012). Management of cancer pain: ESMO clinical practice guidelines. *Annals of oncology*, *23*, vii139-vii154.

Rosen, L. S., Gordon, D., Tchekmedyian, N. S., Yanagihara, R., Hirsh, V., Krzakowski, M., Pawlicki, M., De Souza, P., Zheng, M., & Urbanowitz, G. (2004). Long-term efficacy and safety of zoledronic acid in the treatment of skeletal metastases in patients with nonsmall cell lung carcinoma and other solid tumors: A randomized, phase III, double-blind, placebo-controlled trial. *Cancer*, *100*(12), 2613-2621.

Schweiger, V., Polati, E., Paladini, A., & Varrassi, G. (2013). Interventional Techniques in Cancer Pain: Critical Appraisal. İçinde *Cancer Pain* (ss. 231-247). Springer.

Smith, H. S., & Mohsin, I. (2013). Painful boney metastases. *The Korean journal of pain*, *26*(3), 223.

Vargas-Schaffer, G. (2010). Is the WHO analgesic ladder still valid? Twenty-four years of experience. *Canadian Family Physician Medecin de Famille Canadien*, *56*(6), 514-e205. PubMed.

Wong, R., & Wiffen, P. J. (2002). Bisphosphonates for the relief of pain secondary to bone metastases. *The Cochrane Database of Systematic Reviews*, *2002*(2), CD002068-CD002068. PubMed. https://doi.org/ 10.1002/14651858.CD002068.

In: Musculoskeletal Pain (Common Clinical Presentations) ISBN: 978-1-68507-410-4
Editors: Mehmet Cenk Turgut and Serdar Toy 

*Chapter 33*

# Clinical Management of Neuropathic Pain

***Burcu Bulut Okay**, *MD***
Department of Neurology,
Fatih Sultan Mehmet Education
and Research Hospital, Istanbul, Turkey

## Abstract

Neuropathic pain is defined as burning, stinging, pricking, tingling, squeezing, and chills. Metabolic, infectious, autoimmune, inflammatory and trauma-related diseases of the peripheral and central nervous system may cause neuropathic pain.

Neuropathic pain occurs in 7 - 10% of the population. The quality of life of neuropathic pain patients was found to be low due to the ineffectiveness of neuropathic pain treatments and misdiagnosis.

In neurology practice, we see patients with neuropathic pain very often. The patients with neuropathic pain have chronic diseases and multidrug usage. However, the treatment of neuropathic pain is limited to pharmacological treatments in a daily routine. Alternative non-pharmacological therapies are increasingly being offered to patients in recent years.

* Corresponding Author's E-mail: burcublt@gmail.com.

**Keywords**: Pain, neuropathic pain, chronic pain, neuropathic pain treatment, polyneuropathy

## INTRODUCTION

Neuropathic pain occurs with a direct lesion and/or dysfunction of the somatosensory nervous system. In the ICD 11 classification, it is categorized as peripheral and central neuropathic pain according to the localization of the lesion or disease (Finnerup et al. 2016; Scholz et al. 2019). Neuropathic pain is defined as burning, stinging, pricking, tingling, squeezing, and chills. Metabolic, infectious, autoimmune, inflammatory and trauma-related diseases of the peripheral and central nervous system may cause neuropathic pain.

In our daily practice, pharmacological treatments are primarily applied in the initial treatment of neuropathic pain. Complementary non-pharmacological treatments such as non-invasive neurostimulation and invasive interventional techniques and psychotherapy have recently started to be applied more frequently. Due to the ineffectiveness of drugs, drug side effects, and avoidance of drug-drug interactions due to polypharmacy in elderly patients, the need for multidisciplinary approaches and personalized medical and interventional treatment combinations has increased (Moisset et al. 2020).

## EPIDEMIOLOGY

Neuropathic pain occurs in 7 - 10% of the population. The quality of life of neuropathic pain patients was found to be low due to the ineffectiveness of neuropathic pain treatments and misdiagnosis (Colloca et al. 2017).

## DIAGNOSIS

Because neuropathic pain symptoms are subjective and clinical signs are minimal or absent, a staging system has been developed. According to this staging system, neuropathic pain is classified as probable, possible, and definite. The diagnosis of neuropathic pain is made by neurological examination and history, anatomical localization of sensory findings, and confirmatory tests (Finnerup et al. 2016).

## DISEASE-BASED AND ANATOMY-BASED CLASSIFICATION

### Peripheral Neuropathies

These are focal neuropathies like phantom pain, trigeminal neuralgia and generalized polyneuropathies caused by diabetes, alcoholism, amyloidosis, infections, drugs and toxins.

### Central Pain Syndromes

These are vascular lesions (especially in the brainstem and thalamus), traumatic brain and spinal cord injury, multiple sclerosis, Parkinson's disease, epilepsy, abscess, tumors, inflammatory diseases, and myelitis caused by viruses and syphilis (Baron et al. 2010).

## SCREENING TOOLS

The most common validated screening tools are the neuropathic pain questionnaire, the doleur neuropathique 4 questions, painDETECT and the Leeds assessment of neuropathic symptoms and signs (Colloca et al. 2017).

## TREATMENT

The treatment of neuropathic pain is challenging. Epidemiological surveys have shown that ≤ 50% of patients experience satisfactory pain relief (Dworkin et al. 2007).

Antidepressants, anticonvulsants, tricyclic antidepressants, opioid analgesics, and local anesthetics are used in the pharmacological treatment of neuropathic pain.

Interventional and non-pharmacological strategies are neurostimulation therapies, nerve blocks, psychotherapy and invasive procedures like surgery.

In this chapter, we focus on the pharmacological treatment of peripheral neuropathic pain.

### First-Line Medications

Antidepressants with both norepinephrine and serotonin reuptake inhibition (SNRIs, duloxetine and venlafaxine) and tricyclic antidepressants (TCAs, amitriptyline, nortriptyline and imipramine) are highly recommended in neuropathic pain (Table 1) (Dworkin et al. 2007).

Calcium channel $\alpha_2$-$\delta$ ligands such as gabapentin and pregabalin are the first-line preferred agents in neuropathic pain. Dosage adjustment may be required in the presence of renal dysfunction and sedation (Table 1). To minimize adverse effects, the "start low, go slow" approach is essential for all orally administered drugs.

Topical lidocaine was found to significantly improve the pain scores of patients with postherpetic neuralgia and allodynia (Dworkin et al. 2007).

## Second-Line Medications

Opioid analgesics such as morphine, fentanyl, oxycodone, methadone and tramadol are generally considered as second-line drugs but can be used for first-line treatment in selected clinical circumstances. Patients with neuropathic pain can use opioid drugs while their first-line medication is being titrated.

Clinicians should be aware of misuse, and use the lowest effective dose.

**Table 1. Pharmacological treatment of Neuropathic pain**

| | **Drugs** | **Daily Dosages** |
|---|---|---|
| First line | TCAs | 25-150mg/day |
| | Duloksetin | 60-120mg/day |
| | Venlafaksine | 150-225mg/day |
| | Gabapentine | 1200-3600mg/day |
| | Pregabalin | 150-600mg/day |
| | Topical Lidocaine | 1-3 plasters for 12h/day |
| | Carbamazepine[a] | 600-1200mg/day |
| | Oxcarbamazepine[a] | 600-1800mg/day |
| Second line | Tramadol | 100-400mg/day |
| | Capsaicin 8% | 1-4 patches/3 months |
| | Botulinum toxin A | 50-300 U/3 months |
| | Combination | TCA or SNRIs + opioids or gabapentinoids or behavioral therapy |
| | Lamotrigine[a] | 100-400mg/day |
| Third line | rTMS | 10Hz, 1500-3000 pulses |
| | Spinal cord stimulation | |
| | Valproate | 600-2400mg/day |
| | Levetiracetam | 1000-3000mg/day |
| | Topiramate | 100-400mg/day |
| | Morphine and oxycodone | 50-150mg |

a: trigeminal neuralgia.

## Third-Line Medications

Antiepileptic drugs used in the treatment of neuropathic pain include carbamazepine, oxcarbazepine, lamotrigine, lacosamide, gabapentin and pregabalin. Antiepileptics act by stabilizing neuronal membranes, increasing synaptic inhibition or reducing synaptic excitation. Carbamazepine and oxcarbazepine cause voltage-dependent sodium channel inactivation, further reducing excitatory neurotransmitter release. The side effects and drug interactions of carbamazepine are obvious, as it causes autoinduction. Oxcarbazepine has fewer side effects. Both agents can be used in diabetic neuropathy, postherpetic neuralgia, and trigeminal neuralgia.

The use of cannabinoids such as transmural nabiximols and oral tetrahyrocannabinol is inconclusive in neuropathic pain. High concentration capsaicin patches are considered for the treatment of neuropathic pain but there is insufficient evidence to support the usefulness of oral/intravenous ketamine, intravenous lidocaine, subcutaneous botulinum toxin A, NMDA antagonists, mexiletine and topical clonidine (Moisset et al. 2020).

## Interventional Therapies

### *Neural Blockade and Steroid Injections*

Epidural/perineural steroid and lidocaine injections are recommended for the treatment of cervical/lumbar radiculopathies and acute zoster-associated and compression-related peripheral neuropathic pain (Dworkin et al. 2013).

### *Peripheral and Central Neurostimulation Therapy*

There is insufficient evidence to support the usefulness of transcutaneous electrical nerve stimulation (TENS), repetitive transcranial magnetic stimulation (rTMS), epidural motor cortex stimulation (ECMS), pulsed radiofrequency, spinal cord stimulation, deep brain stimulation and intrathecal therapies in neuropathic pain.

### *Physical Therapies*

Exercise and mirror therapy can be used in neuropathic pain but need further investigation.

### *Psychological Therapies*

Cognitive-behavioral therapy and a mindfulness-based stress reduction program are reported to be effective when combined with other therapies.

***Other Miscellaneous Non-Drug Treatments***

Aromatherapy, auricular acupuncture, massage, low-level laser therapy, vitamin E supplementation, hypnosis, therapeutic patient education, mirror therapy, musicotherapy, art therapy, mesotherapy, and tai chi can be used in neuropathic pain treatment but the quality of evidence is low and inconclusive (3).

## CONCLUSION

In neurology practice, we see patients with neuropathic pain very often. Patients with neuropathic pain have chronic diseases and multidrug usage. However, the treatment of neuropathic pain is limited to pharmacological treatments in a daily routine. Alternative non-pharmacological therapies are increasingly being offered to patients in recent years.

The management of neuropathic pain is challenging. Neuropathic pain is a burden for patients, caregivers, and physicians. To relieve pain and improve quality of life in patients with neuropathic pain we need multidisciplinary approaches, personalized medical and interventional treatment combinations and further investigations.

## REFERENCES

Baron, R., Binder, A. and Wasner, G. (2010). Neuropathic pain: Diagnosis, pathophysiological mechanisms, and treatment. *The Lancet Neurology*, 9(8), 807 - 819.

Colloca, L., Ludman, T., Bouhassira, D., Baron, R., Dickenson, A. H., Yarnitsky, D., Freeman, R., Truini, A., Attal, N., Finnerup, N. B., Eccleston, C., Kalso, E., Bennett, D. L., Dworkin, R. H. and Raja, S. N. (2017). Neuropathic pain. *Nature Reviews. Disease Primers*, 3, 17002 - 17002. PubMed. https://doi.org/10.1038/nrdp.2017.2.

Dworkin, R. H., O'connor, A. B., Backonja, M., Farrar, J. T., Finnerup, N. B., Jensen, T. S., Kalso, E. A., Loeser, J. D., Miaskowski, C. and Nurmikko, T. J. (2007). Pharmacologic management of neuropathic pain: Evidence-based recommendations. *Pain*, 132(3), 237 - 251.

Dworkin, R. H., O'Connor, A. B., Kent, J., Mackey, S. C., Raja, S. N., Stacey, B. R., Levy, R. M., Backonja, M., Baron, R. and Harke, H. (2013). Interventional management of neuropathic pain: NeuPSIG recommendations. *PAIN®*, 154(11), 2249 - 2261.

Finnerup, N. B., Haroutounian, S., Kamerman, P., Baron, R., Bennett, D. L., Bouhassira, D., Cruccu, G., Freeman, R., Hansson, P. and Nurmikko, T. (2016). Neuropathic pain: An updated grading system for research and clinical practice. *Pain*, 157(8), 1599.

Moisset, X., Bouhassira, D., Couturier, J. A., Alchaar, H., Conradi, S., Delmotte, M., Lanteri-Minet, M., Lefaucheur, J., Mick, G. and Piano, V. (2020). Pharmacological and non-pharmacological treatments for neuropathic pain: Systematic review and French recommendations. *Revue neurologique*, 176(5), 325 - 352.

Scholz, J., Finnerup, N. B., Attal, N., Aziz, Q., Baron, R., Bennett, M. I., Benoliel, R., Cohen, M., Cruccu, G. and Davis, K. D. (2019). The IASP classification of chronic pain for ICD-11: Chronic neuropathic pain. *Pain*, 160(1), 53.

In: Musculoskeletal Pain (Common Clinical Presentations) ISBN: 978-1-68507-410-4
Editors: Mehmet Cenk Turgut and Serdar Toy 

*Chapter 34*

# MERALGIA PARESTHETICA

***Onur Yıldız*, MD***
Department of Neurology, Health Sciences University,
Erzurum Regional Health Application and Research Hospital, Erzurum, Turkey

## ABSTRACT

Meralgia paresthetica (MP) is an entrapment neuropathy caused by damage to the lateral femoral cutaneous nerve (LFCN). Typical clinical manifestations of MP are numbness, tingling, pain, and dysesthesia in the anterolateral thigh area. The disease course can be spontaneous or iatrogenic. Reduction of paresthesia after local anesthetic agent injection and nerve conduction tests are the most commonly used diagnostic methods. Conservative methods should be tried first in treatment, and surgery should be chosen for resistant cases.

## INTRODUCTION

MP is a painful mononeuropathy caused by damage to the LFCN. It is most commonly entrapped under the inguinal ligament and causes loss of sensation, paresthesia, and pain in the anterolateral region of the thigh. Bernhardt first described this clinic a century ago (Freud, 1895), and Hager was the first to demonstrate its association with the LFCN (Hager, 1885). Studies have shown that it has an incidence of 43 per 100,000, and it is most commonly seen in the 30-40 age group (van Slobbe et al., 2004). Furthermore, there are claims that the disease is inherited as autosomal dominant (Richer

* Corresponding Author's E-mail: dronuryildiz@hotmail.com.

et al., 2002). In this section, after briefly mentioning LFCN anatomy, the etiology, clinic, diagnostic procedures, and treatment methods of MP will be explained.

## Anatomical Characteristics

The LFCN is a pure sensory nerve that originates from the L1, L2, and L3 spinal nerve roots and leaves the lumbar plexus. The LFCN passes under the inguinal ligament and anterior to the anterior superior iliac spine (ASIS), innervating the anterolateral region of the thigh. Despite many variations, it most often passes 1 cm medial to the ASIS at the level of the inguinal ligament. The LFCN is most commonly squeezed when exiting the pelvis, and 5 types of anatomic variations can be seen in this region. Among these variations shown in a cadaver study, the most common types A, B, and C were shown to be susceptible to mechanical trauma (Aszmann et al., 1997).

## Etiology

LFCN damage can occur due to idiopathic or iatrogenic reasons. Idiopathic causes can also be divided into mechanical or metabolic, and for this diagnosis, there should be no history of surgery that may damage the LFCN (Grossman et al., 2001). Mechanical factors include obesity (Parisi et al., 2011), pregnancy, wearing tight pants or underwear, wearing tight belts and corsets, wearing seat belts (Blake & Treble, 2004), and tumors (iliac crest, uterine). Because of their uniforms, professions such as the military and police are in the risk group (Korkmaz & Ozçakar, 2004). Alcoholism, diabetes mellitus, and lead poisoning are metabolic risk factors for MP (Philip et al., 2009). Diabetes mellitus is thought to be a risk factor because of nerve swelling (Nahabedian & Dellon, 1995). Iatrogenic causes may develop due to orthopedic and non-orthopedic surgical procedures. Operations such as total hip replacement (Ahsan & Curtin, 2001), pelvic osteotomy, acetabular fracture surgery, posterior spine surgeries, bone graft removal from the iliac crest (van den Broecke et al., 1998), inguinal hernia repair (Ger et al., 1993), hysterectomy (Hutchins et al., 1998), and cesarean can lead to iatrogenic MP. The LFCN extends at a significant angle to the inguinal ligament, and hip hyperextension during surgeries also increases the risk of MP.

## Clinical Presentation

Typical clinical manifestations of MP are numbness, tingling, pain, and dysesthesia in the anterolateral thigh area. Complaints usually subside while sitting. Walking and movements that cause hip hyperextension aggravate the pain. The clinic is usually unilateral, but bilateral complaints may occur in 20% of the patients (Ecker & Woltman, 1938). Pain occurs with compression on the medial side of the ASIS and Tinel's sign may be found in this area. Hair loss on the anterolateral thigh is a common finding. If the patient has urogenital and gastrointestinal complaints, the diagnosis of MP is doubtful. In such a situation, different pathologies should be investigated by abdominal and retroperitoneal imaging methods. Since the LFCN is a pure sensory nerve, motor weakness and reflex abnormalities are not expected in MP. The accompanying motor weakness should suggest lumbar disc disease or lumbosacral plexopathy. In such cases, nerve block application does not relieve symptoms.

## Diagnosis

Generally, the diagnosis can be made by typical anamnesis, physical examination, and general neurological examination. Additional diagnostic procedures can be performed for patients who cannot be diagnosed clearly with clinical and physical examination findings.

### Pelvic Compression Test

The pelvic compression test was first described by Nouraei et al. The examiner applies a downward compression force to the pelvis and if symptoms alleviate the test is considered positive. The pelvic compression test has a sensitivity of 95% and a specificity of 93% (Nouraei et al., 2007).

### LFCN Block Test

Showing improvement of symptoms by performing the LFCN block test with local anesthetic helps in the diagnosis of MP. A decrease in symptoms within 30-45 minutes after the injection of 0.25% 8 mL bupivacaine (Dureja et al., 1995) or 1% lidocaine (Haim et al., 2006) at an entry point 1 cm medial to the ASIS is considered to be diagnostic.

### Nerve Conduction Studies

MP patients are frequently referred to the electrophysiology laboratory for nerve conduction studies (NCS). Bilateral LFCN sensory studies should be performed during NCS. However, the sensory response potential may not be obtained on the normal side due to obesity and the variational anatomy of the nerve. Therefore, failure to obtain the LFCN sensory response is not always a pathological result and should be compared with the opposite extremity values. More than a 50% reduction in sensory response amplitude between the two sides or abnormal sensory latency delay supports the diagnosis of MP. In addition, somatosensory evoked potentials can also be used for diagnostic purposes and are more sensitive than sensory nerve conduction tests (el-Tantawi, 2009; Po & Mei, 1992; Seror, 1999).

### Magnetic Resonance Imaging

Magnetic resonance imaging (MRI) can be used to exclude diseases such as lumbar disc disease or lumbosacral plexopathy that can cause thigh pain. Also, the LFCN can be visualized by obtaining high-resolution images with MRI.

## Treatment

Although MP does not cause motor function loss, it causes pain that affects daily life due to severe paresthesias, and therefore treatment is required. MP treatment methods divide into two main groups as non-surgical and surgical methods. Unfortunately, the level of evidence for treatment strategies for MP is low because there has not yet been a good randomized-controlled study.

### Non-Surgical Interventions

Most MP cases have a good prognosis and recover without the need for surgical procedures. Up to an 85% improvement has been reported with conservative methods (Dureja et al., 1995; Ecker & Woltman, 1938). While preventing recurrent traumas and losing weight accelerate the healing process, pain control is provided with nonsteroidal anti-inflammatory and neuropathic pain agents. Antiepileptics, tricyclic antidepressants, and serotonin noradrenaline reuptake inhibitors are used in the treatment of neuropathic pain. Antiepileptic agents such as pregabalin and gabapentin are recommended as first-line therapy for neuropathic pain. Topical capsaicin (Puig et al., 1995) and lidocaine (Devers & Galer, 2000) have also been shown to be effective in treating resistant neuropathic pain in MP. Repeated nerve blockade with local anesthetics and steroids may be required for pain control. The entry point for the blockage is usually 1 cm medial to the ASIS and it is helpful for injection in determining the place where the sensitivity is highest. Performing the blockage with ultrasound increases the efficiency (Khalil et al., 2012). Pulsed radiofrequency is a newly emerging treatment method for MP and its effectiveness has been reported with case reports (Philip et al., 2009). It has been shown that most cases of iatrogenic origin are almost entirely resolved within three months by conservative methods. Similarly, pregnancy-related MP is expected to recover spontaneously within a few months due to weight and fluid loss (Ghent, 1961).

### Surgical Interventions

The complaints of some patients may continue despite conservative methods, and surgical methods may be required in these patients. Neurolysis and transection are the most commonly used and studied surgical methods, and whether neurolysis or transection is the procedure of choice is still controversial. With neurolysis, the LFCN is decompressed and the nerve is brought into medial transposition. Studies have shown the efficacy of neurolysis is between 44% and 78% in resistant MP cases (Macnicol & Thompson, 1990; Nahabedian & Dellon, 1995). Although resection of the nerve by transection is mainly effective in controlling the pain, the LFCN creates permanent anesthesia in the sensory area. In a study of 21 patients comparing neurolysis and transection, a higher rate of complete recovery was observed with transection (van Eerten et al., 1995). In another study, recurrence was observed in all four resistant MP cases who underwent neurolysis within two years, and these patients achieved a permanent improvement in pain with transection (Ivins, 2000). Generally, the first recommended type of surgery is decompression with neurolysis. If the treatment fails despite this surgery, nerve resection with transection is recommended as a second operation (Emamhadi, 2012).

## Conclusion

Patients with MP have only sensory symptoms and a history and physical examination are essential in making the diagnosis. In addition, the LFCN can be used with a block for both diagnostic and therapeutic purposes. Surgical methods can be used in patients who do not benefit from conservative management.

## REFERENCES


Ahsan, M. R., & Curtin, J. (2001, Apr-Jun). Meralgia paresthetica following total hip replacement. *Ir. J. Med. Sci.,* 170(2), 149. https:// doi.org/10.1007/bf03168832.

Aszmann, O. C., Dellon, E. S., & Dellon, A. L. (1997, Sep). Anatomical course of the lateral femoral cutaneous nerve and its susceptibility to compression and injury. *Plast. Reconstr. Surg.,* 100(3), 600-604. https://doi.org/10.1097/00006534-199709000-00008.

Blake, S. M., & Treble, N. J. (2004, Nov). Meralgia paraesthetica - an addition to 'seatbelt syndrome.' *Ann. R Coll. Surg. Engl.,* 86(6), W6-7. https://doi.org/10.1308/14787080456.

Devers, A., & Galer, B. S. (2000, Sep). Topical lidocaine patch relieves a variety of neuropathic pain conditions: an open-label study. *Clin. J. Pain,* 16(3), 205-208. https://doi.org/10.1097/00002508-200009000-00005.

Dureja, G. P., Gulaya, V., Jayalakshmi, T. S., & Mandal, P. (1995, May). Management of meralgia paresthetica: a multimodality regimen. *Anesth. Analg.,* 80(5), 1060-1061. https://doi.org/10.1097/00000539-199505000-00043.

Ecker, A. D., & Woltman, H. W. (1938). Meralgia paraesthetica: a report of one hundred and fifty cases. *Journal of the American Medical Association,* 110(20), 1650-1652.

El-Tantawi, G. A. (2009, Jul). Reliability of sensory nerve-conduction and somatosensory evoked potentials for diagnosis of meralgia paraesthetica. *Clin. Neurophysiol.,* 120(7), 1346-1351. https://doi.org/ 10.1016/j.clinph.2009.04.014.

Emamhadi, M. (2012). Surgery for Meralgia Paresthetica: neurolysis versus nerve resection. *Turk. Neurosurg.,* 22(6), 758-762. https://doi. org/10.5137/1019-5149.Jtn.6068-12.4.

Freud, S. (1895). Ueber die Bernhardtsche Sensibilitaetsstoreung. *Neurol. Centralbl.,* 14, 491-492. [About Bernhardt's sensitivity disorder]

Ger, R., Mishrick, A., Hurwitz, J., Romero, C., & Oddsen, R. (1993, Jan-Feb). Management of groin hernias by laparoscopy. *World J. Surg.,* 17(1), 46-50. https://doi.org/10.1007/bf01655704.

Ghent, W. R. (1961, Oct 14). Further studies on meralgia paresthetica. *Can. Med. Assoc. J.,* 85(16), 871-875.

Grossman, M. G., Ducey, S. A., Nadler, S. S., & Levy, A. S. (2001, Sep-Oct). Meralgia paresthetica: diagnosis and treatment. *J. Am. Acad. Orthop. Surg.,* 9(5), 336-344. https://doi.org/10.5435/00124635-200109000-00007.

Hager, W. (1885). Neuralgia femoris. Resection des Nerv. cutan. femoris anterior externus. Heilung. *DMW-Deutsche Medizinische Wochenschrift,* 11(14), 218-219. [Femoral neuralgia. Resection of the Nerve. cutan. femoris anterior externus. Cure. *DMW-German Medical Weekly*]

Haim, A., Pritsch, T., Ben-Galim, P., & Dekel, S. (2006, Jun). Meralgia paresthetica: A retrospective analysis of 79 patients evaluated and treated according to a standard algorithm. *Acta Orthop.,* 77(3), 482-486. https://doi.org/10.1080/17453670610046433.

Hutchins, F. L., Jr., Huggins, J., & Delaney, M. L. (1998, Aug). Laparoscopic myomectomy-an unusual cause of meralgia paresthetica. *J. Am. Assoc. Gynecol. Laparosc.,* 5(3), 309-311. https:// doi.org/10.1016/s1074-3804(98)80039-x.

Ivins, G. K. (2000, Aug). Meralgia paresthetica, the elusive diagnosis: clinical experience with 14 adult patients. *Ann. Surg.,* 232(2), 281-286. https://doi.org/10.1097/00000658-200008000-00019.

Khalil, N., Nicotra, A., & Rakowicz, W. (2012, Dec 12). Treatment for meralgia paraesthetica. *Cochrane Database Syst. Rev.,* 12(12), Cd004159. https://doi.org/10.1002/14651858.CD004159.pub3.

Korkmaz, N., & Ozçakar, L. (2004, Sep 15). Meralgia paresthetica in a policeman: the belt or the gun. *Plast. Reconstr. Surg.,* 114(4), 1012-1013. https://doi.org/10.1097/01.prs.0000138706.86633.01.

Macnicol, M. F., & Thompson, W. J. (1990, May). Idiopathic meralgia paresthetica. *Clin. Orthop. Relat. Res.* (254), 270-274.

Nahabedian, M. Y., & Dellon, A. L. (1995, Dec). Meralgia paresthetica: etiology, diagnosis, and outcome of surgical decompression. *Ann. Plast. Surg.,* 35(6), 590-594.

Nouraei, S. A., Anand, B., Spink, G., & O'Neill, K. S. (2007, Apr). A novel approach to the diagnosis and management of meralgia paresthetica. *Neurosurgery,* 60(4), 696-700; discussion 700. https:// doi.org/10.1227/01.Neu.0000255392.69914.F7.

Parisi, T. J., Mandrekar, J., Dyck, P. J., & Klein, C. J. (2011, Oct 18). Meralgia paresthetica: relation to obesity, advanced age, and diabetes mellitus. *Neurology,* 77(16), 1538-1542. https://doi.org/10.1212/ WNL.0b013e318233b356.

Philip, C. N., Candido, K. D., Joseph, N. J., & Crystal, G. J. (2009, Sep-Oct). Successful treatment of meralgia paresthetica with pulsed radiofrequency of the lateral femoral cutaneous nerve. *Pain Physician,* 12(5), 881-885.

Po, H. L., & Mei, S. N. (1992, Jan). Meralgia paresthetica: the diagnostic value of somatosensory evoked potentials. *Arch. Phys. Med. Rehabil.,* 73(1), 70-72.

Puig, L., Alegre, M., & de Moragas, J. M. (1995). Treatment of meralgia paraesthetica with topical capsaicin. *Dermatology,* 191(1), 73-74. https://doi.org/10.1159/000246496.

Richer, L. P., Shevell, M. I., Stewart, J., & Poulin, C. (2002, Apr). Pediatric meralgia paresthetica. *Pediatr. Neurol.,* 26(4), 321-323. https://doi.org/10.1016/s0887-8994(01)00397-6.

Seror, P. (1999, Jul-Aug). Lateral femoral cutaneous nerve conduction v somatosensory evoked potentials for electrodiagnosis of meralgia paresthetica. *Am. J. Phys. Med. Rehabil.,* 78(4), 313-316. https://doi. org/10.1097/00002060-199907000-00004.

van den Broecke, D. G., Schuurman, A. H., Borg, E. D., & Kon, M. (1998, Sep). Neurotmesis of the lateral femoral cutaneous nerve when coring for iliac crest bone grafts. *Plast. Reconstr. Surg.,* 102(4), 1163-1166. https://doi.org/10.1097/00006534-199809040-00038.

van Eerten, P. V., Polder, T. W., & Broere, C. A. (1995, Jul). Operative treatment of meralgia paresthetica: transection versus neurolysis. *Neurosurgery,* 37(1), 63-65. https://doi.org/10.1227/00006123-199507000-00009.

van Slobbe, A. M., Bohnen, A. M., Bernsen, R. M., Koes, B. W., & Bierma-Zeinstra, S. M. (2004, Mar). Incidence rates and determinants in meralgia paresthetica in general practice. *J. Neurol.,* 251(3), 294-297. https://doi.org/10.1007/s00415-004-0310-x.

# EDITORS' CONTACT INFORMATION

***Mehmet Cenk Turgut, MD***
Orthopedic Specialist, Erzurum City Hospital,
Erzurum Şehir Hastanesi, Ortopedi Servisi, Turkey
m.cenkturgut@hotmail.com

***Serdar Toy, MD***
Orthopedic Specialist,
Ağrı Training and Research Hospital,
Ağrı Eğtim ve Araştırma
Hastanesi, Ortopedi Servisi, Turkey
serdartoy737@gmail.com

# INDEX

## A

## B



## C

## D

## E

## F



## G



## H

## I



## J



## K



## L

## M

## N



## O



## P

## Q



## R

## S

## T

## U



## V



## W



## X



## Y